Self-Assessment (

T0231484

Small A̲_____
Orthopedics,
Rheumatology, &
Musculoskeletal
Disorders

Second Edition

Daniel D. Lewis
DVM, DACVS
Professor Small Animal Surgery
Jerry & Lola Collins Eminent Scholar Canine Sports Medicine and
Comparative Orthopedics
Department of Small Animal Clinical Sciences
College of Veterinary Medicine, University of Florida
Gainesville, Florida, USA

Sorrel J. Langley-Hobbs
MA, BVetMed, DSAS(Orth), DECVS, FHEA, MRCVS
European Specialist in Small Animal Surgery
Professor in Small Animal Orthopaedic Surgery
University of Bristol
School of Veterinary Sciences
Langford, Bristol, UK

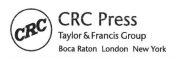

CRC Press
Taylor & Francis Group
Boca Raton London New York

CRC Press is an imprint of the
Taylor & Francis Group, an **informa** business

CRC Press
Taylor & Francis Group
6000 Broken Sound Parkway NW, Suite 300
Boca Raton, FL 33487-2742

© 2014 by Taylor & Francis Group, LLC
CRC Press is an imprint of Taylor & Francis Group, an Informa business

No claim to original U.S. Government works

Printed on acid-free paper
Version Date: 20160302

International Standard Book Number-13: 978-1-4822-2492-4 (Paperback)

Library of Congress Cataloging-in-Publication Data

Self-assessment colour review of small animal orthopaedics.
    Small animal orthopedics, rheumatology, and musculoskeletal disorders : self-assessment color review / editors, Daniel D. Lewis, Sorrel J. Langley-Hobbs. -- Second edition.
        pages cm -- (Veterinary self-assessment color review)
    Preceded by Self-assessment colour review of small animal orthopaedics / [edited by] Daniel D. Lewis, Robert B. Parker, Mark S. Bloomberg. 1997.
    Includes bibliographical references and index.
    ISBN 978-1-4822-2492-4 (hbk. : alk. paper)
    1. Veterinary orthopedics--Examinations, questions, etc.. 2. Veterinary rheumatology--Examinations, questions, etc.. 3. Musculoskeletal system--Diseases--Examinations, questions, etc.. I. Lewis, Daniel D., editor. II. Langley-Hobbs, S. J. (Sorrel J.), editor. III. Title. IV. Series: Veterinary self-assessment color review (Series)
    [DNLM: 1. Orthopedic Procedures--veterinary--Examination Questions. 2. Fractures, Bone--veterinary--Examination Questions. 3. Musculoskeletal Diseases--veterinary--Examination Questions. SF 910.5]

    SF910.5S35 2014
    636.089'6723--dc23   2014013365

Visit the Taylor & Francis Web site at
http://www.taylorandfrancis.com

and the CRC Press Web site at
http://www.crcpress.com

Preface

The original version of the *Self-Assessment Color Review of Small Animal Orthopedics* was published in 1998. The practice of small animal orthopedics has advanced considerably in the 15 years that have transpired since that initial volume went to press. Advanced diagnostic imaging and minimally invasive orthopedic surgery were in their infancy and formal development of the disciplines of canine sports medicine and rehabilitative therapy were only taking root. Diagnostic procedures, instrumentation, implant systems, and surgical techniques for the treatment of orthopedic disorders in the dog and cat have changed and advanced considerably in the new millennium. Building on the precedent established in the late 20th century, continued experimental and clinical research has expanded our understanding of bone and fracture biology, musculoskeletal tumor development and treatment, and the pathophysiology and management of arthropathies, and new interests were founded with regard to non-surgical rehabilitative therapies. This new expanded text has been designed to keep pace with the rapidly expanding practice of small animal orthopedics while embracing the developing fields of canine sports medicine and rehabilitative medicine.

As with the original version, this book is not intended to be an all-encompassing, comprehensive text reviewing every facet of small animal orthopedics. This book is one in a series of self-assessment guides designed to facilitate active learning by presenting selected clinical case scenarios or applied research material. The clinical practice of all aspects of veterinary medicine is a balance of science, art, experience, and judgement. The reader may give a different answer to individual questions to those provided in this text. The contributors and editors have made a conscientious effort to make the information in this book as current and accurate as possible; however, the reader should be cognizant that appropriate alternative answers to many questions, particularly clinical case scenarios, exist. Our intent was to provide an illustrative, self-directed educational tool containing current information of value to veterinary students, interns and residents in training, and general and specialist small animal practitioners with specific interests in orthopedics, canine sports medicine, and rehabilitative medicine. In response to feedback relating to the original version, references have been provided for each question to allow the reader the opportunity to delve more into the topic by reading the referenced journal articles if they so desire.

An international group of 46 clinicians and investigators have contributed to this publication. Orthopedic surgeons, radiologists, internists, neurologists, and anesthesiologists, as well as veterinarians engaged in rehabilitative medicine, have provided their diverse expertise and experience to make this text a comprehensive review of the expanding fields relating to small animal orthopedics.

Finally, we would be remiss if we did not acknowledge the passing of Robert Bennett Parker, one of the co-editors of the original *Self-Assessment Color Review of Small Animal Orthopedics*. Rob's tragic demise, like that of Mark Bloomberg, who was also a contributing editor to the original volume, came much too early, but his memory and legacy serve as a source of inspiration for those of us who had the privilege of working with Rob.

Daniel D. Lewis
Sorrel J. Langley-Hobbs

Broad classification of cases

Contributors

A. Rick Alleman, DVM, PhD, DABVP, DACVP
Professor Clinical Pathology
Department of Physiological Sciences
College of Veterinary Medicine
University of Florida
Gainesville, Florida, USA

Nicholas J. Bacon, MA, VetMB, DECVS, DACVS, MRCVS
ACVS Founding Fellow Surgical Oncology
Imparoto Associate Clinical Professor of Small Animal Surgical Oncology
Department of Small Animal Clinical Sciences
College of Veterinary Medicine
University of Florida
Gainesville, Florida, USA

Clifford Berry, DVM, DACR
Professor Diagnostic Imaging
Department of Small Animal Clinical Sciences
College of Veterinary Medicine
University of Florida
Gainesville, Florida, USA

Sherman O. Canapp Jr., DVM, MS, CCRT, DACVS, DACVSMR
Director and Staff Surgeon
Veterinary Orthopedic & Sports Medicine Group
Annapolis Junction, Maryland, USA

Christina J. Choate, DVM
Small Animal Orthopedic Research Fellow
Collaborative Orthopedics and Biomechanics Laboratory
University of Florida
Gainesville, Florida, USA

Christi R. Cook, DVM, MS, DACR
Teaching Assistant Professor Radiology
Veterinary Medical Teaching Hospital
College of Veterinary Medicine
University of Missouri
Columbia, Missouri, USA

James L. Cook, DVM, PhD, DACVS, DACVSMR
William & Kathryn Allen Distinguished Professor in Orthopaedic Surgery
Director Comparative Orthopedic Laboratory
Comparative Orthopedic Laboratory
University of Missouri
Columbia, Missouri, USA

Eithne J. Comerford, MVB, PhD, CertVR, CertSAS, PGCertHE, DECVS, MRCVS
School of Veterinary Science
University of Liverpool
Neston, Cheshire, UK

Alan R. Cross, DVM, DACVS
Staff Surgeon
Georgia Veterinary Specialists
Atlanta, Georgia, USA

Laura C. Cuddy, MVB, MS, DACVS
Lecturer Small Animal Surgery
School of Veterinary Medicine
University College Dublin
Dublin, Ireland

Nicole Erhart, VMD, MS, DACVS
ACVS Founding Fellow Surgical Oncology
Professor Surgical Oncology
Director Laboratory of Comparative Musculoskeletal Oncology and Traumatology
Flint Animal Cancer Center
College of Veterinary Medicine & Biomedical Sciences
Colorado State University
Fort Collins, Colorado, USA

James P. Farese DVM, DACVS
ACVS Founding Fellow Surgical Oncology
Staff Surgeon
VCA Animal Care Center of Sonoma County
Rohnert Park, California, USA

Cassio R. Ferringo, DVM, MS, PhD
Professor Small Animal Surgery
Department of Surgery
College of Veterinary Medicine
University of São Paulo
University City, São Paulo, Brazil

Noel M. Fitzpatrick, MVB, CertVR, DSAS(Orth), DACVSMR, MRCVS
Professor of Veterinary Orthopaedics
University of Surrey Veterinary School
Director, Fitzpatrick Referrals
Godalming, Surrey, UK

Steven M. Fox, MS, DVM, MBA, PhD
President, Securos – A Division of MWI
Fiskdale, Massachusetts, USA

Krista-Britt Halling DVM, CCRT, DACVS
Staff Surgeon
Mississauga-Oakville Veterinary Emergency &
Referral Hospital
Oakville, Ontario, Canada

Graham M. Hayes, VetMB, MA, CertSAS,
DECVS, MRCVS
Department of Veterinary Medicine
University of Cambridge
Cambridge, UK

Caleb C. Hudson, DVM, MS, DACVS
Staff Surgeon
Gulf Coast Veterinary Specialists
Houston, Texas, USA

Kenneth A. Johnson, MVSc, PhD, FACVSc,
DACVS, DECVS
Director of Orthopaedics, Associate Dean
University Veterinary Teaching Hospital
University of Sydney
Sydney, New South Wales, Australia

Amy S. Kapatkin, BS, DVM, MS
Associate Professor Surgical and Radiological
Sciences
School of Veterinary Medicine
University of California Davis
Davis, California, USA

Sharon C. Kerwin, DVM, MS, DACVS
Professor Small Animal Surgery
Department of Small Animal Clinical Sciences
College of Veterinary Medicine
Texas A&M University
College Station, Texas, USA

Stanley E. Kim, BVSc, MS, DACVS
Assistant Professor Small Animal Surgery
Department of Small Animal Clinical Sciences
College of Veterinary Medicine
University of Florida
Gainesville, Florida, USA

Kristin A. Kirkby Shaw, DVM, MS, CCRT,
DACVS, DACVSMR
Senior Professional Services Veterinarian
Northwest District
Novartis Animal Health
Seattle, Washington, USA

Sorrel J. Langley-Hobbs, MA, BVetMed,
DSAS(Orth), DECVS, FHEA, MRCVS
European Specialist in Small Animal Surgery
Professor in Small Animal Orthopaedic Surgery
University of Bristol
School of Veterinary Sciences
Langford, Bristol, UK

Daniel D. Lewis, DVM, DACVS
Professor Small Animal Surgery
Jerry & Lola Collins Eminent Scholar
Canine Sports Medicine and Comparative
Orthopedics
Department of Small Animal Clinical Sciences
College of Veterinary Medicine
University of Florida
Gainesville, Florida, USA

Ron M. McLaughlin, DVM, DVSc, DACVS
Professor and Chief Small Animal Surgery
Department Head Small Animal Sciences
Department of Clinical Sciences
College of Veterinary Medicine
Mississippi State University
Mississippi State, Mississippi, USA

Andy Moores, BVSc, DSAS(Orth), DECVS,
MRCVS
Anderson Sturgess Veterinary Specialists
Winchester, Hampshire, UK

Martin Owen, BVSc, BSc, PhD, DSAS(Orth),
DECVS, MRCVS
Dick White Referrals
Six Mile Bottom Veterinary Specialist Centre
Six Mile Bottom, Suffolk, UK

Ross H. Palmer, DVM, MS, DACVS
Professor Small Animal Surgery
Department of Clinical Sciences
College of Veterinary Medicine & Biomedical
Sciences
Colorado State University
Fort Collins, Colorado, USA

Alessandro Piras, DVM, ISVS, MRCVS
Oakland Small Animal Veterinary Clinic
Banbridge, Northern Ireland, UK

Simon R. Platt, BVM&S,
DACVIM(Neurology), DECVN, MRCVS
Department of Small Animal Medicine & Surgery
College of Veterinary Medicine
University of Georgia
Athens, Georgia, USA

Antonio Pozzi, DMV, MS, DACVS,
DACVSMR
Associate Professor Small Animal Surgery
Department of Small Animal Clinical Sciences
College of Veterinary Medicine
University of Florida
Gainesville, Florida, USA

Robert M. Radaasch, DVM, MS, DACVS
Staff Surgeon
Dallas Veterinary Surgical Center
Dallas, Texas, USA

Heidi Radke, Dr. Med. Vet., DECVS, MRCVS
Surgery Lecturer
Department of Veterinary Medicine
University of Cambridge
Cambridge, UK

Rick A. Read, BVSc, PhD, FACVSc, FNZCVSc
Adjunct Professor Small Animal Surgery
School of Veterinary & Life Sciences
College of Veterinary Medicine
Murdoch University
Murdoch, Western Australia, Australia

David J. Reece, DVM, DACVR
Senior Lecturer Diagnostic Imaging
School of Veterinary & Life Sciences
College of Veterinary Medicine
Murdoch University
Murdoch, Western Australia, Australia

Colin W. Sereda, DVM, MS, DACVS
Staff Surgeon
Guardian Veterinary Center
Edmonton, Alberta, Canada

Chris Seymour, MA, VetMB, DVA, DECVAA,
MRCVS
Lecturer in Veterinary Anaesthesia
Department of Veterinary Clinical Sciences
Royal Veterinary College
Hatfield, Hertfordshire, UK

G. Diana Shelton, DVM, PhD, DACVIM
Professor, Department of Pathology
Comparative Neuromuscular Laboratory
University of California – San Diego
La Jolla, California, USA

Thomas Sissner, MS, DVM, CertSAS,
DECVS, MRCVS
Staff Surgeon
Calgary Animal Referral and Emergency Center
Calgary, Alberta, Canada

Jane E. Sykes, BVSc, PhD, DACVIM
Professor Medicine and Epidemiology
School of Veterinary Medicine
University of California Davis
Davis, California, USA

Kelley M. Thieman DVM, MS, DACVS
Clinical Assistant Professor, Small Animal
Surgery
Department of Small Animal Clinical Sciences
College of Veterinary Medicine
Texas A&M University
College Station, Texas, USA

Ricco Vannini, Dr. Med. Vet., DECVS
Bessy's Kleintierklinik
Watt, Switzerland

Aldo Vezzoni, Med. Vet., SCMPA, DECVS
Clinica Veterinaria Vezzoni
Cremona, Italy

Katja Voss, Dr. Med. Vet., DECVS
Small Animal Surgery Specialist
Head of Small Animal Surgery
University Veterinary Teaching Hospital
University of Sydney
Sydney, New South Wales, Australia

Matthew D. Winter, DVM, DACVR
Assistant Professor Diagnostic Imaging
Department of Small Animal Clinical Sciences
College of Veterinary Medicine
University of Florida
Gainesville, Florida, USA

Abbreviations

Image acknowledgements

31b	Reproduced with permission from *Clean Run Magazine*, March 2007, Non-responsive hindlimb lameness in agility dogs – iliopsoas strain.
39a, b	From Cook JL, Renfro DC, Tomlinson JL *et al.* (2005) Measurement of angles of abduction for diagnosis of shoulder instability in dogs using goniometry and digital image analysis. *Vet Surg* 34:463–468, with permission.
53a, b, 74a, 116	Courtesy Anne Raines
71a, b	Courtesy Dr. Natasha Arzi
73	Courtesy Dr. Natasha Arzi
88	Courtesy Dr. Rebecca Parker©
96a, b	Courtesy Dr. Mike Targett
108	Courtesy Dr. Heather Wamsley
125	Reproduced with permission from the *BSAVA Manual of Canine and Feline Musculoskeletal Disorders.* © BSAVA.
126a, b	From Voss K, Geyer H, Montavon PM (2003) Antebrachiocarpal luxation in a cat. A case report and anatomical study of the medial collateral ligament. *Vet Comp Orthop Traumatol* 16:266–70, with permission.
134b, c	Courtesy Dr. Gordon Brown
148	Courtesy Dr. George Papadopoulos
206a, b	Courtesy Dr. Joy Archer

We would like to acknowledge the contribution of Ms. Debby Sundstrom and her expertise in helping to prepare many of the images for this book.

1 Two radiographic views of the left elbow of a 33 kg, 6-month-old male Dogue De Bordeaux that had bilateral forelimb lameness are shown (1a, b). On physical examination there was a palpable effusion of the dog's left elbow, while pain was elicited on extension of both elbows.

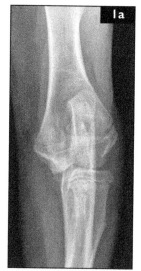
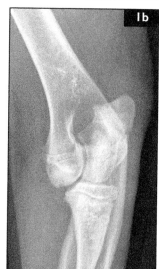

i. What is the diagnosis?
ii. Describe the two radiographic views shown and discuss the value of these two views relative to establishing a diagnosis of the condition affecting this dog.

2 An 11-month-old male cat was referred for treatment after it sustained a right tibial fracture after jumping off a bed. The cat had previously sustained a left tibial fracture, which had been managed with external coaptation. The owner was unaware of any prior trauma or lameness. A ventrodorsal radiograph of the pelvis and hindlimbs, obtained at the time of this most recent presentation, is shown (2).

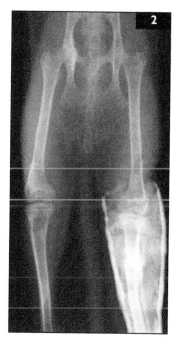

i. Give a list of differential diagnoses for potential underlying causes of the fractures observed in this cat.
ii. What diagnostic tests can be done to further investigate the etiologies of those fractures?

Answers: 1, 2

1 i. This dog has a well-demarcated subchondral bone defect of the trochlea of the humeral condyle consistent with an osteochondrosis lesion. Although a mineralized cartilage flap is not evident, it is reasonable to assume that this defect represents an osteochondritis dissecans lesion, as there is effusion in the left elbow and pain can be elicited on manipulation of the joint. The possibility of this dog having a fragmented coronoid process in the left or both elbows should also be considered. **ii. 1a** is a well-positioned craniocaudal radiograph. **1b** is a craniolateral-caudomedial oblique (CrLCaMO) radiograph, which is made by angling the radiographic beam 15° off the cranial midline of the joint. Although subchondral bone sclerosis can be appreciated in both images, the subchondral bone defect is more obvious on the CrLCaMO radiograph, as this view avoids superimposition of the trochlea with the medial coronoid process of the ulna. A recent study assessing the efficacy of five radiographic views for identifying osteochondritis dissecans lesions affecting the humeral condyle found the CrLCaMO view to have the greatest sensitivity for detecting these lesions. An earlier prospective study also documented that the CrLCaMO view was the most likely projection to identify fragmentation of the medial coronoid process, although identification of fragments was only possible in 62% of the elbows assessed. CT has greater sensitivity and provides more information when evaluating dogs with elbow dysplasia, but its availability is generally limited to referral institutions.

2 i. When a young cat is evaluated for multiple fractures with a history of only minor or no accompanying trauma, the primary differential diagnoses should include nutritional or metabolic bone disease, physical abuse (non-accidental injury) and osteogenesis imperfecta.
ii. Nutritional secondary hyperparathyroidism is the most common cause of pathologic fracture in young animals, but this cat had been fed a normal balanced diet. With no history of dietary imbalance and serum concentrations of ionized calcium, phosphorus, vitamin D, and parathormone within reference ranges, a diagnosis of osteogenesis imperfecta must be considered. Osteogenesis imperfecta is a heritable disease characterized by brittle bones. Results of studies using cultured skin fibroblasts indicate that most humans affected with osteogenesis imperfecta have a mutation in the type I collagen genes (*COL1A1* and *COL1A2*). Osteogenesis imperfecta has been identified in dogs. Radiographic findings included multiple fractures in various stages of healing and generalized osteopenia. Cultured fibroblasts from skin biopsy specimens were used to diagnose osteogenesis imperfecta. Structural abnormalities were found in type I collagen from each dog. This cat was euthanized after sustaining fractures to both humeri while hospitalized overnight. A provisional diagnosis of osteogenesis imperfecta was made given the cat's normal blood results, normal diet, and multiple atraumatic fractures.

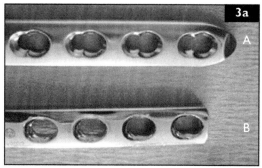

3 Two 3.5 mm bone plates are shown (3a).
i. Name the implants.
ii. Explain why plate B must be accurately contoured to the shape of the underlying bone prior to application.
iii. Why is it not essential to accurately contour plate A prior to application?
iv. Describe the differences in the mechanism of screw failure for these two types of plates.

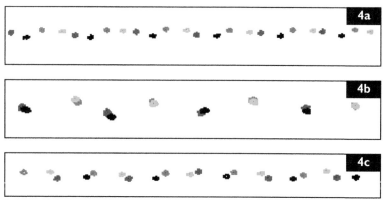

4 A 3-year-old male Labrador retriever has developed a gait abnormality that is observed when performing obedience. The owner and trainer describe a gait pattern in which the ipsilateral forelimb and hindlimb are contacting the ground at the same time.
i. What type of gait pattern has this dog developed, and what adverse implications are associated with this type of gait pattern?
ii. Describe the gait patterns iillustrated in the images shown (4a–c).
iii. What is the correct order of paw placement for a dog at a walk?
iv. What is the correct paw placement pattern for a trotting dog? Why is the trot the preferred gait pattern for evaluating lameness and for conditioning dogs?

Answers: 3, 4

3 i. B is a dynamic compression plate. A is a locking compression plate.

ii. For a dynamic compression plate, stability is achieved by the head of the screws compressing the plate against the bone's cortex, creating friction. The plate must be accurately contoured to conform to the surface of the bone in order to provide multiple contact points between the implant and the bone.

iii. A locking plate functions as an 'internal fixator'. Stability is afforded by the fixed position of the screws, which lock into the threaded holes in the plate. While the screws engage both the bone and locking plate, the plate is not compressed against the bone's cortex and the distance between the plate and the bone is maintained during screw tightening. The locking mechanism thus obviates the requirement for accurate plate contouring.

iv. Screw failure in conventional plates occurs from cyclical loading and backing out of screws from the bone. Minor screw loosening results in loss of friction and reduction. Loosening of individual locking screws is unusual and if failure does occur, the failure mechanism is complete construct pull-out (**3b**) or breakage of multiple screws at the screw–plate interface.

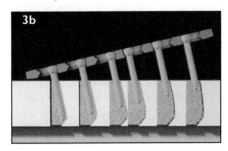

4 i. Pace, a symmetric gait in which support is maintained by the animal by paired ipsilateral limbs (**4c**). The animal moves by swinging the ipsilateral forelimb and hindlimb while bearing weight on the contralateral limbs. Pacing is a gait used in long-legged dogs (e.g. Salukis); it allows the animal to move forward without the interference between the fore- and hindlimbs that may occur at a trot. Pacing is also seen in dogs that are fatigued, out of condition, or have an orthopedic problem. Pacing causes the dog's center of gravity to shift from side to side, which wastes energy and stresses muscles and ligaments. In addition, only two paws are in contact with the ground at any given time.

ii. a, walk; b, trot; c, pace.

iii. The correct order is right hind, right fore, left hind, left fore. Three paws should be in contact with the ground at any time.

iv. Contralateral, diagonal fore- and hindlimbs move forward at the same time. The hind paw should fall into the paw print of the ipsilateral fore paw. Ipsilateral limbs should be straight, forming a V-shape as the paws converge towards the midline. Trotting is the only gait in which a dog's movement is symmetrical. It is the ideal gait for conditioning, as trotting will build symmetrical muscle strength.

5 A 9-month-old German shepherd dog is presented for hip evaluation (5a).

i. What type of radiographic examination was performed?

ii. Describe how this radiograph is obtained and what quantitative parameter can be derived from this radiograph.

iii. For the parameter alluded to in ii, what is the value below which dogs are considered to be at a low risk for developing osteoarthrosis?

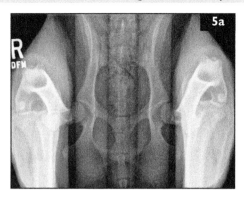

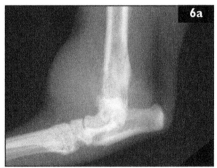

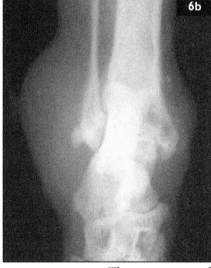

6 A 10-year-old male shorthaired cat presented with a non-weight-bearing lameness of the left hindlimb of 2 weeks' duration. On physical examination, swelling and pain were localized to the distal left tibia. Radiographs of the left crus were obtained (6a, b). An aspirate of the mass confirmed that the lesion was an osteosarcoma. The cat was staged and there was no evidence of metastasis found. The owner elected to have an amputation performed, but asked if the entire limb needed to be removed.

i. Would performing a mid-femoral amputation be appropriate for this cat?

ii. Discuss the advantages of performing a coxofemoral disarticulation (amputation) in this cat.

iii. What is the prognosis for a cat with an appendicular osteosarcoma treated by amputation without administering adjunctive chemotherapy?

Answers: 5, 6

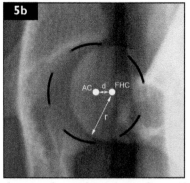

5 i. A PennHIP (Pennsylvania Hip Improvement Program) distraction radiograph.
ii. This radiograph is made with the dog positioned in dorsal recumbency with a PennHip distraction device placed within the dog's inguinal region. The examiner holds the dog's stifles symmetrically in flexion with both femora aligned perpendicular to the radiographic table. Once the limbs are aligned, the examiner adducts the hindlimbs and a radiographic exposure is made. This maneuver produces a radiograph with the coxofemoral joints in distraction. The distraction index (DI) is calculated to quantitate coxofemoral joint laxity. The DI represents the relative displacement of the femoral head from the acetabulum ($DI = d/r$, where DI is the distraction index, d represents the distance between the center of the femoral head (FHC) and the center of the acetabulum (AC), and r represents the radius of the femoral head) (5b).
iii. The DI is predictive of the dog's potential for developing degenerative joint disease and is breed specific; however, for breeds commonly affected with hip dysplasia, a dog with a DI of <0.3 has been shown be at low risk for developing osteoarthrosis.

6 i. A mid-femoral amputation could be done because the tumor is located distal to the stifle. This is a relatively quick, technically simple surgery compared with coxofemoral disarticulation. Mid-femoral amputation provides a cosmetically more appealing short-term result, as the muscles of the proximal femur still give the hindquarters some contour and bulk.
ii. Coxofemoral disarticulation achieves wider surgical margins compared with amputation via a mid-femoral osteotomy. Also, the hindlimb musculature can atrophy over time after mid-femoral amputation. Amputation via coxofemoral disarticulation avoids potential late cosmetic issues and might be preferable to the owner once the long-term benefits are explained.
iii. In one study, four out of five cats with appendicular osteosarcoma that underwent amputation were alive at 26 months following surgery. In another study of 11 cats that underwent amputation and had available follow-up information, five were deceased with a median survival of 49 months. The other six cats were still alive, with survival times ranging from 13–64 months, with four being 5 years beyond surgery. A third study evaluated 30 cats with appendicular osteosarcoma and reported a mean survival of 11.8 months, although some cats included underwent incisional biopsy only and not amputation.

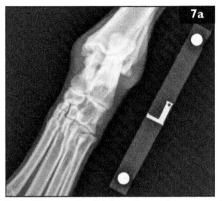
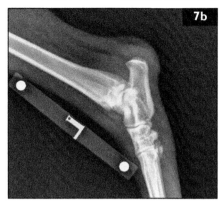

7 A 10-month-old female entire rottweiler is presented with a 3-month history of left hindlimb weight-bearing lameness, which was refractory to conservative management. Clinical examination revealed swelling associated with the medial and lateral aspects of the left tarsocrural joint, more prominent medially, and pain on manipulation. Radiographs (7a, b) were taken on presentation.
i. Describe the radiographic abnormalities.
ii. What is the most likely diagnosis?
iii. What further diagnostic modalities could be utilized to support your diagnosis?
iv. What treatment options exist for this condition?

8 A right lateral radiograph of the skull of an 8-month-old West Highland white terrier with a history of being reluctant to eat and drink for several weeks is shown (8). The dog has refused to eat for the past several days and pain is elicited when the owner attempts to open the dog's mouth. On physical examination the dog is febrile and a hard palpable swelling is noted along the caudal angle of the mandible bilaterally.

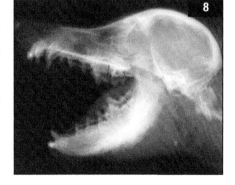

i. Describe the radiographic abnormalities.
ii. Given the dog's signalment and history, as well as the clinical and radiographic abnormalities, what is the most likely diagnosis?
iii. What is the pathogenesis of the condition?
iv. Describe appropriate treatment for this dog.

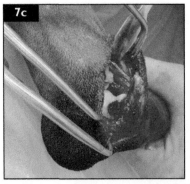

7 i. There is radiolucency with disruption of the contour of the subchondral bone of the medial ridge of the talus and associated swelling in the region of the medial collateral ligament on the dorsoplantar radiograph. The mediolateral radiograph reveals flattening of the outline of the subchondral bone on the caudal aspect of the medial talar ridge.

ii. Osteochondritis dissecans of the medial trochlear ridge of the talus.

iii. CT allows improved lesion visibility without effects of superimposition. MRI is useful in determining the depth of subchondral pathology and the presence of bone marrow lesions. Arthroscopy is indicated for assessment of synovial inflammation and cartilage or subchondral bone pathology.

iv. Conservative management is an option, although a salvage surgical procedure may eventually be required due to progressive degenerative joint disease. Lesion debridement, via arthrotomy or arthroscopy, is associated with poor long-term clinical outcomes. Osteochondral transplantation can be employed; however, surface contour matching of the talar ridge using an autograft is technically demanding. A medial malleolar osteotomy using a 6-mm diameter synthetic osteochondral resurfacing graft is shown (7c) with the surface topography trimmed to match the articular contour of the medial talar ridge. Pantarsal arthrodesis can be employed for salvage if suboptimal function persists or occurs after any treatment option.

8 i. There is a moderately severe, irregular periosteal reaction with associated soft tissue swelling extending along the caudal margin of both hemimandibles. There is smoothly marginated osseous proliferation noted along the ventral margins of the osseous bulla and ventral aspect of the temporal bones at the level of the temporomandibular joints.

ii. Craniomandibular osteopathy (CMO), sometimes referred to as 'lion jaw'.

iii. CMO is an osteoproliferative disorder primarily confined to the bones of the skull, specifically the mandibles, occipital, and temporal bones. The tympanic bullae can become markedly thickened. While the pathology is typically symmetric, osseous proliferation can be asymmetric or even unilateral in some dogs. Atrophy of the temporalis and masseter muscles often develops in dogs that are reluctant or incapable of masticating.

iv. Treatment is supportive, focusing on providing analgesia and maintaining the dog's hydration and nutrition. NSAIDs should be administered to mitigate pain. Since this dog has been reluctant to eat or drink, consideration should be given to placing an esophagostomy tube. As this dog is febrile, thoracic radiographs are warranted to ensure that the dog has not developed aspiration pneumonia. CMO is typically self-limiting and will abate or resolve after the dog has reached skeletal maturity; however, ankylosis of the temporomandibular joint can be a sequela in severely affected dogs.

9 A 7-month-old, 55 kg male pedigree dog was presented because of concerns related to the dog's forelimb conformation. The dog had conformational abnormalities of both antebrachii, but was not overtly lame, and musculoskeletal pain could not be elicited during the physical examination. A medio-lateral radiograph of the right antebrachium is shown (**9**).
i. Describe the radiographic abnormalities.
ii. What is the pathogenesis of the distal ulnar lesion?
iii. Describe typical clinical abnormalities associated with this lesion.
iv. Which breeds of dogs are most commonly affected?

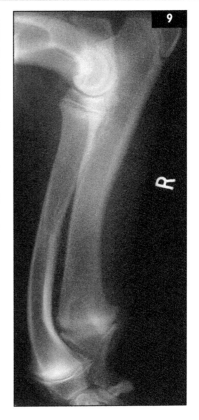

10 Describe the pattern of the four fractures shown (**10A–D**) and speculate as to what force would have been expected to cause each of these fractures.

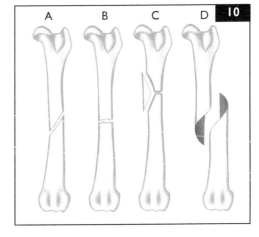

9 i. There is a flame-shaped radiolucency extending proximally from the distal ulnar physis. This radiographic lesion represents a retained cartilage core. While the radial growth plate still appears to be open, the distal ulnar physis appears abnormal and there is procurvatum of the distal radius associated with retarded ulnar growth.

ii. Retained cartilage cores are a permutation of osteochondrosis in which there is a failure in the normal process of physeal endochondral ossification. Histopathologic examination of retained cartilage cores has revealed an accumulation of hypertrophic chondrocytes that have failed to undergo the usual process of development and subsequent degeneration. These lesions can be associated with oversupplementation of calcium and the owner should be queried regarding the dog's dietary history.

iii. Affected dogs can be asymptomatic, but retained cartilage cores can result in longitudinal bone growth abnormalities. This dog's ulna is disproportionately short and restricts normal longitudinal growth of the radius, resulting in procurvatum. Valgus deviation and external rotation of the distal antebrachium, as well as proximal radioulnar subluxation resulting in elbow incongruency, can also develop. These abnormalities can cause pain and lameness.

iv. Great Danes and Irish wolfhounds are commonly affected.

10 A. Oblique fracture, likely caused by axial compression. When cortical bone is axially loaded, the fracture tends to propagate along shear planes, resulting in an oblique fracture because cortical bone is weakest when loaded in shear and strongest when loaded in compression.

B. Transverse fracture, typically caused by bending forces that produce tensile forces along the convex cortex and compressive forces on the opposite, concave cortex. Since bone is weaker when loaded in tension and strongest when loaded in compression, the fracture initiates in the cortex loaded under tension and propagates transversely toward the cortex loaded in compression.

C. Comminuted fracture. The bone is fractured into more than two pieces and the fracture lines communicate. Likely caused by both axial compressive and bending loads. Similar to a fracture produced by bending forces alone, this fracture initiates on the tensile surface of the bone, but as the fracture propagates toward the surface of the bone loaded in compression, the fracture line divides both proximally and distally along shear planes, resulting in a third, separate butterfly fragment.

D. Spiral fracture, most likely to have been sustained during torsional loading. The fracture is initiated as a longitudinal fissure in the cortex, which spirals around the bone's circumference along shear stress planes at an approximately 45° angle until the crack returns to its origin, completing the spiral fracture.

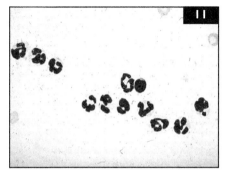

11 A six-year-old female Doberman pinscher presented because the dog was reluctant to exercise and had a symmetrical generalized stilted gait. On physical examination there was effusion of both carpi and tarsi. Radiographs of the right carpus and tarsus were obtained, and the only radiographic abnormality noted was soft tissue swelling associated with involved joints. Synovial fluid obtained from the right carpus had decreased viscosity and a nucleated cell count of 39 × 10^9/l. An image of the cytologic preparation is shown (**11**). Synovial fluid obtained from the left carpus and both tarsi had a similar cytologic appearance.
i. Describe how to perform arthrocentesis of the carpus.
ii. Interpret this dog's cytology.
iii. Discuss possible etiologies for this dog's arthropathy.

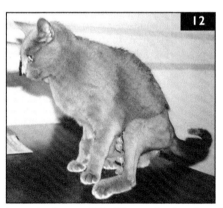

12 A 6-year-old female cat is shown (**12**). The cat had a chronic stifle luxation that was managed by stifle arthrodesis with a transarticular external skeletal fixator, after surgical reduction of the luxation had failed.
i. What is the recommended angle for stifle arthrodesis in cats?
ii. What type of hindlimb function should be expected from a cat following stifle arthrodesis?

11 i. The most accessible joint space is the radiocarpal articulation. When the carpus is flexed slightly, a depression is palpable along the craniomedial aspect of the articulation, between the distal articular margin of the radius and the proximal aspect of the radiocarpal bone. The needle should be inserted cranially, parallel to the articular surface of the distal radius, to enter the joint space.

ii. The eosinophilic, slightly granular background indicates the synovial fluid has decreased mucin content. The nucleated cell population is predominantly non-degenerate neutrophils containing nuclei with dark chromatin and clear cytoplasm. A single lymphocyte is present. Infectious agents are not visualized. This dog has non-septic, inflammatory joint disease. Normal synovial fluid from dogs should contain $<3 \times 10^9$ nucleated cells/l, with the majority being mononuclear cells including lymphocytes, monocytes, macrophages, and an occasional synovial lining cell. Neutrophils are only occasionally present ($<10\%$) in normal joint fluid.

iii. Since this dog did not have erosive changes on radiography, the suppurative polyarthropathy is likely immune-mediated caused by either antibodies directed against joint tissue or the deposition of circulating immune complexes in synovial membranes. Etiologies such as systemic lupus erythematosus, drug-induced poly-arthritis, and idiopathic polyarthritis should be considered. Immune complex deposition may also be secondary to chronic infections such as heartworm disease, pyometra, pyorrhea, or septicemia. Infectious agents such as *Anaplasma* spp., *Ehrlichia* spp., and *Borrelia* spp. can also infect joints directly, and typically are non-erosive. This dog was being treated for bacterial pyoderma with a sulfa-methoxazole–trimethoprim compound. The clinical signs subsided after antibiotic administration was discontinued.

12 i. The stifle should be arthrodesed at an angle of 120–125° in most cats, which is a more acute (flexed) angle than for dogs. The ideal fusion angle for each cat is determined preoperatively by measuring the normal standing angle of the contralateral stifle joint. To compensate for bone excision performed during surgery, 5° is added to the measurement obtained.

ii. While stifle arthrodesis does not restore normal limb function, acceptable, pain-free function can be expected if the procedure is performed properly. Results are best if the ipsilateral coxofemoral and talocrural joints are normal and the stifle is fused such that the paw contacts the ground without requiring excessive flexion or extension in the joints of the contralateral hindlimb.

13 A 6-year-old spayed female beagle presented with a 7-day progressive history of left fore-limb monoparesis (**13a**). The dog would not bear weight on the affected limb, but ambulated without apparent problems on the other three limbs. Mild muscle atrophy was present over the left scapula. The flexor withdrawal reflex and postural reaction in the left forelimb were

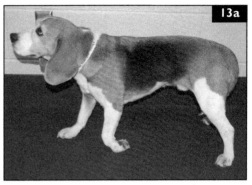

reduced. Reflexes in the other three limbs were intact, but the postural reactions were reduced in the left hindlimb. Extension and flexion of the left scapulohumeral joint elicited a mild pain response. There was a mild anisocoria noted with the left eye being miotic and accompanied by mild protrusion of the third eyelid, suggestive of Horner's syndrome.

i. Where would the responsible lesion be localized based on this dog's appendicular reflex abnormalities?

ii. Explain the relevance of this dog's ocular abnormalities.

iii. What differential diagnoses should be considered in this dog?

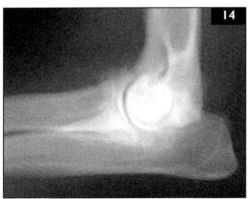

14 A 7-year-old spayed female Labrador retriever is presented for mild intermittent right forelimb lameness. Physical examination reveals pain isolated to the right elbow. Radiographs taken of the dog's right elbow revealed moderate osteoarthritis (**14**). A polysulfated glycosaminoglycan (PSGAG) was administered as part of this dog's therapeutic protocol. Why would PSGAG administration be an appropriate component in the management of this dog's osteoarthritis?

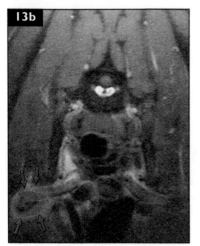

13 i. The responsible lesion would be localized to the left side of spinal cord segments C6–T2, the associated nerve roots and spinal or peripheral nerves. Ipsilateral postural reaction abnormalities in the hindlimbs suggest a spinal cord or proximal nerve root lesion. Intact reflexes in the forelimbs of a tetraparetic dog suggests a lesion cranial to the 6th cervical spinal segment. Hyporeflexia in the left forelimb, as was noted in this dog, indicates a pathologic process of the lower motor units originating in the C6–T2 spinal cord segments. The presence of concurrent ipsilateral hindlimb postural reaction abnormalities supports this localization.

ii. The abnormalities are consistent with Horner's syndrome, in this dog likely a lesion affecting the C6–T2 spinal cord segments, more specifically involving the T1–T2 spinal cord segments or nerve roots. Unilateral Horner's syndrome can develop if the cranial thoracic nerve roots are affected by a tumor or with cord compression at this location.

iii. Differentials should include lateralized disc herniation or neoplasia. An MRI was performed which showed an enlarged nerve exiting the left C7/T1 intervertebral foramen (13b, arrows). Following contrast administration the enlarged nerve enhanced and was seen coursing to the level of the cranial mediastinum. Histopathology confirmed this as a malignant peripheral nerve sheath tumor.

14 PSGAG is most appropriately administered in the early stages of osteoarthritis, as hyaline cartilage does not regenerate once depleted or damaged. The strategy in administering this chondroprotective agent is to mitigate the progression of osteoarthritis and delay the onset of instituting constant, daily administration of an NSAID. Experiments conducted *in vitro* have shown that PSGAGs inhibit prostaglandin E synthesis and certain catabolic enzymes, which have increased activity in inflamed joints. PSGAGs inhibit serine proteinases, which play a role in the interleukin-1-mediated degradation of cartilage proteoglycans and collagen. PSGAGs also inhibit catabolic enzymes such as elastase, stromelysin, matrix metalloproteinases, cathepsin G and B, and hyaluronidases, which degrade collagen, proteoglycans, and hyaluronic acid. PSGAGs also enhance the activity of some anabolic enzymes. PSGAGs have shown a specific potentiating effect on hyaluronic acid synthesis by synovial membrane cells *in vitro*. Although not recognized as an analgesic, clinical investigations have revealed analgesic effects ascribed to PSGAG administration in dogs afflicted with hip dysplasia.

15 A 4-year-old, otherwise healthy, 75 kg Irish wolfhound presented for a presumptive diagnosis of a distal radial osteosarcoma. After obtaining images to stage this dog's tumor there was no overt evidence of metastasis to lung or other skeletal sites. The owners did not wish to pursue amputation.

i. Based on the results of the staging tests and the radiograph shown (**15a**), list the criteria that make this dog a suitable candidate for limb salvage surgery.

ii. What advantages are there for using a metal endoprosthesis (**15b**) rather than an allograft when performing limb salvage?

iii. What are the disadvantages of using a metal endoprosthesis when performing a limb salvage procedure?

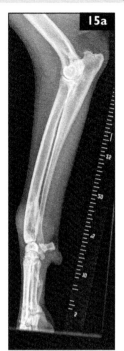
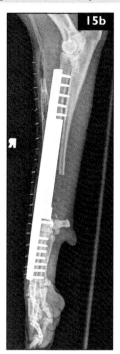

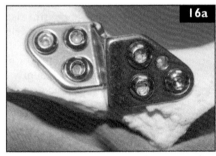

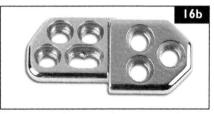

16 Two plates developed for a specific application in dogs are shown (**16a, b**).
i. What is the intended use for these plates?
ii. Name each implant.
iii. What advantages are associated with use of plate **b** compared with plate **a**?

15 i. The tumor involves less than half the longitudinal length of the radius, there is no evidence of pathologic fracture, and the dog is free of overt metastatic disease or other co-morbidities that would preclude survival for at least 9 months. This dog would therefore be a suitable candidate for limb salvage surgery.
ii. Advantages include: the implants are readily available negating the need for an allograft from a bone bank; metal endoprostheses do not require shaping to fit into a defect – the osseous defect is created to conform to the endoprosthesis; and a endoprosthesis is biomechanically stronger than allograft bone.
iii. Disadvantages include: there are limited sizes of implants – tumors that are small may not require such a large ostectomy to accommodate the smallest implant and tumors that are very large may exceed the length of the available endoprostheses; metal has a very different modulus of elasticity than bone and mismatching the moduli of elasticity creates unique biomechanical challenges that can lead to implant failure; and there is little or no osteointegration of the implant, therefore the overall strength of the construct is completely dependent on the integrity of the implants.

16 i. To stabilize pelvic osteotomies, specifically triple pelvic osteotomies in young dogs affected with hip dysplasia. The angular step in the central portion of the plate produces ventrolateral rotation of the secured acetabular segment: the resultant acetabular ventroversion can effectively increase dorsal acetabular coverage of the femoral head, thereby negating coxofemoral subluxation when performed appropriately.
ii. Slocum canine pelvic osteotomy plate (**16a**). This plate has six non-locking screw holes and is available in 20°, 30°, and 40° options. The plate accepts conventional 3.5 mm cortical or 4.0 mm cancellous screws. The cranial portion of the plate contains two asymmetrically positioned round screw holes and one elongated hole, which has an inclined plane that can be used to compress the ilial osteotomy. The caudal portion of the plate has three asymmetrically positioned round holes, as well as a fourth, smaller hole, designed to accept a hemicerclage wire.
New Generation Devices triple pelvic osteotomy plate (**16b**). This plate is a seven hole locking plate available in 15°, 20°, 25°, 30°, and 40° options. The plate also accepts conventional 3.5 mm cortical or 4.0 mm cancellous screws as well as 3.5 mm and 4.0 mm locking cortical screws. The cranial portion of the plate has four screw holes; three are round locking holes while the fourth is an elongated locking combined-hole design. The elongated hole has an inclined plane, which can be used to compress the ilial osteotomy. The caudal portion of the plate has three symmetrically positioned, round locking screw holes.
iii. The New Generation Devices plate is associated with a lower incidence of postoperative screw loosening (0.4%) and an overall lower incidence of complications than previously reported with the Slocum plate (6–23%). Other advantages include the symmetric design of the caudal portion of the plate, which avoids impingement of the implant on the origin of the rectus femoris muscle during plate application.

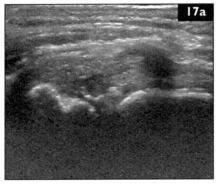

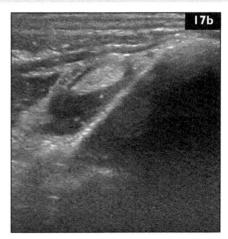

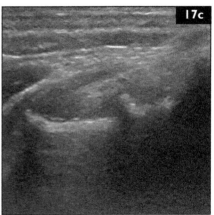

17 A 5-year-old, 29 kg male castrated Labrador retriever, which competes in frisbee competitions, presented with a 1-month history of intermittent left forelimb lameness that developed during and following these activities. During the physical examination, pain was elicited when digital pressure was applied to the cranial aspect of the dog's left scapulohumeral joint. Radiography of the left scapulohumeral joint revealed mild enthesophyte formation on the supraglenoid tubercle of the scapula. Ultrasonographic evaluation of the dog's left biceps brachii tendon was performed. Images of the biceps brachii tendon, one sagittal (**17a**) and two transverse (**17b, c**), are shown.

i. What is the diagnosis?
ii. Describe the pertinent ultrasonographic abnormalities.
iii. How could adhesions, if present, be identified with ultrasound?

18 The Ortolani examination is a clinical diagnostic test used to evaluate hip conformation in dogs and a screening tool for detecting canine hip dysplasia.
i. Briefly describe how the Ortolani maneuver is carried out to test for the presence of a positive Ortolani sign.
ii. For the clinician performing this procedure, what signifies a positive Ortolani sign?
iii. What does a positive Ortolani sign reveal about the conformation and/or stability of the affected coxofemoral joint?

17 i. Bicipital tenosynovitis with interstitial fiber tearing.

ii. There is an increased volume of hypoechoic fluid surrounding the tendon of origin of the biceps brachii muscle (evident in **17a** and **17c**). The biceps brachii tendon is thickened and heterogenous in appearance with loss of the tendon fibers and fiber alignment (best appreciated in the sagittal image). There is a small area of calcification within the biceps tendon just distal to the supraglenoid tubercle (evident in **17a**). The proximal joint capsule is thickened and hyperechoic consistent with chronic injury. There is a small osteophyte along the intertubercular groove (evident in **17c**).

iii. Adhesions will commonly form secondary to bicipital tenosynovitis. These adhesions, identified as hyperechoic thickening of the joint capsule, occur primarily between the cranial margin of the biceps brachii tendon and the joint capsule. The tendon is in close proximity to the joint capsule, which is typically thickened in affected dogs, and separating the two structures can be difficult. To differentiate isolated capsular thickening from an actual adhesion, the tendon can be imaged while moving the scapulohumeral joint through a range of motion. The joint capsule and biceps brachii tendon will normally glide past each other during flexion and extension of the shoulder. When adhesions are present, the joint capsule and biceps tendon do not move independently, as a result of the joint capsule being tethered by the adhesed portion of the tendon.

18 i. The dog should be anesthetized or deeply sedated. The Ortolani maneuver is best performed with the dog in lateral recumbency with the femora parallel and the coxofemoral joint positioned in a standing angle. The uppermost stifle is grasped and a compressive force directed proximally up the shaft of the femur while the clinician's other hand is used to hold the pelvis stationary. While maintaining the compressive force, the stifle is slowly abducted, keeping the pelvis stable.

ii. A positive Ortolani sign is defined as a palpable or audible 'click' or 'clunk' when the hip is abducted under compression during the Ortolani maneuver. This click is the point at which the subluxated femoral head slides off the acetabular rim and relocates into the acetabulum. The degree of coxofemoral joint abduction at the point of reduction can be measured using a goniometer to obtain the angle of reduction.

iii. A positive sign indicates passive coxofemoral laxity. This passive laxity may correlate to the functional laxity (or subluxation) that occurs during normal weight bearing. The angle of reduction provides information regarding the extent to which the dorsal acetabular rim is able to contain the femoral head under compression: the higher the angle, the more open the acetabulum, suggesting reduced acetabular support.

19 A 4-year-old male castrated miniature pinscher was stepped on by the owner and would not place weight on its right hindlimb following the incident. The dog was evaluated later that day. The right metatarsus was swollen and painful. Crepitus and instability were elicited on manipulation of the paw. Radiographs revealed that the dog had fractures of metatarsal bones II–IV (**19a, b**). The fractures were reduced and immobilized in a splint.
i. What method of fracture reduction would be appropriate considering that the fractures were managed in a splint?
ii. What principles would need to be adhered to in order to properly immobilize these fractures with external coaptation?

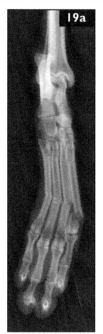
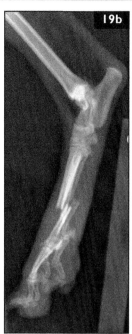

20 A 5-month-old male neutered Labrador retriever was presented because of an intermediate mild weight-bearing left forelimb lameness of 4 weeks' duration. During the orthopedic examination, pain could be elicited on extension of the left elbow. No abnormalities were observed on orthogonal radiographs of this joint. A CT scan was obtained. Transverse sections through both elbows are shown (**20**).
i. What is the diagnosis?
ii. What other diagnostic modalities could have been used to establish this diagnosis?
iii. Which dog breeds are predisposed to this condition?

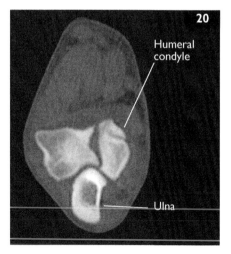

19 i. Closed reduction should be performed if the fractures are to be managed exclusively with external coaptation. This is typically accomplished under general anesthesia using indirect manipulation of the fracture segments, including traction, countertraction, or toggling. In this dog, a towel clamp was placed through the third phalanx of each fractured digit and traction applied sequentially to each digit while countertraction was applied to the crus. A splint was applied once reduction, assessed by palpation and fluoroscopy, was considered adequate (**19c**).

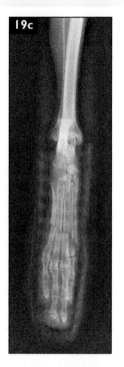

ii. When applying external coaptation, the joint proximal (tarsometatarsal) and distal (metatarsophalangeal) to the fracture must be immobilized. In this dog, the splint extended to the mid-calcaneus, but not to the calcaneal tuber, to avoid potential issues with pressure sores in this region. Splints typically extend distally to the digits to avoid potential distal limb constriction. The very distal portions of the digits are left exposed to allow assessment for developing complications. A Mason metasplint, fashioned using thermoplastic splint material, was molded to conform to the contour of the dog's paw and positioned plantar to maintain reduction and allow weight bearing. The splint was maintained for 9 weeks until the fractures healed.

20 i. This condition is known as incomplete ossification of the humeral condyle (IOHC), and can result in a persistent remnant of cartilage separating the medial and lateral portions of the humeral condyle. The condition is ascribed to failure of fusion of the ossification centers of the medial and lateral portions of the humeral condyle during development. The ossification centers of the humeral condyle are normally fused in dogs by 8–12 weeks of age. While some affected dogs may not have any associated lameness, dogs with incomplete ossification of the humeral condyle are at risk of sustaining fractures of the capitulum of the humeral condyle. The condition has also been ascribed to a stress fracture.

ii. The fissure can usually be detected on high-quality craniocaudal radiographs of the elbow; however, indentification requires the x-ray beam to be directed parallel to the fissure. It might require multiple radiographs at slightly different angles of rotation to make a diagnosis. CT, MRI, and arthroscopy are also used to diagnose IOHC. The condition can be missed during arthroscopy if the articular cartilage is intact across the fissure.

iii. Springer and cocker spaniels are overrepresented, but this condition has been described in other breeds including Labrador retrievers and rottweilers.

21 A 5-year-old male lurcher pre-sented with a 6-week history of right hindlimb lameness (**21a**), which was acute in onset and occurred after the dog had chased a rabbit.
i. What is the most likely diagnosis?
ii. What difficulties should be antici-pated when attempting repair in this dog?
iii. How might this dog have been managed surgically?

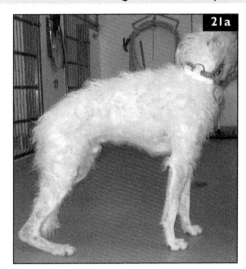

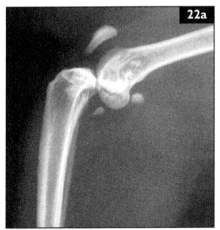
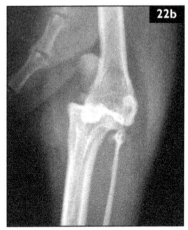

22 An 11-year-old male neutered domestic shorthaired cat presented with an acute left hindlimb lameness. The left stifle was swollen and painful, crepitus and instability were palpable on orthopedic examination. Mediolateral and cranio-caudal view radiographs were taken of the left stifle (**22a, b**).
i. What is the diagnosis?
ii. What anatomic structures are commonly involved with this injury?
iii. What surgical options are available for stabilization of this injury?

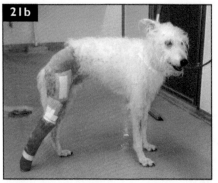

21 i. This dog has hyperflexion of the right tarsus resulting in a somewhat plantigrade stance. The digits on the right hind paw are in a slightly extended position compared with the digits on the forefeet. This dog's lameness is likely due to a rupture of all of the muscles that contribute to the common calcaneal tendon (Achilles tendon complex) – the paired tendon of the gastrocnemius muscle, the combined tendon of the semitendinosus, gracilis and biceps femoris muscles, and the superficial digital flexor tendon.

ii. The injury is chronic in this dog so the tendon ends will be widely distracted and fibrosis may make the ends difficult to identify. Tendon healing is notoriously slow so the repair will need protection from excessive force for a prolonged period of time. After tendon rupture, rather than disruption due to a sharp laceration, the ends are often frayed and poorly identifiable, and suture holding is poor.

iii. A 3.5 mm calcaneotibial screw was placed with the hock in extension prior to tendon repair. Three-loop pulley sutures were applied to realign the tendons in close apposition and a free fascia lata graft was applied around the tendons to augment the repair. A bivalved cast was applied (**21b**).

22 i. Stifle dislocation with cranial displacement of the tibia and fibula. This injury is also referred to as disrupted or deranged stifle.

ii. Traumatic stifle joint disruption results in complete dislocation of the tibiofemoral joint and severe instability. Damaged structures typically include a combination or three or more of: the medial and lateral collateral ligaments, CrCL and CaCL, joint capsule, and medial and lateral menisci. The tendon of origin of the long digital extensor muscle can also be damaged.

iii. The objective of surgery is to repair or replace all disrupted structures and achieve anatomic reduction, which should yield adequate long-term stability. The joint must be thoroughly explored to identify which structures are injured. Damaged portions of menisci are typically resected and avulsed menisci are sutured back into position on the joint capsule. Frayed ends of the collateral ligaments and joint capsule are sutured with a slowly absorbable suture material and the primary collateral ligament repair is augmented with a prosthesis anchored with screws and washers or bone anchors. A lateral tibiofabellar suture of slowly absorbable or non-absorbable material is used to neutralize cranial drawer. Temporary immobilization of the stifle joint is necessary to protect the repair during the first 3–4 weeks after surgery: a transarticular pin or external skeletal fixator is commonly used.

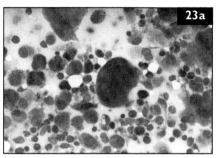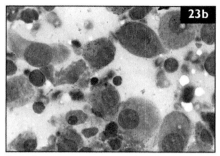

23 A 9-year-old male Irish setter presented with an acute onset of right forelimb lameness. Radiographs showed that there was a spiral fracture of the right proximal humerus. Bone lysis was present at the fracture site. An FNA of the lesion was performed and the retrieved material was evaluated cytologically (**23a, b**).
i. Give a cytologic description of the retrieved material.
ii. What is the diagnosis?
iii. What is the diagnostic accuracy of FNA for this lesion?

24 A 6-month-old female golden retriever is presented because the owner felt the dog had a 'clumsy' hindlimb gait and heard an audible clicking when the dog walked. Observation of the dog at a walk revealed that the dog 'bunny hopped' on both hindlimbs, with dramatic side-to-side swaying of the pelvis. On orthopedic examination, both coxofemoral joints had a positive Ortolani sign and pain was elicited on extension and abduction of both coxofemoral joints. A radiograph of the pelvis is shown (**24**). There is subluxation of both coxofemoral joints, with inadequate acetabular coverage of both femoral heads. Bilaterally, the acetabula are shallow, with blunted cranial margins and marked incongruity between the articular surfaces of the femoral heads and the

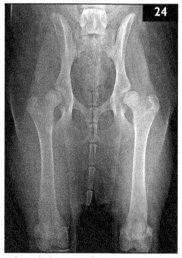

acetabula. The left femoral neck is mildly thickened and there is the impression of mild left hindlimb muscle atrophy. This dog has bilateral hip dysplasia with very early, bilateral secondary degenerative joint disease.
i. Why is this dog painful on coxofemoral joint manipulation?
ii. Which of the following terms – linear, exponential, or biphasic – best describes the relationship between age and discomfort in dogs affected with hip dysplasia?

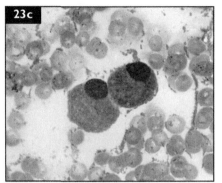

23 i. There is a predominance of individually arranged, round-to-oval cells, with low numbers of large, multinucleated giant cells (**23a**). A dense, amorphous, pink material consistent with osteoid is seen extracellularly (**23a, b**). The majority of cells contain variable amounts of moderately basophilic cytoplasm, often containing granular, eosinophilic material. Nuclei are usually eccentrically located within the cytoplasm. Many nuclei exhibit anaplastic features of malignancy (anisokaryosis, clumped chromatin, multiple or prominent nucleoli, variable nuclear to cytoplasmic ratio). Inflammatory cells are not observed.

ii. Possible etiologies for a pathologic fracture with evidence of bone lysis include infection, inflammation, and neoplasia. The lack of neutrophils and/or macrophages makes infection unlikely. The monomorphic population of cells is indicative of neoplasia. The anaplastic nuclear features are typical of malignancy and the arrangement of the cells is most suggestive of a sarcoma (osteosarcoma, fibrosarcoma, chondrosarcoma, hemangiosarcoma, giant cell sarcoma). The cytologic features of round-to-oval cells with eccentrically located nuclei reminiscent of osteoblasts (normal osteoblasts, **23c**), multinucleated giant cells, and the presence of extracellular pink material, as well as intracytoplasmic granules, is consistent with osteoid, substantiating a tentative diagnosis of osteosarcoma.

iii. In one study osteosarcoma was accurately diagnosed from 85% of FNAs and 95% of core biopsies. There was no significant difference between the two techniques.

24 i. At this age, discomfort is related to inflammation within the joint, progressive stretching of the joint capsule, tearing of Sharpey's fibers, as well as osteochondral damage within the coxofemoral joint. Subluxation of the femoral head alters load distribution in the joint. The altered contact mechanics results in cartilage damage and microfractures within the subchondral bone of the dorsal acetabular rim and femoral head. As the fractures heal, the bone becomes harder and less efficient with respect to load transfer. This propagates further osteochondral damage, which can lead to complete loss of articular cartilage and eburnation of the underlying subchondral bone.

ii. Biphasic. Many dogs exhibit subtle characteristic clinical abnormalities, due to the pain from joint laxity, at 4–5 months of age. Pain and dysfunction tend to increase until 12–16 months of age. At that point, in most dogs, pain and dysfunction begin to subside as the progressive intra- and periarticular changes, most notably the thickening of the joint capsule, lead to improved coxofemoral joint stability. Affected dogs typically become more comfortable and exhibit less lameness. Unfortunately, clinical signs and discomfort tend to recur as the dogs become older and osteoarthritis progresses.

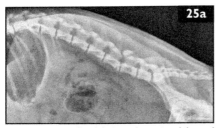

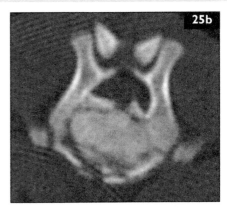

25 A 6-month-old female mixed-breed dog weighing 10 kg was presented after being hit by a car. The dog had hindlimb paraplegia, and a Schiff–Sherrington posture. Hindlimb reflexes were depressed or absent, but superficial and deep pain sensation was retained in both hindlimbs. Two fractures (T12/13; L5/6) were identified on radiographs of the thoracolumbar vertebral column (25a) and CT was performed to further characterize these lesions: 25b is a transverse view of the cranial aspect of the body of T13 and 25c is a transverse view of the cranial aspect of L6. Although paraplegic, retention of superficial and deep pain sensation suggests that this dog has a fair-to-good prognosis for recovery.

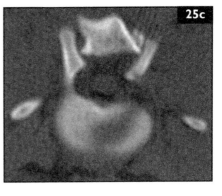

i. List criteria that would justify surgical intervention predicated on this dog's history, clinical examination findings, and images.
ii. List possible surgical options for stabilizing either vertebral injury.

26 An implant system used to manage coxofemoral abnormalities in dogs is shown (26).
i. Name this specific implant system.
ii. What materials are used in manufacturing the individual implant components?
iii. How does this system differ from the more traditional systems used for this application in dogs?

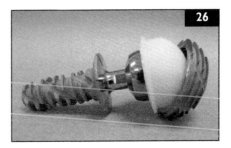

25 i. The objective of treatment is to limit further damage associated with continued instability and to relieve spinal cord or nerve root compression. Advanced imaging (CT or MRI) can be helpful. Instability can be demonstrated, using standard radiography or fluoroscopy, by obtaining dynamic flexion and extension views of the vertebral column. The efficacy, accuracy, and risk of this approach are not well established. Many surgeons use a 'three column system' to characterize instability. In this system, the dorsal column consists of the laminae, spinous processes, and associated ligaments. The dorsal longitudinal ligament, dorsal annulus, and dorsal cortex of the vertebral bodies constitute the middle column. The ventral column consists of the ventral longitudinal ligament, the ventral annulus, and the ventral cortex of the vertebral bodies. If more than one column is affected, instability is likely, increasing the need for surgical intervention. Consideration could be given to surgical stabilization of both of this dog's fractures.

ii. Spinal stapling; dorsal spinous process plating using lubra plates (fractured dorsal spinous processes would preclude application to the caudal fracture); pins or screws used in conjunction with PMMA; vertebral body plating (particularly to stabilize the T12/13 fracture) using either a conventional or string of pearls plate(s); or an external fixator (particularly to stabilize the lumbar fracture), which could be applied in an open or closed (fluoroscopy-assisted) fashion.

26 i. Helica hip prosthesis system. This system consists of a hip stem screw, an acetabular cup with an inlay, and a femoral head.

ii. The hip stem and the acetabular screw cup are made from a titanium alloy. The acetabular inlay is made from high molecular weight polyethylene. The femoral head is made from 316L stainless steel with a titanium nitride coating. Both the hip stem screw and acetabular screw cup have a rough blasted surface to encourage osteointegration of the implant.

iii. The femoral component of most traditional hip replacement systems has a stem that is inserted into the intramedullary canal of the proximal femur after reaming. In the intact femur the stress is distributed over the entire cross section of the bone. After hip replacement this pattern of stress distribution is altered because of the manner in which load is transferred from the prosthesis to the bone, which may result in fracture of the femur or bone resorption. A more proximal osteotomy, made through the femoral neck, is done when implanting a Helica hip prosthesis. The available bone stock in the femoral neck is utilized for anchoring the hip stem screw. Securing the femoral component in the neck also allows relatively simple revision by placement of larger implants or, alternatively, conversion to a traditional hip replacement system can be done if necessary.

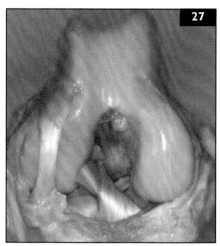

27 An image obtained during dissection of a dog's stifle is shown (27).
i. Name the two bands that form the CrCL.
ii. What are the anatomic features of the two bands of the CrCL?

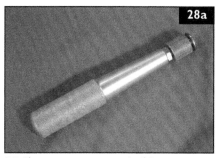
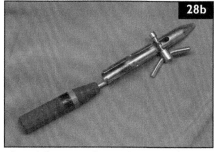

28 Shown are two surgical instruments used to tighten cerclage wire (28a, b).
i. Describe the configuration of cerclage wire that each of these instruments is designed to produce.
ii. What are the advantages and disadvantages of the two types of cerclage produced with these instruments?

27 i. The CrCL is one of the four femorotibial ligaments that provide primary ligamentous support to the stifle. The CrCL is divided into craniomedial and caudolateral bands.

ii. The CrCL originates in a fossa on the caudomedial aspect of the lateral femoral condyle. The ligament courses craniomedially through the intercondylar fossa and inserts on the cranial intercondyloid area of the tibial plateau subjacent to the intermeniscal ligament and the cranial horn of the medial meniscus. The CrCL is grossly divided into a thinner craniomedial band and a larger caudolateral band. The craniomedial band has a more caudoproximal origin on the lateral femoral condyle and inserts on the craniomedial aspect of the cranial articular surface of the tibial plateau. As the CrCL courses from proximal to distal, the fascicles of the craniomedial band are oriented in an outward spiral arrangement. During flexion these fascicles are deformed around the larger fascicles of the caudolateral band. The caudolateral band is shorter and straighter than the craniomedial band and inserts along the caudolateral aspect of the tibial attachment.

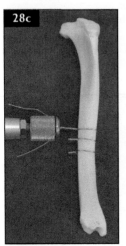

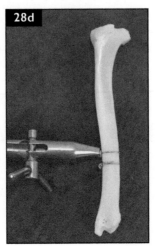

28 i. The instrument in **28a** is used to tighten twist-type cerclage wires. The two free ends of the wire are inserted into holes in the head of the instrument, which is then tightened. The instrument is rotated while applying tension to ensure that an even braid will be formed as the wire is twisted (**28c**). The instrument in **28b** is used to tighten loop-type cerclage wires. The free end of the wire is passed through the preformed eye at the other end of the wire, then fed through the oval hole in the end of the instrument and finally through the cannulation in the crank handle. The crank is placed in one of the slots in the instrument. Turning the crank tightens the wire. When the wire is tight, it is secured by bending the wire through a 180° angle in the plane parallel to the loop (**28d**).

ii. The static tension of loop-type wires is greater than that of twist-type wires. Twist-type wires have a greater ultimate strength and greater resistance to knot failure, due to the increased area of contact in the twist-type knot. The loop-type wires have less potential for traumatizing adjacent soft tissue structures than protruding twist-type wires. Twist-type wires, however, lose significant tension if the twist is bent over to lie flat against the cortex.

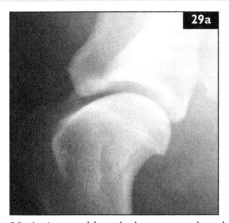
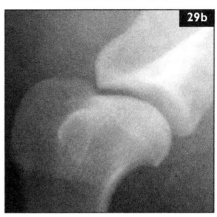

29 A 4-year-old male large cross-breed dog presented with a 3-month history of left forelimb lameness. The lameness occurred acutely while exercising. Some improvement was noted following exercise restriction and administration of an anti-inflammatory medication, but the dog remained moderately lame. The lameness was exacerbated by exercise. On orthopedic examination the dog had swelling and pain in the region of the origin of the biceps brachii tendon and pain was elicited on flexion of the scapulohumeral joint with the elbow extended. Mediolateral radiographs of the left (29a) and right scapulohumeral joints (29b) are shown.
i. Describe the radiographic abnormalities.
ii. What type of contrast agent, and what volume and concentration, should be used to perform shoulder arthrography in this dog?

30 A 6-year-old female neutered cat went missing overnight. When the cat returned home it would not place weight on the left forelimb. On presentation, the cat held the left elbow in slight flexion. Palpation revealed soft tissue swelling proximal to the olecranon and the area was very painful. A mediolateral radiograph of the left elbow is shown (30).
i. What is the most likely diagnosis based on the clinical and radiographic findings?
ii. What conditions or circumstances have been reported that predispose cats and dogs to this injury?
iii. Describe appropriate treatment and aftercare for this cat.

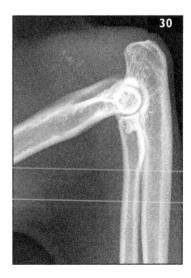

29 i. There is a slightly irregular appearance to the most cranial margin of the left supraglenoid tuberosity due to enthesophyte formation, and the bone is slightly sclerotic when compared with the right shoulder.

ii. A water-soluble non-ionic contrast, such as Omnipaque (iohexol), is most commonly used to perform arthrography in dogs. Water-soluble ionic contrast such as Urografin (sodium diatrizoate and meglumine diatrizoate) can also be used. The concentration of iohexol used for arthrography varies between 100 and 150 mg I/ml: 3–5 ml are typically injected into the scapulohumeral joint in an average sized dog.

30 i. Avulsion of the insertion of the triceps tendon. The radiograph reveals marked soft tissue swelling proximal to the olecranon. Several small, irregularly shaped, mineral opaque structures are visible within the swelling. The margin of the olecranon is smooth, suggesting the opacities represent mineralization, rather than avulsed osseous fragments, and that this cat had a pre-existing triceps tendinopathy (see also **ii.**). In animals with a complete rupture of the triceps tendon, the animal is unable to actively extend the elbow and a gap in the tendon can often be palpated proximal to the olecranon.

ii. Pre-existing tendinopathy of the triceps tendon has been reported. Intra-tendinous mineralization may be caused by previous or repetitive trauma or a disturbance in the local blood supply. Triceps tendon rupture has been described in two dogs as a sequela to local corticosteroid injection.

iii. Surgery is indicated to restore limb function. In this cat the avulsed tendon was debrided and reattached to the olecranon (through a series of tunnels) using a modified three-loop pulley suture. The tenorrhaphy was oversewn with a series of horizontal mattress sutures. The limb was placed in a Spica splint for 3 weeks to maintain the elbow in extension. Alternatively, a transarticular external fixator could have been used to protect the repair. Cage confinement was imposed for 6 weeks, followed by a gradual return to normal activity.

31 At a recent agility trial a 5-year-old male castrated Border collie splayed out when the dog landed after a jump. The right hindlimb went into extension and abduction. The dog subsequently would not place weight on the right hindlimb and was pulled from the trial. On physical examination, obvious discomfort was elicited when the right coxofemoral joint was

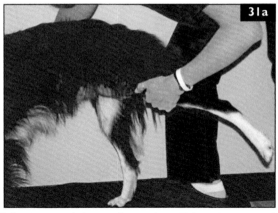

placed into extension with abduction and internal rotation (**31a**). Spasm and discomfort were also noted during palpation of the right groin region.
i. What is the diagnosis, and how are these injuries typically sustained?
ii. Describe the anatomy of the injured structure.

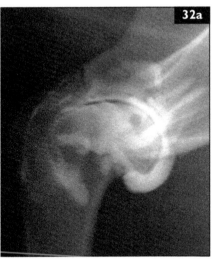

32 A left shoulder arthrogram was performed on the dog described in case **29**. The mediolateral view of the arthrogram is shown (**32a**).
i. What abnormalities are seen on the arthrogram, and what might these abnormalities indicate?
ii. Describe appropriate treatment options for this dog.

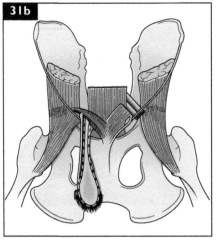

31 i. This dog has likely sustained an iliopsoas strain resulting from excessive force acting on this muscle. These injuries are commonly incurred during highly athletic activities such as agility. The musculotendinous junction, which is the weakest segment of the myotendinous unit, is the area usually affected. Eccentric contraction, in which the muscle is activated during stretch, is often the cause of acute strain injuries. Traumatic incidents that result in active eccentric muscle contraction (e.g. slipping into a splay-legged position, jumping out of a vehicle, aggressive agility training) often precipitate acute lameness.

ii. The iliopsoas muscle represents the fusion of the psoas major and the iliacus muscles (**31b**). The psoas major muscle arises from the transverse processes of the lumbar vertebrae of the lower spinal column at L2 and L3 and the bodies of L4–7. The iliacus muscle arises from the ventral or lower surface of the ilium. The two muscles conjoin and have a common insertion on the lesser trochanter of the femur. The action of this muscle is to advance the hindlimb relative to the trunk via coxofemoral joint flexion.

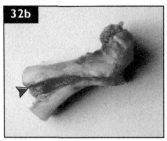

32 i. There is a longitudinal linear filling defect in the region of the origin of the biceps brachii tendon. The outline of the distal portion of the tendon is indistinct. There is leakage of contrast shown as linear streaks superimposed on the caudal shoulder joint. These abnormalities are indicative of bicipital tenosynovitis and the filling defect suggests that there may be a longitudinal tear in the tendon.

ii. Some dogs with bicipital tenosynovitis can be managed effectively with conservative treatment. As conservative treatment had not been effective in alleviating this dog's lameness, surgical exploration was performed though a craniomedial approach to the scapulohumeral joint. The tendon was partially ruptured from the supraglenoid tuberosity. A tenectomy was performed (**32b** shows the excised segment of the origin of the biceps brachii tendon). The longitudinal tear that was apparent as a filling defect on the arthrogram is visible (arrowhead) and there is pronounced fraying, fibrillation, and loss of normal gross tendon structure. After resection of the damaged portion of tendon, a tenodesis was performed using a spiked staple to secure the remaining tendon to the proximal humerus.

33 With regard to the dog in case **31**:
i. What diagnostic procedure(s) can be performed to confirm the diagnosis?
ii. What are the treatment options for iliopsoas strains?

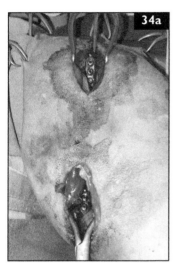 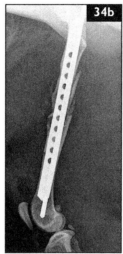 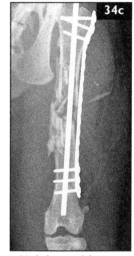

34 A 2-year-old female cat sustained a comminuted diaphyseal left femoral fracture. The fracture was stabilized with a plate-rod construct applied using the minimally invasive plate osteosynthesis (MIPO) technique (**34a**). Immediate postoperative radiographs are shown (**34b, c**).
i. What type of reduction technique is generally used when performing MIPO?
ii. What are the potential advantages of employing a MIPO technique?
iii. List potential problems and complications associated with MIPO.

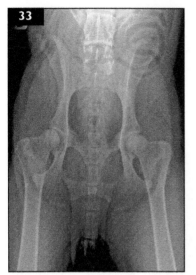

33

33 i. Several different diagnostic imaging modalities can be used. Radiography is of little value in acute injuries, but may reveal mineralization just cranial to the lesser trochanter in chronic cases (33). Ultrasonography is a relatively inexpensive, non-invasive imaging modality for dogs with more chronic injuries, but it is dependent on the expertise of the operator, which may limit its application in some settings. CT and MRI may be used to identify iliopsoas strains and both are used extensively to diagnose acute, stretch-induced, muscle injuries in people. Although CT is valuable for imaging soft tissue lesions, MRI has greatly increased the ability to detect more subtle lesions.

ii. Iliopsoas strains often respond favorably to conservative treatment. Skeletal muscle relaxants may be administered in severe cases to reduce pain and muscle spasms. Medical management typically includes NSAIDs, cryotherapy, and controlled activity. Rehabilitation can be very effective. Rehabilitation therapy programs typically utilize modalities such as laser therapy, manual therapy, and a therapeutic exercise program. One study demonstrated that 33% of dogs improved with rest and administration of NSAIDs compared with 63% that improved with rehabilitation therapy.

34 i. Indirect fracture reduction is generally used. Highly comminuted fractures are often non-reducible, as the bone column cannot be anatomically reconstructed. The objective of reduction is focused primarily on restoring normal limb alignment (i.e. correct axial alignment of the adjacent joints and restoration of bone length). This is achieved by realigning the proximal and distal articular portions of the major fracture segments without exposing or disturbing the intercalary fracture fragments. Tension in the soft tissue surrounding the fracture will often align the comminuted fragments as the fracture is distracted out to length.

ii. MIPO offers the potential advantages of limiting iatrogenic tissue trauma and minimizing further disruption to the osseous blood supply. These attributes should lessen the risk of infection, decrease postoperative pain, and allow for faster recovery and earlier rehabilitation, all of which should accelerate fracture healing. Decreased operative times should be expected from surgeons experienced in the MIPO technique.

iii. In human patients, MIPO is greatly facilitated by the use of intraoperative fluoroscopy, which is not routinely available in veterinary institutions. Thus, intraoperative assessment of bone orientation and accurate implant placement are challenging. Potential problems with this technique include poor fracture reduction, which can result in malalignment and fracture malunion, or a large fracture gap leading to delayed or non-union.

35 Immediate postoperative radiographs of a short oblique mid-diaphyseal tibial fracture with a concurrent fibular fracture in a 7-month-old male cat are shown (35a, b). The fracture was reduced and stabilized with an intramedullary pin and a unilateral uniplanar (type Ia) external skeletal fixator.

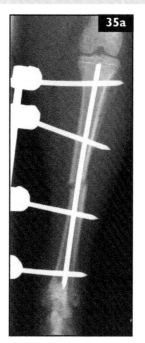
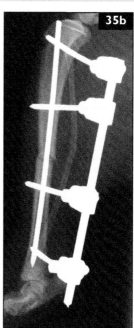

i. Describe the techniques for normograde and retrograde insertion of an intramedullary pin in a cat's tibia.
ii. When placing an intramedullary pin in a cat's tibia, should the pin be inserted in a normograde or retrograde fashion?

36 A mode of manual postoperative therapy is being applied to the surgical incision over a dog's hip joint (36).
i. Name this mode of therapy.
ii. Describe the mechanisms of action of this therapeutic modality.
iii. What are common clinical indications for using this therapeutic modality in dogs and cats?
iv. What precautions should be taken with the application of this modality in order to prevent iatrogenic tissue injury?

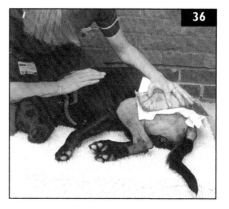

35 i. Normograde technique: the pin is inserted in the proximal tibia midway between the tibial tuberosity and the medial tibial condyle on the medial ridge of the tibial plateau via a medial parapatellar approach. The tip of the pin is seated just cranial to the intermeniscal ligament, the stifle flexed to 90°, and the pin advanced into the medullary cavity. Once the pin emerges at the fracture, the fracture segments are aligned and the pin is advanced into the distal tibial segment. Retrograde technique: the pin is inserted into the medullary cavity from the fracture site and directed proximally. The pin is aimed slightly craniomedial as it is advanced. Once the pin emerges proximally, the chuck is attached to the protruding pin and the distal end of the pin is withdrawn into the proximal fracture segment. The fracture is aligned and the pin is advanced and seated in the distal tibial segment. With either method, caution is used to avoid advancing the pin too far distally and penetrating the tarsus. Once seated distally, the proximal end of the pin is cut short, preferably using a counter sinking technique, to minimize soft tissue impingement.

ii. A feline cadaveric study found that retrograde pins could be directed to emerge cranial to the intermeniscal ligament, avoiding articular penetration. Pins, however, often impaled the patellar tendon and thus normograde pin insertion is advocated when stabilizing tibial fractures in cats.

36 i. Cryotherapy: in this instance a cold pack is being applied to the dog's thigh.
ii. Cryotherapy is a physical method of local pain control, which is achieved by decreasing each of the following at the site of application: tissue perfusion (via vasoconstriction), edema formation, hemorrhage, histamine release, local metabolism, muscle spindle activity, nerve conduction velocity, spasticity, and acute inflammation.
iii. Cryotherapy can be used in dogs and cats to treat the following conditions: acute inflammation, particularly inflammation associated with trauma including post-surgical trauma, cutaneous burns, and cutaneous hemorrhage.
iv. If applied incorrectly or under the wrong circumstances, cryotherapy can result in congelatio (frostbite). Cryotherapy should therefore not be applied to ischemic or poorly perfused tissues and the cold pack should not be applied directly to the skin; rather a damp cloth should be placed between the cryotherapy agent and the animal's skin. The cloth will prevent direct contact of the cryotherapy unit with the animal's soft tissues, and the moisture will facilitate heat conduction. Cryotherapy should be applied for a maximum of 15 minutes per treatment.

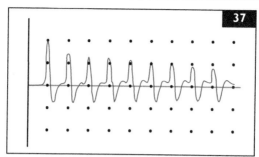

37 The results of repetitive peripheral nerve stimulation obtained during electro-diagnostic evaluation of a 7-year-old female German short-haired pointer are shown (37). The owner reported that the dog had a 4-month history of exercise intolerance, but no specific lameness. No abnormalities were noted during the orthopedic examination other than the dog tired quickly and subsequently refused to ambulate when walked outside to assess its gait.

i. What abnormality is apparent on the repetitive peripheral nerve stimulation evaluation?

ii. What is the most likely diagnosis?

iii. Describe the etiopathogenesis of this condition.

iv. What additional diagnostic evaluations could be done to substantiate the diagnosis?

38 A 1-year-old black Labrador retriever sustained a non-weight-bearing lameness after being kicked by a horse. The dog's shoulder was swollen and marked pain was elicited on gentle manipulation of this joint. A radiograph of the shoulder region is shown (38). Describe and classify this fracture.

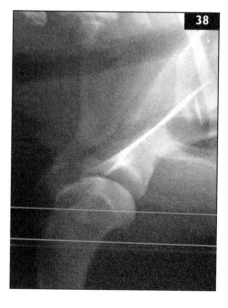

37 i. There is a decremental response of the evoked muscle action potentials as the amplitude of the waves progressively decreases with successive stimulation.
ii. Generalized myasthenia gravis (MG), most likely the acquired form given the dog's age and history. Large breed dogs are most commonly affected. A familial basis has been suggested in Great Danes and Newfoundlands.
iii. Acquired MG, an immune disorder of unknown origin, is caused by the production of autoantibodies that bind to postsynaptic membrane acetylcholine receptors, preventing the binding of endogenous acetylcholine released from the terminal axon in response to efferent neuronal impulses. Receptors bound by antibodies become dysfunctional and must be replaced by new receptors; however, the large number of receptors typically ensures some functional receptors are active. Exercise-induced fatigue or paresis occurs as the remaining functional receptors are stimulated, but they do not have sufficient time to recover and be reactivated during periods of sustained activity.
iv. Intravenous administration of the short-acting cholinesterase inhibitor edrophonium chloride, the so-called 'Tensilon test', will often transiently improve an affected dog's exercise tolerance or eliminate a dog's decremental response to repetitive nerve stimulation. Edrophonium blocks the degradation of acetylcholine, increasing the concentration of available acetylcholine molecules to bind to receptors that have not been inactivated by antibodies. Immunoprecipitation radio-immunoassay testing for serum acetylcholine receptor antibody titers is considered the definitive means of diagnosing MG. Acetylcholine receptor antibodies can also be identified by incubating an affected dog's serum on histologic preparations of sections of normal dog muscle. The preparation is subsequently incubated with staphylococcal protein A that has been conjugated with horseradish peroxidase and will detect serum acetylcholine receptor antibodies that have bound to the neuromuscular junctions of the normal muscle.

38 This dog has sustained a comminuted fracture of the scapula. The fracture has a Y-shaped configuration with one arm extending from the supraglenoid tuberosity proximally into the scapular body cranial to the scapular spine. The other arm of the Y extends through the distal third of the scapular spine. There is proximal displacement of the glenoid, acromion process, and distal scapular spine. Traditional classification schemes classify scapular fractures as type I, II, or III. Fractures that can be included in more than one category should be classified according to the most severe category involved. This dog would be categorized as a type III, the most severe type, as the fracture involves the scapular neck and supraglenoid tubercle. Type I fractures involve the scapular body and type II the scapular spine and acromion. An alternative classification system considers biomechanical principles. Fractures are classified as stable extra-articular, unstable extra-articular, and intra-articular. The fracture in this dog would likely be considered as an unstable extra-articular, as the fragments are liable to displace with weight bearing or avulsive muscular forces. Intra-articular fractures in this classification scheme are considered the most severe fractures.

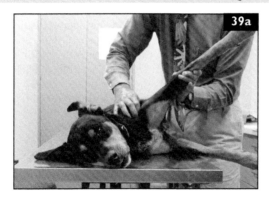

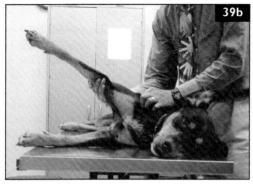

39 A 3-year-old male neutered mixed-breed agility dog was evaluated for a chronic weight-bearing lameness of the left forelimb. On examination, abnormalities were isolated to the left shoulder, which was painful on abduction. Mild atrophy of the left infraspinatus and supraspinatus muscles was also noted. Palpation of both the right (**39a**) and the left (**39b**) scapulohumeral joint with the dog sedated is shown.
i. What test is being performed in these images?
ii. What anatomic structures does this test evaluate?
iii. What is the most likely diagnosis for the cause of this dog's lameness?
iv. What arthroscopic findings would be expected in this dog's left shoulder?

40 i. Why should the fracture in case **38** be addressed surgically rather than with conservative or non-surgical management?
ii. Describe the surgical approach that would allow open reduction and stabilization of this fracture.

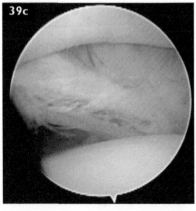

39 i. A shoulder abduction angle test.
ii. Measuring abduction angles with a goniometer is useful for diagnosing medial shoulder instability. This test evaluates the integrity of the medial support structures of the scapulohumeral joint. The images show a much higher abduction angle (greater laxity) in the left than in the right scapulohumeral joint. Reference range reported for abduction angles of normal shoulders of large-breed dogs is 32.6° $\pm$ 2.0°, while shoulders affected with medial instability had abduction angles of 53.7° $\pm$ 4.7°.

iii. The structures most commonly affected in dogs with medial shoulder instability include the subscapularis tendon, the medial glenohumeral ligament, and the craniomedial joint capsule. In dogs with chronic injuries, the articular cartilage, biceps tendon, and supraspinatus tendon may become affected due to instability and compensatory changes.
iv. A craniolateral arthroscopic portal should be used to evaluate the medial compartment of the scapulohumeral joint. Tearing of the medial glenohumeral ligament, fiber separation of the subscapularis tendon, joint capsule laxity, fibrillation of the labrum along the medial rim of the glenoid of the scapula, and localized synovitis would be expected and were found during arthroscopy of this dog's left shoulder (39c).

40 i. Surgical management would be advantageous because the cranial fracture segment is displaced distally, suggesting distraction by the biceps tendon. The glenoid segment is shifted proximally due to weight-bearing forces and muscle disruption. The fracture configuration, specifically the cranial fragment, may also interfere with shoulder extension.
ii. A wide exposure is often necessary to allow for accurate fracture reduction. In this dog, an osteotomy of the greater tubercle was done to allow proximal reflection of the supraspinatus tendon and muscle. An osteotomy of the acromion process was also done to reflect the acromion head of the deltoid muscle distally. After the fracture was reduced and stabilized, the greater tubercle was replaced and stabilized with pin and tension band fixation. The acromion osteotomy was stabilized with wire sutures; alternatively, pin and tension band fixation could have been used. An intermuscular approach to the supraglenoid tuberosity has been described, avoiding osteotomies, but affords limited exposure. The latter approach has been used for repair of isolated avulsion fractures of the supraglenoid tubercle.

41 A 4-year-old, 23 kg mixed-breed dog presented with a 1-month history of mild lameness and a large firm palpable mass over the left proximal femur. A ventrodorsal radiograph of the pelvis is shown (41a).
i. Describe the radiographic abnormalities.
ii. What is the most likely diagnosis?
iii. What additional diagnostic procedure should be done to establish a definitive diagnosis?

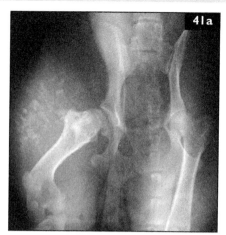

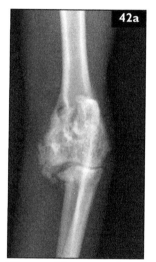

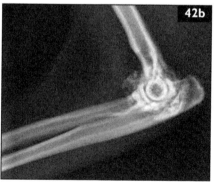

42 A 17-year-old castrated male Abyssinian cat presented for evaluation of a chronic left forelimb lameness that had progressively increased in severity. On orthopedic examination, the cat had an obvious weight-bearing lameness of the left forelimb. The left elbow was thickened and crepitus and pain could be elicited during elbow flexion and extension. Mediolateral and craniocaudal radiographs of the left elbow are shown (42a, b).
i. Describe the radiographic abnormalities.
ii. What are the differential diagnoses for the condition affecting this cat's elbow?
iii. Describe the pathophysiology of this disease.

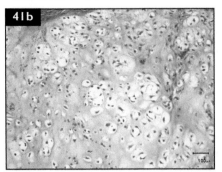

41 i. There is unilateral left coxofemoral degenerative joint disease and a large osteoproliferative mass associated with the lateral aspect of the left proximal femur. Cortical lysis is not apparent.
ii. Primary bone tumor, most likely either an osteosarcoma, possibly a parosteal or periosteal osteosarcoma, or a chondrosarcoma.
iii. An incisional biopsy should be obtained. In this dog, a wedge of tissue was obtained via a small skin incision in a location that would allow the biopsy tract to be completely excised at the time of any definitive surgery. Histologic examination yielded a diagnosis of chondrosarcoma (**41b**). A wedge biopsy was done, rather than needle core biopsies obtained with an instrument such as a Jamshidi needle, because a large biopsy specimen could be procured without inducing cortical trauma, which might predispose this dog's femur to a pathologic fracture. Clinicians must be wary of a diagnosis of chondrosarcoma based on small biopsy specimens as the tumor could in fact be a chondroblastic osteosarcoma. Osteoid must be identified to establish a diagnosis of osteosarcoma and core biopsy specimens may be too small to demonstrate the presence of osteoid. This dog was treated by amputation and the diagnosis of chondrosarcoma confirmed.

42 i. There are multiple, irregular, well-marginated discrete mineralized opaque bodies located circumferentially within this cat's elbow. Small, well-defined osteophytes are noted in association with the humeral condyle, the ulna, and the lateral margin of the radius. Enthesophyte formation is also seen on both humeral epicondyles. The subchondral bone of the ulnar trochlear notch is sclerotic.
ii. These radiographic abnormalities are most compatible with synovial osteochondromatosis (synovial chondrometaplasia) with secondary degenerative joint disease (DJD). This must be differentiated from feline osteochondromatosis, fragmented osteophytes in conjunction with severe DJD, hypervitaminosis A, fibrodysplasia ossificans, and myositis ossificans. Osteochondritis dissecans is very uncommon in cats, but has been reported.
iii. Synovial osteochondromatosis is an uncommon disease characterized by formation of chondral or osteochondral nodules within the synovial tissue of a joint, tendon sheath, or bursa. Discrete, subsynovial nodules of collagen, fibro-cartilaginous metaplasia, or hyaline cartilage form, and some of these metaplastic nodules undergo endochondral ossification. Lesions can develop in articular, periarticular, or juxta-articular locations. Initially, the radiographic appearance may reflect only soft tissue swelling due to the presence of the non-mineralized bodies and effusion. As the disease progresses, the lesions may mineralize and become visible radiographically, along with various degrees of DJD.

43 A 2-year-old female racing greyhound was presented 2 days after a race for evaluation of a unilateral hindlimb lameness. The owner reported that the dog had slowed down on the last bend. Lameness was not obvious immediately after the race, but had become more noticeable over the

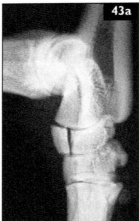

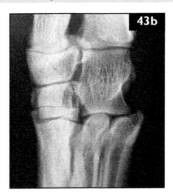

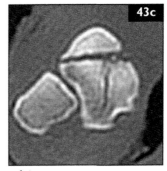

subsequent 24 hours. Physical examination revealed marked swelling affecting the dorsal aspect of one of the tarsi. Pain was elicited on full flexion and extension of the affected hock and when firm digital pressure was applied to the dorsal aspect of the talocentral joint. Radiographs (orthogonal mediolateral, plantarodorsal) (43a, b) and a CT scan (43c) were obtained.

i. What is the diagnosis?
ii. Which hock is typically affected in racing greyhounds?
iii. Which three additional bones are commonly fractured concurrently in racing dogs that sustain this injury?
iv. How would this fracture be classified?
v. What is the most common etiopathogenesis for this type of injury?
vi. What treatment would most likely allow this dog to return to racing?

44 A dog is shown receiving treatment that is commonly used in both human physical therapy and canine rehabilitation therapy (44).
i. Name the therapeutic modality being used in this dog and list the common indications for its use in dogs with orthopedic injuries.
ii. Describe the purported therapeutic mechanism of this modality.
iii. List potential contraindications for the use of this therapeutic modality.

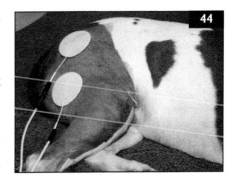

43 i. Fracture of the central tarsal bone, one of the most common fractures sustained by racing greyhounds.
ii. The right hock is affected in 96% of racing dogs with this injury.
iii. Tarsal bone IV, the calcaneus, and tarsal bone III.
iv. Fractures of the central tarsal bone have been classified into five types. Based on the radiographs, this appears to be a simple displaced dorsal slab fracture, which would be classified as a type II fracture. The CT scan reveals a second incomplete fracture line, making this a type IV fracture.
v. These fractures are stress related in racing dogs. The repetitive bone loading, generated by the anticlockwise racing around a track, initiates a site-specific adaptive remodeling response. Remodeling is characterized by thick, compacted trabeculae with reduced marrow space and microcrack formation in the dorsal region of the bone. Fractures occur when the adaptive response is inadequate or does not respond fast enough to cyclic loading stress.
vi. Type IV fractures should be treated with open reduction and internal fixation with screws placed in lag fashion. Traditionally, a 4.0 mm partially threaded cancellous screw is inserted from the medial fragment into tarsal bone IV. A 2.7 mm or 2.0 mm cortical screw is inserted, again in lag fashion, from the dorsal fragment to engage the plantar process of the central tarsal bone. The prognosis for return to pre-injury racing form is generally good.

44 i. Transcutaneous electrical nerve stimulation (TENS) – involves the therapeutic application of an electric current to stimulate neuromuscular activity. In dogs, TENS can be used to decrease postoperative joint pain and effusion, for the treatment of osteoarthritis, or to manage chronic musculoskeletal pain.
ii. The precise mechanism of action of TENS has yet to be clearly elucidated, but there are two current theories. The first is the gate control theory, which states that small-diameter, slow-conducting, nociceptive nerve fibers, with little or no myelin (A-delta, C fibers), transmit painful stimuli to the spinal cord and the brain. These fibers can be inhibited by electrical stimulation of large-diameter, fast-conducting, highly myelinated proprioceptive sensory nerve fibers (A-beta fibers), thereby reducing the transmission of pain. The second is the opiate-mediated control theory. Endogenous opiates, produced in the pituitary gland as beta-endorphins and in the spinal cord as enkephalins, are released by electrical stimulation of sensory nerves. The opiates then bind to receptor sites in the central and peripheral nervous systems where these substances block the perception of pain. It is most likely that both mechanisms function *in vivo*, depending on which method is applied and the exact settings of the electrical stimulation.
iii. TENS should not be used in dogs with demand-type pacemakers, in pregnant bitches or in dogs with epilepsy, on areas of infection or over the carotid sinus.

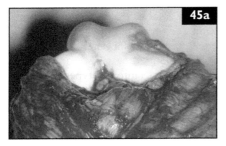

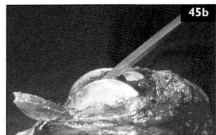

45 A 12-month-old female, Labrador mixed-breed dog had a history of intermittent left hindlimb lameness and occasional hesitation when rising from a sitting position. On examination, the dog had a left grade II/IV lateral patellar luxation; the patella typically luxated when the dog assumed a sitting posture as the stifle flexed. When the dog extended the stifle to stand, the patella would spontaneously reduce. The radiologist's report stated that, 'the length of the patellar ligament is 1.3 times the length of the patella on the

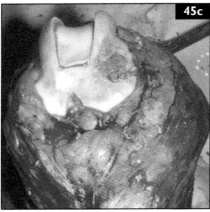

lateral radiographic image'. The dog was surgically treated for grade II/IV lateral patellar luxation.

i. What co-morbidity of the femoropatellar joint, typical of dogs with lateral patellar luxation, was noted on the radiographic report that accounts for the fact that the dog's patella typically luxates during stifle flexion?

ii. What morphologic abnormalities are evident in **45a**?

iii. What procedure is being performed in **45b, c**?

iv. Discuss the merits of this specific procedure for improving this dog's femoro-patellar joint conformation.

46 Eccentric, concentric, and isometric exercises are common techniques used during both physical therapy in human patients and rehabilitation therapy in dogs.

i. Define concentric, eccentric, and isometric contractions.

ii. Describe how these contractions would be completed in relation to motion of the elbow.

iii. Give an example of a forelimb or hindlimb isometric exercise used in dogs.

45 i. Patella baja. Several indices have been used to describe the vertical (proximal-to-distal) position of the patella. The most commonly reported index in veterinary medicine is the L:P ratio (patellar ligament length:patellar length). This index is a derivation of the Insall–Salvati index used in humans. In large-breed dogs, L:P ratio <1.45 is a useful criterion for patella baja (low patella) and >1.97 for patella alta (high patella). Dogs with a lateral patellar luxation commonly have concurrent patella baja. This condition accounts for lateral luxation during stifle flexion (as in sitting) because the distally positioned patella is no longer constrained by the trochlear ridges.
ii. A shallow trochlear sulcus and hypoplasia of the lateral trochlear ridge are present. There is also complete erosion of the tendon of origin of the long digital extensor, which is a relatively common finding in large-breed dogs with chronic lateral patellar luxation.
iii. A block recession trochleoplasty.
iv. Recession trochleoplasty techniques were developed to preserve hyaline cartilage. The block recession more effectively increases proximal trochlear depth, increases patellar articular contact with the recessed trochlea, recesses a larger percentage of the trochlear surface area, and results in greater resistance to patellar luxation when the stifle is positioned in extension as compared with the wedge recession trochleoplasty.

46 i. During concentric contraction, muscles shorten while generating force. During eccentric contraction, the muscle elongates while under tension due to an opposing force. Rather than working to pull a joint in the direction of the muscle contraction, the muscle acts to decelerate the joint at the end of a movement or otherwise control the repositioning of a load. Isometric contraction of a muscle generates force without changing length.
ii. Concentric contraction of the biceps brachii muscle causes flexion of the elbow. Concentric contraction of the triceps muscles extends the elbow. During eccentric contraction of the biceps muscle the elbow starts movement flexed and then straightens. During eccentric contraction of the triceps muscle the elbow starts straight and then flexes as the paw moves towards the shoulder.
iii. Three-leg standing is an isometric exercise performed by lifting and holding the contralateral fore- or hindlimb off the ground. It engages the isometric contraction of the muscles of the affected, standing limb and is used to strengthen the limb. The stance is typically held for 5–60 seconds and 5–10 repetitions of this exercise are performed twice a day. Three-leg standing should be initiated 2 weeks after surgery.

47 A 4-year-old male pit bull dog was presented with a non-weight-bearing right forelimb lameness sus-tained when the dog was hit by a car earlier in the day. The dog held the right forelimb with the elbow abducted and in slight flexion with the right antebrachium externally rotated. The right elbow was markedly swollen with a decreased range of motion and pain and crepitus were elicited on 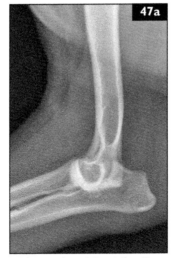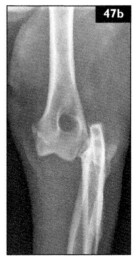 manipulation of this joint. Radiographs of the right elbow were obtained (47a, b).

i. What is the diagnosis?

ii. Describe appropriate non-surgical management of this dog's injury.

iii. What anatomic structures are considered to be primary, secondary, and tertiary stabilizers of the dog's elbow?

iv. How should the integrity of the collateral ligaments be assessed in this dog's elbow?

48 A 2-year-old female large cross-breed dog presented with a 3-week progressive history of pain when climbing the stairs and on rising from a prone position. The discomfort was localized to the lumbosacral region. The dog did not have neurologic deficits and was continent. A lateral radiograph of the lumbosacral verte- 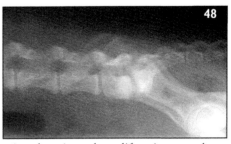 bral column was obtained (48). There is sclerosis and proliferative new bone formation and probable lysis at the endplates of the seventh lumbar and first sacral vertebrae. The lysis of contiguous vertebral endplates is strongly suggestive of discospondylitis.

i. What is the most common etiologic agent that causes discospondylitis in dogs?

ii. How should this dog be managed?

47 i. The dog has a lateral luxation of the elbow. The luxation is not obvious on the lateral view, which demonstrates the importance of obtaining orthogonal view radiographs.

ii. Closed reduction should be initially attempted with the dog anesthetized. Obtaining and maintaining reduction are dependent on relocating the anconeal process (AP) in the olecranon fossa. The elbow needs to be flexed beyond 90° and the antebrachium rotated internally and abducted until the AP is forced under the lateral supracondylar ridge of the humerus and into the fossa. The limb is then extended slightly and the antebrachium abducted and rotated internally as digital pressure is applied to the lateral portion of the radial head to complete the reduction.

iii. When the elbow is examined in pronation, the AP is the only structure considered to be a primary stabilizer. When the elbow is examined in supination, the lateral collateral ligament is considered to be a primary stabilizer, the AP a secondary stabilizer, and the medial collateral ligament a tertiary stabilizer of the elbow.

iv. To assess the integrity of the collateral ligaments, the elbow and carpus should be flexed to 90° and the antebrachium internally and externally rotated. In dogs rotation should not exceed 30° of pronation and 45° of supination. These values will be doubled if the respective ligament is severely damaged.

48 i. *Staphylococcus intermedius*; other bacteria include *Streptococcus* spp., *E. coli*, *Actinomyces* spp., and *Brucella canis*. Discospondylitis frequently develops via hematogenous seeding from distant foci of infection, but can also be caused by direct infection of the disk space or vertebra via penetrating wounds, surgery, or plant material migration, which is usually seen at the level of L2–L4. Immunosuppression due to factors such as diabetes mellitus and hyperadrenocorticism are considered to be potential predisposing causes.

ii. Treatment consists of antibiosis, cage rest, and analgesia. Empirical treatment assuming *S. intermedius* to be the causative organism is often initiated; however, consideration should be given to obtaining specimens for culture prior to administering antibiotics. Intravenous antibiotic administration should be considered in dogs with profound neurologic abnormalities, otherwise oral antibiotic administration is acceptable. Antibiotic administration for a minimum of 8 weeks is recommended even if a dog responds favorably to a shorter course. Resolution of clinical signs (e.g. pain and fever) should be expected within 5 days of initiating therapy; however, complete neurologic resolution may take several months. NSAIDs should be administered initially while awaiting a response to antibiotic administration, but can often be discontinued. Corticosteroids are not considered appropriate for treatment of this disease. Surgical decompression and/or spinal stabilization is rarely needed and should be reserved for refractory cases, dogs that present with profound neurologic abnormalities, dogs that do not respond to initial medical management, and dogs with vertebral subluxation.

49 A 4-year-old neutered male domestic shorthaired cat is presented with multiple pelvic fractures sustained in a road traffic accident (**49**). After stabilization of the cat's condition, surgery to address the pelvic fractures is scheduled for the following day. Describe a suitable immediate perioperative analgesic plan for this cat.

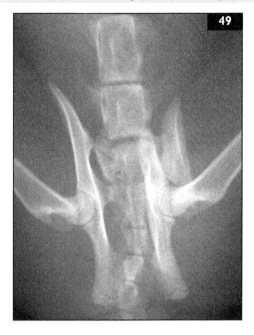

50 A 19-week-old male terrier-cross puppy presented with a bilateral forelimb gait abnormality, worse on the right, that was first noted 6 weeks previously. No pain was apparent on manipulation of the carpal and elbow joints. Antebrachial radiographs did not reveal any abnormalities. A photograph of the dog's forelimbs is shown (**50**).
i. State a diagnosis.
ii. What is the proposed underlying pathogenesis of this condition?
iii. Describe the typical signalment of a dog commonly affected with this condition.
iv. What treatment is recommended?

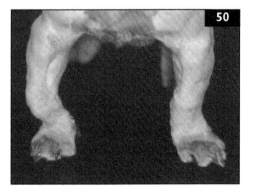

49 Regional trauma might prevent identification of the normal anatomic landmarks necessary to administer epidural analgesia in this cat. Consequently, reliance will necessarily be placed on systemic analgesics. Multimodal analgesia is likely to be more effective, with blockade of the pain pathway at multiple sites. Analgesic drugs have additive or synergistic effects, so that the dose of each individual drug can often be reduced. In this case, a suitable plan would include an opioid, ketamine, and an NSAID. A more stable degree of analgesia can be achieved by using a constant rate infusion (CRI) of ketamine and a short-acting opioid such as fentanyl. A fentanyl patch could be considered, but would need to be in place at least 12 hours before surgery to ensure adequate plasma concentrations. Lidocaine CRIs are not recommended in cats because of concerns regarding cardiovascular depression, toxicity, and lack of efficacy. Following surgery, administration of a ketamine CRI may be continued at a lower rate provided it does not cause dysphoria, which can also be a problem with opioids, especially pure μ-agonists, in cats. Buprenorphine has been shown to be as effective as morphine in cats undergoing a variety of orthopedic and soft tissue procedures, although its main advantages are longer duration of action (6–8 hours), high efficacy when given by the oral transmucosal route, and infrequent dysphoria. Tramadol may be used, although there is little published information regarding its use in cats. Tapering this cat's analgesic administration must be done based on appropriate pain assessment.

50 i. This puppy has a condition termed flexural deformity or carpal hyperflexion.
ii. A growth imbalance resulting in functional shortening of the flexor muscles of the distal forelimb in comparison with the radius and ulna. Tautness in the flexor carpi ulnaris muscle group (ulnar and humeral heads) results in a tight musculotendinous band on the caudal aspect of the antebrachium inserting on the accessory carpal bone. The problem is often transient and resolves as affected puppies age. The severity of this condition is variable. The deformity can appear to fluctuate, with a tendency for the carpus to 'knuckle' over or hyperflex more when more weight is placed on the limb. Radiographs typically do not reveal any abnormalities.
iii. This condition has been reported most frequently in Doberman pinschers and Great Danes, but many breeds are affected on an individual basis. Affected puppies are generally between 6 and 12 weeks of age.
iv. Mildly affected young puppies are generally managed without surgical intervention and the condition often spontaneously resolves with time. In older puppies in which the condition is persistent, surgery involving transection of either or both the humeral and ulnar heads of the flexor carpi ulnaris muscle tendon provides rapid resolution of the problem. Surgery was undertaken in this puppy and both ulnar and humeral heads of the flexor carpi ulnaris tendons were transected. The dog's gait abnormality resolved immediately after surgery.

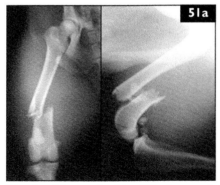

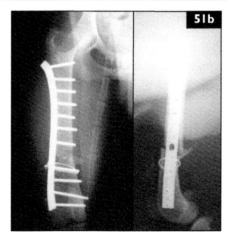

51 A 16-month-old, 35 kg male Labrador retriever was involved in a road traffic accident and sustained a comminuted fracture of the distal third of the diaphysis of the right femur (**51a**). The fracture was stabilized using a 12 hole, 3.5 mm dynamic compression plate (DCP) applied laterally with a single cerclage wire placed to stabilize one of the butterfly fragments (**51b**). The dog began to use the limb immediately following surgery, but 2 weeks postoperatively became acutely

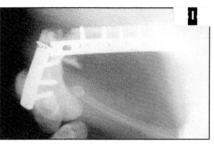

non-weight bearing on the limb. Physical examination and radiographs revealed that the plate had broken (**51c**).

i. Why did the plate fail?

ii. What could have been done differently when plating this fracture to prevent implant failure?

iii. How should this fracture be managed at this point in time?

52 A plate and some of the components of that plating system are shown (**52**).

i. Name the implant system and explain how the components shown in the image function during plate application.

ii. How do the mechanical properties of the 3.5 mm plate in this image compare with the mechanical properties of a 3.5 mm dynamic compression plate?

iii. How many degrees of freedom does this implant allow during contouring?

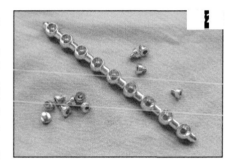

51 i. While this young dog's activity and body weight challenged the fixation, failure occurred because the medial cortices, opposite the plate, were not in contact. This transcortical gap resulted in cyclic bending of the plate, metal fatigue, and ultimately implant failure.

ii. A plate-rod construction would have provided greater resistance to cyclic loading. Alternatively, a stronger plate, such as a 3.5 mm broad DCP, or application of a second plate, positioned orthogonal to the lateral plate on the cranial aspect of the femur, could have been considered.

iii. Revision surgery is necessary, with the application of different implants (see **ii.** above). In addition, cancellous bone grafting should be performed to augment fracture healing. In this dog a 3.5 mm broad DCP was utilized and the fracture was grafted (**51d**). The fracture achieved complete union 6 months following revision surgery without further complications (**51e**).

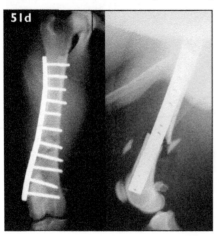
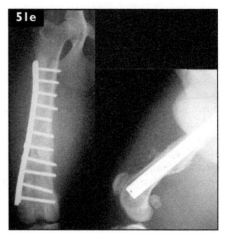

52 i. A String of Pearls (SOP) plate and multiple SOP plate bending tees. A bending tee is inserted into each of the screw holes in the node or 'pearl' of the plate prior to contouring the implant. The bending tees ensure that there will be controlled plastic deformation of the plate as the implant is bent or twisted. The tees also prevent deformation of the screw holes during contouring. Once contouring of the plate is completed, the tees are removed. These plates accept standard cortical bone screws.

ii. The 3.5 mm SOP plate is approximately 50% stiffer and has a bending strength that is 16–30% greater than that of a 3.5 mm dynamic compression plate. Even when bent to 40° or twisted by 20°, a 3.5 mm SOP plate maintains similar strength to an uncontoured 3.5 mm dynamic compression plate.

iii. Six: medial-to-lateral bending, cranial-to-caudal bending, and in either direction of torsion. Properly performed, the deformation resulting from contouring is confined to the cylindrical internode positioned between the nodes.

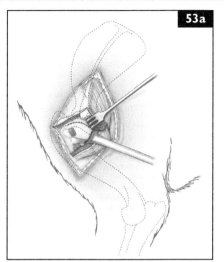

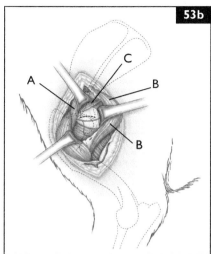

53 These drawings (**53a, b**) illustrate two different approaches to the scapulohumeral joint used for open debridement of osteochondritis dissecans lesions of the humeral head in dogs.

i. A tenotomy of what tendon has been done in the approach in **53a**?

ii. Name the muscles (labeled A, B and C) that are separated to expose the joint capsule in the approach in **53b**.

iii. What neurovascular structures must be avoided when performing an arthrotomy via the the approach in **53b**?

iv. Discuss the potential advantages and disadvantages afforded by each of these approaches for open debridement of an osteochondritis dissecans lesion of the humeral head.

54 i. How does the function of the String of Pearls (SOP) plate shown in case **52** differ from that of a dynamic compression plate?

ii. When using this plate to stabilize a long-bone fracture, how many screws should be inserted in each of the two major fracture segments?

53 i. The tendon of insertion of the infraspinatus muscle has been incised. Using a craniolateral approach to the scapulohumeral joint, a craniolateral arthrotomy is done to expose the articular cartilage of the humeral head. The tenotomy generally allows sufficient exposure for debridement of an osteochondritis dissecans lesion if the shoulder is markedly flexed and internally rotated.

ii. The intermuscular septum between the caudal border of the scapular portion of the deltoideus muscle (A) and the long head of the triceps muscle (B) is incised and separated when performing a caudal approach to the scapulohumeral joint. This reveals the teres minor muscle (C), which is retracted craniodorsally to expose the caudal joint capsule.

iii. The axillary nerve, as well as the caudal circumflex humeral artery and vein, which lie directly on the joint capsule, must be identified and protected.

iv. Craniolateral approach: simple to perform, especially if the surgeon is operating alone, and affords greater exposure of the articular surface of the humeral head, but it is associated with a reasonable degree of postoperative morbidity. Subluxation of the scapulohumeral joint is often required to gain sufficient exposure for debridement of osteochondritis dissecans lesions, resulting in transient postoperative lameness. Seroma formation is a common problem associated with this approach. Caudal approach: requires more elaborate retraction and does not yield as extensive an articular exposure, but the arthrotomy is positioned to afford sufficient focused exposure since most lesions develop in the caudal aspect of the humeral head. There is generally less morbidity associated with this approach because muscles are separated along their fascial planes, and the joint is not subluxated. In addition, seroma formation is less common.

54 i. The SOP plate is a locking plate in which standard cortical screws are rigidly retained within the holes in the plate. There is a section of standard thread in the terminal depth of the screw holes, subjacent to the section into which the head of the screw recedes. As the screw head recedes into the node, it comes into contact with a ridge, causing the screw to press fit into the 'pearl'. This press fit prevents screw loosening during the cyclic loading of weight bearing, resulting in a rigid fixed angle construct. SOP plates cannot be used to generate interfragmentary compression and therefore can only function as neutralization or buttress plates.

ii. Theoretical considerations suggest that at least four screws should be placed in each major fracture segment to protect the screws from fatigue failure. Placement of some unicortical screws is acceptable. There is a distinct stress riser at the interface between the screws and the plate where forces are transferred from a less stiff element (the screw) to a much stiffer element (the plate). The cross-sectional area of the 3.5 mm SOP plate is 20 mm^2, while the cross-sectional area of the core of a 3.5 mm cortical screw is approximately 5 mm^2. Therefore, by placing four screws in a fracture segment, the shear area of the screws will approximate that of the SOP plate.

55 A 7-month-old, 35 kg male Russian terrier presented with a 2-month history of left forelimb lameness that had not responded to rest and administration of NSAIDs. Clinical examination revealed marked effusion and pain on extension of the left elbow. A radiograph of the left elbow is shown (55a).

i. What is the diagnosis?

ii. What would be the advantage of obtaining a flexed lateral view radiograph in this dog?

iii. What are the treatment options, and what is the expected outcome for dogs affected by this condition?

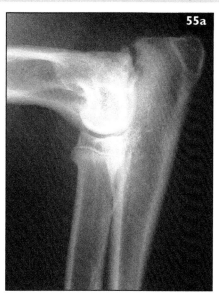

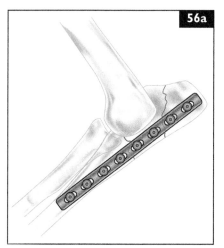

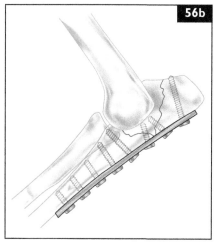

56 Two different plate positions for the stabilization of olecranon fractures are illustrated (56a, b).

i. When is plate fixation indicated for olecranon fractures?

ii. Explain the biomechanical advantages and disadvantages of the two plating methods illustrated.

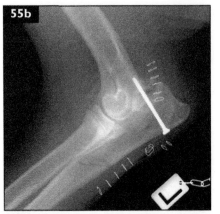

55 i. Ununited anconeal process. In many large-breed dogs the anconeal process has been shown to develop from a separate center of ossification. The cartilaginous anlage begins to mineralize around 12 weeks of age and confluent ossification of the anconeal process with the remainder of the ulna is normally completed by 18–20 weeks of age.

ii. Elbow flexion avoids superimposition of the humeral condyle over the anconeal process, which simplifies identification of the radiolucent separation.

iii. Anconeal process excision is usually reserved for dogs with advanced osteoarthritis or dogs older than 12 months. Excision generally provides an acceptable functional outcome. Other techniques are advocated for dogs diagnosed at younger than 12 months and are aimed at promoting fusion of the anconeal process to the olecranon. Lag screw fixation of the anconeal process alone yielded radiographic fusion in 6/10 elbows in one study. Proximal ulnar diaphyseal osteotomy alone resulted in fusion of the anconeal process in 14/28 dogs in another study, with 80% of the dogs considered to have excellent outcomes. Lag screw fixation in combination with ulnar osteotomy (55b) has been reported to have the most promising result in terms of fusion, function, and mitigating the progression of osteoarthritis.

56 i. Plate fixation is preferable for most olecranon fractures unless the proximal fragment is too small to accommodate at least two screws. Plate fixation is strongly advocated for intra-articular fractures and for comminuted proximal ulna fractures. Plate fixation affords greater stability and is associated with a lower incidence of complications than the use of pin and tension band fixation.

ii. Caudal application positions the plate on the tension surface of the bone. The plate is therefore acting as a tension band and a relatively small plate can be used to stabilize the fracture. Longer screws can be placed if the plate is positioned caudally, providing improved holding power than if the plate was placed laterally. When stabilizing articular fractures, the plate must be slightly overcontoured over the fracture to avoid creating a transcortical gap in the articular surface of the semilunar notch. Screws must be placed judiciously, avoiding penetration of the elbow or contact with the caudal surface of the radius.

Lateral application may be preferable, particularly in smaller dogs and cats, as the caudal ulna is extremely thin, concaved (craniocaudally), and curved (mediolaterally), making accurate plate contouring and screw insertion technically difficult from the caudal aspect. In addition, if the plate has to function in buttress fashion, a laterally positioned plate will have a greater moment of inertia and resist bending forces better than a caudally positioned plate.

57 This is a lateral radiograph of the tibia (57a), which will be used to calculate the tibial plateau angle (TPA) during planning for a tibial plateau leveling osteotomy (TPLO).
i. What are the radiographic landmarks used to calculate the TPA as described by Slocum?
ii. What is considered the normal range for TPAs in large breed dogs such as Labrador retrievers?
iii. What factors can influence the radiographic measurement of the TPA in a dog?

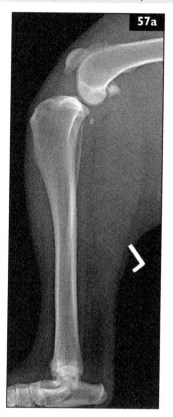

58 A diagram depicting the molecular structure of hyaluronic acid (HA) is shown (58).
i. List the mechanisms of action of HA that may have benefits in treating osteo-arthritis.
ii. What biochemical feature of various commercially available HA products has been reported to affect its efficacy?
iii. Name clinical conditions for which HA has proven efficacy in palliating the symptoms of osteoarthritis in dogs.

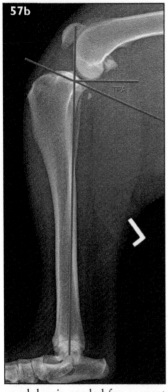

57b

57 i. The apex of the intercondylar tubercles of the proximal tibia and the center of the talocrural joint are identified and a line drawn between these points to identify the functional tibial axis. A second line is drawn from the cranial to the caudal limits of the medial tibial condyle. The TPA is the angle between the second line and a line perpendicular to the functional axis of the tibia (57b).

ii. The TPA varies between individuals, but the mean angle in a cohort of skeletally mature Labrador retrievers without evidence of orthopedic disease was 23.5 degrees (SD +/-3.1). This did not differ significantly from a second similarly sized group of Labrador retrievers with confirmed CrCL insufficiency.

iii. Factors that can influence the radiographic measurement of TPA include inter- and intra-observer variation, osteophyte formation obscuring anatomic landmarks, and limb positioning. Cranial and proximal positioning of the limb relative to the X-ray beam leads to overestimation, while caudal and distal positioning leads to underestimation of the TPA. Proper lateral positioning of the tibia, defined by superimposition of the femoral and tibial condyles, is needed for accurate TPA determination before TPLO.

58 i. The purported benefits of HA are improving viscoelastic properties of synovial fluid, stimulation of endogenous HA production and chondroprotection, as well as anti-inflammatory and analgesic effects.

ii. The molecular weight of HA has been reported to affect efficacy. Clinical studies in horses and humans indicate that high molecular weight (>2 million Da) HA has better clinical efficacy than low molecular weight (<1 million Da) HA; however, other studies have reported no differences based on molecular weight.

iii. While there have not been any studies to date that document clinical efficacy of HA for treatment of naturally occurring osteoarthritis in dogs, several experimental studies have reported efficacy of intra-articular HA for treatment of induced osteoarthritis in research dogs including decreased pain, lameness, osteophytosis, synovitis, and cartilage degradation.

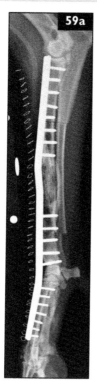

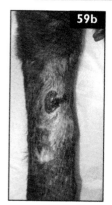

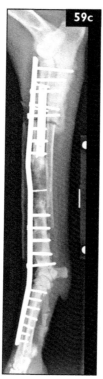

59 A 6-year-old male Labrador retriever originally presented with a right mid-diaphyseal radial osteosarcoma. A limb-sparing procedure was performed using a pasteurization technique and the sterilized radioulnar autograft was stabilized with a plate that extended from the proximal radius to the distal metacarpus (59a). Four months after surgery the dog re-presents because of lameness. Several draining tracts have developed on the cranial aspect of the right antebrachium (59b). Radiographs of the right antebrachium are obtained (59c).
i. What complication has developed?
ii. What radiographic abnormalities support the diagnosis?
iii. Describe an appropriate treatment plan for this dog.

60 A 3-year-old female neutered whippet sustained a traumatic medial dislocation of the tendon of origin of the biceps brachii muscle while racing. At the time of presentation the dog had only a nominal lameness when walking, but became lame when running. On physical examination, a palpable 'popping' sensation was elicited in the craniomedial proximal brachium during flexion of the affected shoulder.
i. What is the diagnosis?
ii. What breeds of dog are most commonly affected by this condition?
iii. Describe the proposed etiology of this condition.
iv. Describe appropriate treatment that would allow this dog to return to racing.

59 i. The limb has become infected and the pasteurized autograft has become a sequestrum.

ii. There is a poorly marginated proliferative periosteal reaction on the caudal border of the proximal ulna extending to the level of the proximal radial and ulnar osteotomies. Bone lysis is also present around the proximal screws. While there is evidence of healing at the distal radial osteotomy, the proximal osteotomies are still sharply demarcated with little to no radiographic evidence of bone union. The original bone lesion in the radial diaphysis has undergone substantial lysis with extensive cortical resorption.

iii. Amputation should be considered, otherwise such a severe infection and loss of diaphyseal bone requires removal of the implants, excision of the sequestrum, and administration of appropriate antibiotic therapy. Representative specimens of non-viable bone and the implants should be submitted for culture and antimicrobial sensitivity testing. The limb segment needs to be supported postoperatively, using either coaptation or external fixation, while the infection is being treated prior to attempting another limb salvage procedure.

60 i. Intermittent displacement of the tendon of origin of the biceps brachii muscle.

ii. Sight hounds, most notably racing greyhounds. This condition has also been reported in a German shepherd dog and a Border collie.

iii. Rupture or avulsion of the transverse humeral ligament is necessary for the tendon to displace from the intertubercular groove. For the ligament to rupture in isolation, the acting force must be localized and extreme. Such a force might develop during acute deceleration or stumbling while running at high speed. Pre-existing hypoplasia of the bicipital groove or pathology of the transverse humeral ligament can often exist.

iv. Surgical intervention is indicated and consists of reconstruction of the transverse humeral ligament with augmentation either with screws and non-absorbable sutures or a surgical staple. The brachiocephalicus muscle is retracted caudally (and either medially or laterally); the insertion of the superficial pectoral muscle is incised and retracted caudally. The supraspinatus and pectoralis muscles are retracted cranially and caudally, respectively (**60a**). In this dog an 'epiphyseal staple' was used to maintain the tendon in the intertubercular groove (**60b**).

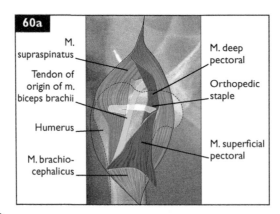

60a

M. supraspinatus

Tendon of origin of m. biceps brachii

Humerus

M. brachio-cephalicus

M. deep pectoral

Orthopedic staple

M. superficial pectoral

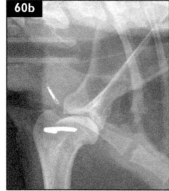

60b

61 A 2-year-old male boxer dog had a mandibular fracture stabilized with an acrylic external skeletal fixator (61).
i. What method of intubation is being used in this dog?
ii. What is the advantage of intubating the dog in this manner?
iii. Which structures are at risk of iatrogenic injury when placing fixation pins in the mandible, and how are such injuries best avoided?

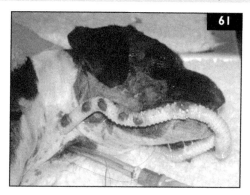

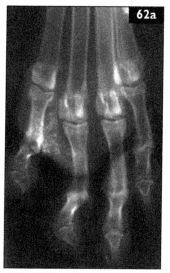 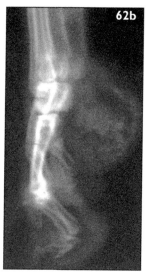

62 A 10-month-old female German shepherd dog presented with a 3-week history of right forelimb lameness. There was an ulcerated area on the metacarpal pad of the right fore paw. The involved portion of the pad was swollen, firm, and painful on palpation. The paw was radiographed (62a, b).
i. What is the diagnosis?
ii. How should this condition be treated?
iii. What is the prognosis for this dog after appropriate treatment?
iv. Where has this condition been most commonly reported to occur?
v. What underlying causes have been reported?

61 i. Intubation is via a temporary tracheostomy.
ii. The tracheostomy allows the surgeon to continuously assess occlusion during surgery. In complex mandibular fractures the maxillary arcade can serve as a template, which assists in aligning the fractured mandible when the jaw is closed. If anesthesia is maintained via oral intubation, the endotracheal tube would need to be removed periodically to assess occlusion. Alternatively, the dog could have also been intubated through a pharyngotomy incision, but a pharyngotomy may have been a more difficult option in this brachycephalic breed.
iii. At-risk structures include the mandibular artery and nerve, the tooth roots, and the soft tissue structures that lie between the two hemimandibles. Damage to the mandibular artery and nerve can be avoided by placing fixation pins in the ventral third of the mandible, ventral to the mandibular canal. Damage to the roots of the teeth can also be avoided by placing fixation pins in the ventral third of the mandible and by aiming the pins away from the perceived location of the tooth roots. Damage to soft tissue structures lying between the two hemimandibles can be avoided by using only half-pins and by not placing implants that transfix both hemimandibles.

62 i. The lesion affecting this dog's metacarpal pad is calcinosis circumscripta, an uncommon syndrome of ectopic idiopathic, dystrophic, metastatic, or iatrogenic mineralization characterized by deposition of calcium salts in soft tissues.
ii. Treatment is by surgical excision for a lesion in this location that is causing lameness. This lesion is small enough to allow marginal excision while still preserving a functional metacarpal pad, which will allow the dog to bear weight on the limb.
iii. Guarded for recurrence. In this dog the lesion did not recur and the lameness resolved once the pad had healed.
iv. In a retrospective study of 77 dogs, lesions occurred most commonly on the hind paws (50%) with the tongue (23%) being the second most common location (**62c**).
v. Calcinosis circumscripta usually develops in young (8–10 months of age), healthy large-breed dogs, but has also been reported in dogs with chronic renal failure, as a reaction to polydioxanone suture material, secondary to an injection of medroxyprogesterone acetate, or secondary to trauma such as use of choke chains.

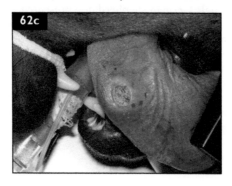

62c

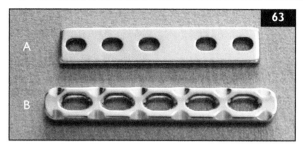

63 The undersurfaces of two Synthes bone plates are shown (63).
i. Name the implants.
ii. What are the benefits of the 'scalloped' underside of the plate in 63?
iii. In comparison with plate A, how does the spacing of the screw holes on plate B influence plate and screw position when stabilizing a diaphyseal fracture?

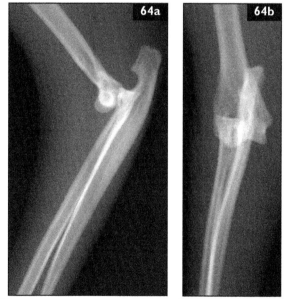

64 A 6-year-old male neutered cat presented with a history of acute-onset lameness after jumping off a roof. On presentation the cat would not bear weight on the right forelimb and the right elbow was painful and swollen. Lateral (64a) and craniocaudal (64b) radiographs of the elbow were obtained.
i. Which ligaments would need to be disrupted to allow this cat's elbow to luxate in this fashion?
ii. Describe the anatomic differences between cats and dogs that have been implicated in the pathogenesis of elbow luxations in each species.

63 i. The upper plate is a dynamic compression plate. The lower plate, with the characteristic 'cut-outs' on the under surface of the implant, is a limited contact dynamic compression plate.

ii. The scalloped underside reduces the contact area between the plate and bone ('plate footprint') by approximately 50%, thereby causing less disruption of the periosteal circulation than a conventional dynamic compression plate. The scalloped surface also reduces the stiffness of the solid sections of the plate between screw holes, which has the benefit of distributing stress more evenly along the implant, eliminating stress risers, and allowing more uniform bending during plate contouring by reducing the tendency to kink at the holes.

iii. Limited contact dynamic compression plates have symmetrical, evenly distributed screw holes, which are inclined at both ends of each hole, allowing compression to be applied in either direction when a screw is placed with an appropriate drill guide. This allows for multifocal axial compression. In addition, the 'scalloped' underside allows greater angulation of plate screws by up to 40° in a longitudinal direction.

64 i. A cadaveric study reported that in cats both the medial and lateral collateral ligaments needed to be transected to induce an elbow luxation; however, the loss of stability associated with transection of both collateral ligaments was only sufficient to induce a luxation in 50% of elbows tested. This cat had a caudolateral luxation and the radius and ulna were substantially displaced, which would likely mean that the olecranon ligament was also disrupted. Since the proximal radioulnar articulation appears congruent, the annular ligament was likely to be intact.

ii. Cats have a very strong olecranon ligament, which is shorter but twice as thick as in dogs. The ligament originates on the lateral surface of the medial epicondyle and inserts at the cranial crest of the olecranon, extending distally to the apex of the anconeal process. This ligament is taut when the elbow is flexed and contributes substantially to the stability of the cat's elbow. Luxation could consistently be induced in cadaver dog elbows following transection of the lateral collateral ligament alone. Luxations could not be induced in dog elbows following transection of the medial collateral ligament, corroborating previous observations that this ligament is not a major stabilizer in dog elbows.

65 The luxation in the cat in case **64** was reduced in a closed fashion, but was extremely unstable, so the cat was taken to surgery. Describe three stabilization options, including potential use of postoperative external coaptation, that would be appropriate for this cat.

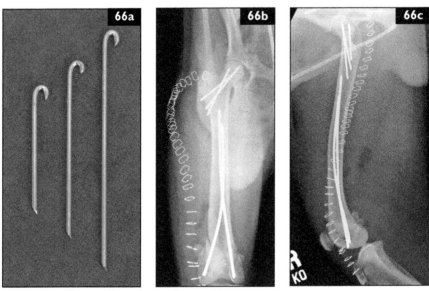

66 i. Name these orthopedic implants (**66a**).
ii. Describe how these implants are intended to function.
iii. Shown are initial postoperative radiographs of a 6-month-old Queensland blue heeler that underwent stabilization of proximal and distal right femoral physeal fractures (**66b, c**). Describe how the implants are functioning to stabilize the distal fracture.

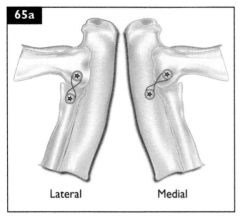

65a

Lateral   Medial

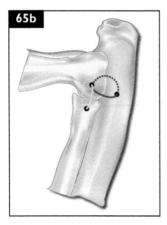

65b

65 (1) Primary collateral ligament repair. Avulsion of the origin of collateral ligaments can be treated by reattachment either by passing a suture through bone tunnels or by the use of screws and washers or bone anchors. Avulsion of the insertion of the collateral ligaments can be treated by suturing the ligament to the annular ligament and associated fibrous tissue. Primary ligament repair alone, however, is frequently not sufficient. (2) Placement of figure-of-eight prosthetic sutures anchored via bone anchors, screws, or bone tunnels. As the caudal part of the medial collateral ligament is wide and inserts on the ulna in cats, the medial collateral ligament should be reconstructed from the humerus to the ulna, not to the radius as is done for the lateral collateral ligament (**65a**). (3) Placement of circumferential suture prostheses passed through humeral transcondylar, transradial and transulnar bone tunnels (**65b**). Following stabilization methods (1) and (2), external coaptation in a Spica splint for 2–3 weeks is recommended. Method (3) can be done as a standalone procedure without external coaptation. Confinement for 6 weeks is advisable, irrespective of the method of stabilization, followed by a gradual return to normal activity.

66 i. Rush pins. The pins have a bevel at one end and a hook at the opposite end: the hook is used to insert and seat the pin.

ii. When properly inserted, Rush pins provide dynamic stabilization of juxta-articular fractures. Rush pins are typically inserted in pairs, at an acute angle to the longitudinal axis of fractured appendicular long bones. During insertion, the beveled end of the pins should deflect off the endosteal cortices and because they are somewhat elastic, the pins should bend slightly and continue to advance within the medullary cavity. The bent shaft of the pins exerts a centrifugal force against the endosteal cortices, conferring dynamic fixation and effectively neutralizing bending and rotational forces.

iii. Although Rush pins are rarely used in small animal practice, small diameter, and thus flexible, Steinmann pins or Kirschner wires (as used in this dog) are often used 'in the manner of Rush pins' to stabilize physeal fractures. The Kirschner wires, with a chisel-point tip, were inserted at an acute angle, deflecting rather than penetrating the endosteal cortex, to achieve dynamic fracture fixation.

67 A 7-year-old, 40 kg intact male Labrador retriever was presented for an open gunshot fracture of the left femur, which was stabilized with a titanium 4.5 mm narrow limited contact dynamic compression plate. The preoperative (67a), immediate postoperative (67b), and 14 months postoperative (67c) craniocaudal view radiographs are shown.

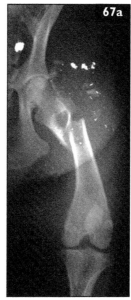

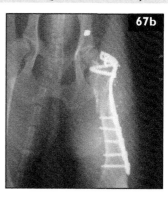

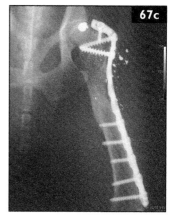

i. How would this plate be described with respect to the implant's functional application?

ii. What type of bone healing has occurred with this fracture?

iii. Describe the progression of tissue differentiation that occurred as this fracture healed. How does the healing process affect interfragmentary strain?

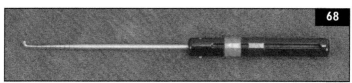

68 A surgical instrument is shown (68).

i. Name the instrument.

ii. Describe how this instrument is utilized during surgical exploration of a CrCL-deficient stifle.

iii. How has this instrument been shown to improve diagnostic accuracy during open surgical or arthroscopic examination of a CrCL-deficient stifle?

67 i. The fracture was stabilized without reconstructing the osseous column in the subtrochanteric region, therefore the plate is functioning in a buttress application mode.

ii. Secondary or indirect bone healing.

iii. The normal progression of tissue differentiation associated with secondary bone healing is: fracture hematoma, granulation tissue, fibrous tissue, cartilage, mineralized cartilage, woven bone, and finally remodeled lamellar bone. These tissues have a descending tolerance for interfragmentary strain within the fracture gap. The fracture hematoma has virtually no tensile strength and thus negligible effect on interfragmentary strain. As the fracture enters the repair phase, granulation tissue replaces the hematoma, reducing strain with a slight increase in strength (up to 0.1 Nm/mm^2). Granulation tissue is subsequently replaced with fibrous tissue, with higher tensile strength collagen fibers, which improves tensile strength from $1-60$ Nm/mm^2 and resisting elongation up to 17%. Local stem cells then differentiate, becoming chondrocytes that produce cartilage, further improving the biomechanics by forming 'soft callus' (ultimate tensile strength of $4-19$ Nm/mm^2, tolerating elongation of $10-13$%). Eventually, the cartilage mineralizes and becomes 'hard callus' and remodels to compact bone (ultimate tensile strength of 130 Nm/mm^2 with an ability to elongate 2%). This dog's fracture is still remodeling 14 months after surgery.

68 i. A meniscal probe.

ii. The tip of the probe is used to palpate the meniscus and identify meniscal pathology that may not be readily apparent either during arthrotomy or arthroscopy. Both the femoral and tibial surfaces of the meniscus are probed to detect incomplete vertical longitudinal tears. The probe is very useful for detecting additional, residual vertical tears, which can easily be missed following excision of more obvious axial lesions. The probe can also be used to apply traction to the caudal horn of the medial meniscus: cranial displacement indicating the presence of a peripheral tear. Meniscal texture can also be assessed. A normal meniscus is firm and resilient, while a soft meniscus is likely degenerate. The meniscus should be probed repeatedly during debridement to confirm that appropriate debridement has been performed.

iii. Accurate identification of meniscal pathology is essential for effective treatment. In a study using cadaver dogs with simulated meniscal tears, meniscal probing was shown to enhance the sensitivity and specificity of diagnosing meniscal tears during both arthroscopy and arthrotomy. Probing doubled the odds of correctly identifying medial meniscal tears via a craniomedial arthrotomy and increased the odds of correctly identifying medial meniscal tears during arthroscopy by 8-fold.

69 This 2-year-old, 41 kg male German shepherd dog is undergoing rehabilitative therapy in an underwater treadmill (**69**). The dog had a tibial plateau leveling osteotomy performed 8 weeks previously.

i. List and describe the advantageous properties afforded by water when using this modality.

ii. What benefits have been shown in dogs that receive early rehabilitative therapy, including underwater treadmill therapy, following tibial plateau leveling osteotomy?

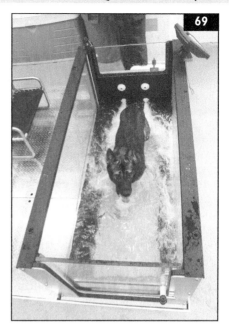

70 A ventrodorsal radiograph of the pelvis of a 7-year-old female cat presented with hindlimb weakness, reluctance to ambulate, and bilateral hip pain is shown (**70**).

i. What is the radiographic diagnosis?

ii. What is the incidence of this condition in cats?

iii. Describe the appropriate treatment for this cat.

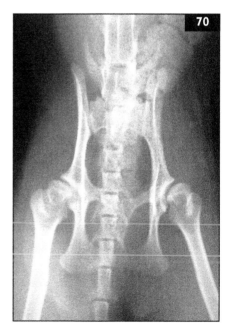

69 i. (1) Buoyancy: the upward thrust of water acting on a body creates a functional decrease in weight. Quantitative thrust is equal to the weight (or mass) of water displaced. The depth of the water in an underwater treadmill can be adjusted to optimize treatment. (2) Viscosity: the resistance caused by the attractive forces between molecules in a liquid making ambulation more difficult than through air. The resistance provided is proportional to the velocity of movement through the water and this can be increased by increasing treadmill speed, water turbulence (by using jets), or water depth. (3) Hydrostatic pressure: the pressure a fluid exerts on the body's surface; is dependent on the fluid's depth and density and can help resolve limb and joint swelling as well as decrease pain during exercise. (4) Surface tension: water molecules are cohesive and adhere to one another, particularly at the water's surface. This phenomenon increases resistance when ambulating through the water's surface.

ii. One study assessed the benefits of early intensive postoperative rehabilitative therapy in dogs following tibial plateau leveling osteotomy. Dogs began underwater treadmill exercise 10 days after surgery as a component of an intensive therapy program. Dogs that received intensive postoperative rehabilitation had a significantly greater increase in muscle mass and a superior range of motion during the postoperative convalescent period and at 6 weeks there were no significant differences in hindlimb muscle mass or range of stifle motion.

70 i. Advanced bilateral degenerative joint disease typical of feline hip dysplasia. Common radiographic abnormalities in dysplastic cats may include femoral head subluxation, shallow acetabula, and mild remodeling of the craniodorsal acetabular margin. Hip laxity is associated with the development of osteoarthritis and may be confirmed using distraction radiography, particularly in younger cats. Alternatively, measuring Norberg angles on a hip-extended ventrodorsal radiographic view can be used to assess coxofemoral conformation. The mean Norberg angle in normal cats is 92.4°. These radiographic assessments are unnecessary in older cats with marked degenerative changes.

ii. Hip dysplasia is less common in cats than in dogs, but overall incidence in the general cat population is undetermined. Cats with hip dysplasia do not always display overt clinical abnormalities, therefore diagnosis of hip dysplasia in cats is often based on radiographic findings of coxofemoral joint laxity, osseous remodeling, and osteoarthritis. Clinical abnormalities, when present, may include reduced activity, reluctance to ambulate or jump, mild lameness, and pain on manipulation of the coxofemoral joints.

iii. Cats with clinical abnormalities referable to hip dysplasia can often be effectively managed with 2–3 weeks cage confinement. Medical management (NSAIDs) may be used, but long-term administration is rarely necessary. Femoral head and neck excision or possibly total hip replacement may be necessary in cats with persistent clinical signs that do not respond to appropriate medical therapy.

71 A 4-year-old female spayed Dalmatian was referred for evaluation of pleural and abdominal effusion. The owner noted that the dog was lethargic and anorexic and on physical examination the dog had obvious ascites and jugular pulses. The dog also had a 2-year history of a weight-bearing left hindlimb lameness and the limb was atrophied with firm swelling centered over the left tarsus. Radiographs of the dog's left hock obtained 20 months prior to referral revealed abnormalities ascribed to osteoarthritis. The lameness had been treated with herbal medi-

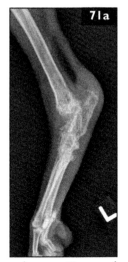
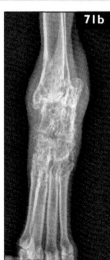

cations with an equivocal response to therapy. Upon referral the dog was suspected of having restrictive pericarditis with right-sided congestive heart failure based on abnormalities present on thoracic and abdominal radiographs and an echocardiogram. Cytologic evaluation of joint fluid retrieved via arthrocentesis of the left tarsus revealed suppurative arthritis. Radiographs of the left tarsus were obtained (71a, b).
i. Describe the radiographic abnormalities.
ii. What differential diagnoses should be considered when evaluating the radiographs of this dog's hindlimb?
iii. What historical information should be solicited from this dog's owner?

72 A craniocaudal radiograph is shown of a dog that has sustained a traumatic hip luxation (72a). What physical examination findings are supportive of the clinical diagnosis of a craniodorsal coxofemoral luxation?

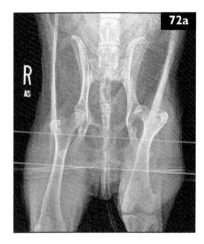

71 i. There is soft tissue swelling surrounding the left hock with aggressive osteolytic lesions affecting the distal left tibia and the left tarsus as well as the proximal metatarsal bones. There is moderate-to-severe periarticular osteophytosis associated with the intertarsal joints.
ii. Differential diagnosis would include osteomyelitis from a bacterial, a fungal (cryptococcosis, coccidioidomycosis, blastomycosis, histoplasmosis, hyalohyphomycosis, aspergillosis, osteoarticular sporotrichosis) or an algal infection (protothecosis), or neoplasia (primary or metastatic).
iii. Given that this dog has severe systemic clinical abnormalities in addition to aggressive destructive osseous pathology that crosses multiple joints, the potential for fungal disease must be considered. Many fungal diseases have regional distributions and owners should be queried regarding locations they have lived or visited with their dog. The owner of the dog had previously lived in the southwestern United States where coccidioidomycosis is endemic.

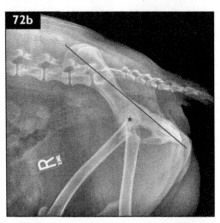

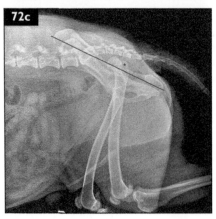

72 The luxated femoral head displaces cranial and dorsal to the acetabulum, resulting in external rotation of the femur and, consequently, the entire limb. Dogs with an acute luxation will not bear weight and the limb is characteristically adducted and the stifle and paw rotated externally. Palpation of the position of the greater trochanter is useful in establishing the diagnosis. Normally, the greater trochanter is located distal to a line extending cranially from the tuber ischii and bisecting the wing of the ilium (**72b**). In a dog with a craniodorsal luxation, the greater trochanter will be located proximal to this line (**72c**). In addition, the distance between the greater trochanter and the tuber ischii is increased in comparison with the contralateral normal limb and the examiner can place a thumb in the depression situated caudal to the greater trochanter and cranial to the tuber ischii. In a dog with a normal hip, the examiner's thumb is displaced from the depression when the femur is externally rotated. If the hip is luxated, the thumb will not be displaced by external rotation of the femur.

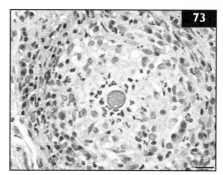

73 The tentative diagnosis for the dog in case **71** was systemic coccidioidomycosis.
i. What additional non-invasive diagnostic test could be used to substantiate the diagnosis of coccidioidomycosis?
ii. The dog underwent a minimally invasive thoracoscopic partial pericardiectomy to address the restrictive pericarditis. A histopathologic section of the pericardial biopsy is shown (**73**). Do the histopathologic abnormalities substantiate the tentative diagnosis of coccidioidomycosis?
iii. How should this dog be treated?
iv. What is this dog's prognosis?

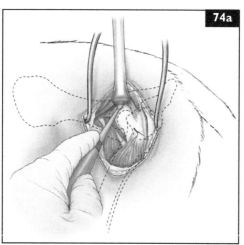

74 This is an illustration (**74a**) of a surgeon using a bone curette to perform a surgical procedure advocated for the treatment of dogs affected with hip dysplasia.
i. What procedure is being performed?
ii. Describe the purported therapeutic effect of this procedure.
iii. What is the reported clinical efficacy of this procedure?

73 i. *Coccidioides* gel immunodiffusion antibody test.
ii. Yes. The section shows multiple regions of fibrous tissue that are replaced by multifocal to coalescing inflammatory nodules composed of central regions of macrophages and degenerate neutrophils surrounded by epithelioid macrophages and an outer zone of plump fibroblasts mixed with lymphocytes and plasma cells. At the center of these pyogranulomas there is a single *Coccidioides* spp. spherule. The radiographic abnormalities (see case **71**) are also compatible with the dog having fungal osteomyelitis. *Coccidioides* commonly disseminates from the lungs to other tissues, with the pericardium and bone being predilection sites in dogs.
iii. Dogs should be treated with a combination of an azole antifungal drug (keto-conazole, itraconazole, fluconazole, voriconazole) and deoxycholate or lipid-complexed amphotericin B. Treatment must be continued for at least 6 months. Decisions to discontinue treatment are based on the results of serial radiography and monitoring of the *Coccidioides* antibody titer. Surgery (amputation) may be required for osseous lesions that are refractory to treatment.
iv. Guarded. The prognosis is best for dogs with localized pulmonary coccidioido-mycosis. Complete recovery in dogs with disseminated coccidioidomycosis and extensive bone involvement is uncommon.

74 i. Hip denervation. The periosteum can be debrided adjacent to the coxofemoral joint in a semicircular pattern, beginning at the craniodorsal margin of the acetabulum and progressing toward the cranial and ventral borders of the ilium (**74b**, red shaded area), or the dorsal aspect of the acetabulum can be included (**74b**, blue shaded area).
ii. Periosteal debridement produces coxofemoral analgesia, derived from resultant neurotomy of the afferent sensory nerve fibers in the pericapsular region.
iii. Denervation was performed in 17 dogs affected with hip dysplasia and 91% of the treated dogs became more comfortable on coxofemoral joint manipulation, with 56% of dogs (**74b**, red shaped area) having improved lameness scores 3 days after the surgery. Most dogs remained free of clinical abnormalities at the time of long-term evaluation. In another study of 96 dogs with a larger area of denervation (**74b**, blue shaded area), most (96%) dogs had a reduction or resolution of coxofemoral joint pain and lameness, as well as an improved quality of life.

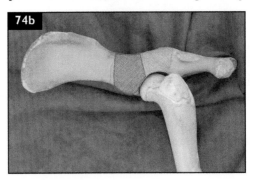

75 A 9-month-old male neutered Pug became acutely lame and would not bear weight on the right hindlimb after falling off a couch. On physical examination a pain response was elicited on manipulation of the right coxofemoral joint. A radiograph of the pelvis is shown (75).

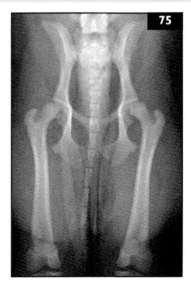

i. Describe the radiological abnormalities.

ii. Explain the mechanics involved to create this type of injury.

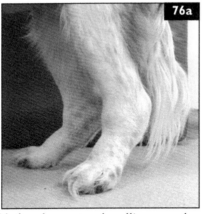

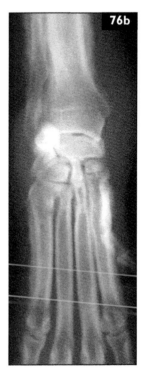

76 A 12-year-old female neutered collie-cross dog presented with a history of swelling and edema in all four limbs. Diffuse, firm, painful swelling of all four distal limbs was found on physical examination (76a). Radiographs of the limbs were obtained and a radiograph of the left distal forelimb is shown (76b).

i. State the diagnosis.

ii. List some underlying disorders that have been reported to produce these osseous changes in dogs.

75 i. There is a minimally displaced, complete, intra-articular fracture of the right femoral head. There is also poor acetabular coverage of the femoral head bilaterally with mild joint incongruity, consistent with hip dysplasia. Degenerative changes of the coxofemoral joints are minimal.

ii. This dog has an avulsion fracture of the right femoral head, with the round ligament attached to the small capitular fragment. The fall may have induced subluxation of the coxofemoral joint because of the underlying joint laxity associated with hip dysplasia. Excessive tension generated in the round ligament would have been transmitted to the bone. Osseous failure occurs more frequently than ligamentous rupture in young skeletally mature dogs (1–3 years of age) due to the bone's inferior mechanical strength. If this dog was older (>4 years of age) at the time of trauma, elongation or tearing of the round ligament with or without coxofemoral luxation would have been more likely. If this dog was younger with open femoral capital physes at the time of trauma, the dog would have likely sustained a Salter–Harris type I or II fracture.

76 i. This dog has hypertrophic osteopathy, also known as hypertrophic pulmonary osteopathy, hypertrophic osteoarthropathy, or Marie's disease. Affected animals have increased circulation to the extremities, resulting in periosteal new bone formation. Characteristic radiographic changes include diffuse palisading periosteal reaction affecting the abaxial aspects of metacarpal and metatarsal bones II and IV, the radius, and the tibia; less commonly, the proximal long bones and pelvis may also be affected.

ii. Hypertrophic osteopathy develops most commonly in dogs with primary or metastatic pulmonary tumors. This dog had multiple soft tissue nodules of various sizes throughout the lung fields, some of which were cavitating (**76c**). These lesions were suspected to be neoplastic, but this was not confirmed. Other neoplasms in the abdomen have been implicated in hypertrophic osteopathy, such as renal carcinoma, urinary bladder rhabdomyosarcoma, and prostatic carcinoma. Non-neoplastic diseases reported to cause hypertrophic osteopathy include *Spirocerca lupi*, *Dirofilaria immitis*, eosinophilic bronchitis, pulmonary abscessation, intrathoracic foreign body, and congenital or acquired cardiac disease.

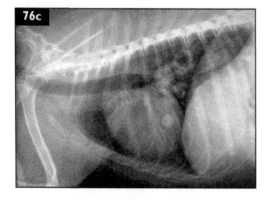

76c

77 A 2-year-old, 38 kg castrated male German shepherd dog was presented with a closed, transverse mid-diaphyseal fracture of the right humerus. Pre-operative radiographs (77a, b) and images obtained immediately following surgery (77c, d) are shown.

i. What implant system was utilized to stabilize this fracture?

ii. List advantages afforded by this implant system.

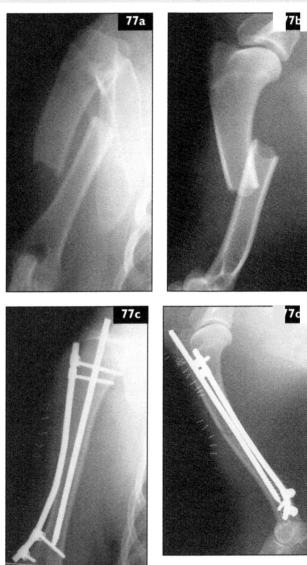

78 Describe the treatment options for the dog in case 75.

77 i. The fracture was anatomically reduced via a limited open reduction. An intramedullary Steinmann pin was placed to maintain alignment and a 3.5 mm clamp-rod internal fixator (CRIF; Synthes) applied to the lateral humerus. The CRIF is composed of specially made clamps designed to engage a standard screw and a rod. The system is available with clamps and rods that accommodate 2.0, 2.4/2.7, 3.5, or 4.5 mm screws.

ii. The CRIF is advantageous because maintenance of an extensive inventory is not required, as a variable number of clamps can be placed on each rod and the rods can be cut to length as needed. The rods can be contoured in three dimensions, simplifying stabilization of bones with complex conformation, such as stabilizing a fracture of the distal femur in a dachshund. The design of the fixator affords internal stability with minimal contact between the fixation device and the periosteal surface of the bone, thus favoring vascularity and, possibly, indirect bone healing. The clamps can be placed on either side of the rod, facilitating divergent fixation of short fracture segments. The narrow width of the device allows for placement of a second CRIF if deemed necessary in larger dogs or other situations where additional stabilization is desirable.

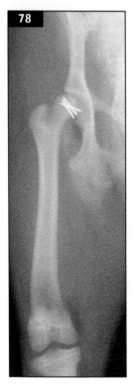

78 Although the fracture appears minimally displaced, surgical intervention is warranted. Intra-articular fractures should be anatomically reduced and stabilized with rigid fixation. A routine craniolateral approach to the hip was considered; however, exposure of the fracture site for manipulation of the avulsed fragment and placement of implants would have been difficult. Instead, a ventral approach to the hip was performed. For ventral exposure, the dog was positioned in dorsal recumbency with the hindlimbs in a 'frog-leg' position. An incision was made over the cranial border and parallel to the pectineus muscle. The origin of the pectineus muscle was transected at the pubis then reflected distally. Retraction of the iliopsoas muscle cranially and the adductor muscle caudally exposed the joint capsule. The fracture was anatomically reduced and stabilized with divergent 0.8 mm Kirschner wires (**78**). Fragment excision was not considered, as the avulsion fragment was large and attached to the round ligament, which is a primary stabilizer of the coxofemoral joint. Alternatively, a femoral head and neck ostectomy or possibly a total hip replacement could have been performed given the dysplastic nature of the affected joint.

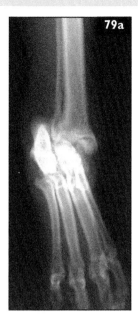

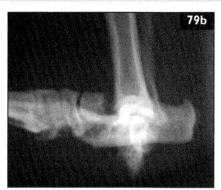

79 A 5-year-old female domestic shorthaired cat presented after being missing for 48 hours; it was non-weight bearing on the right hindlimb. Radiographs of the right tarsus were obtained (**79a, b**).
i. Describe the cat's fracture.
ii. What additional structures must be damaged to allow for the degree of displacement seen on the radiographs?
iii. How should this injury be managed?

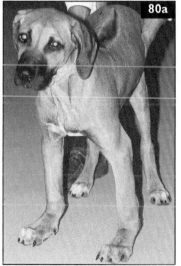

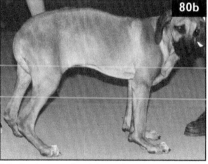

80 A 4-month-old male Great Dane puppy, which had been purchased by the owners as a potential show dog, was presented for examination due to concerns about the dog's conformation (**80a, b**).
i. What is the normal standing angle of the carpus for dogs?
ii. List two causes of carpal hyperextension in skeletally immature dogs.
iii. What would be the recommended treatment be for this dog?

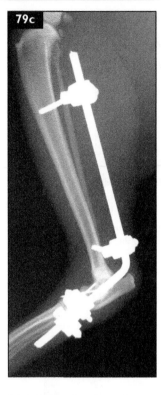

79 i. There is a short oblique fracture of the talar neck, with proximal and lateral displacement of the talar head.

ii. This cat also has a concurrent talocalcaneal luxation, which implies that there must be disruption of the proximal talocalcaneal ligament to allow the calcaneus to displace proximolaterally. The talocalcaneal articulation is a synovial diarthrodial joint. There are three pairs of cartilage-covered articular facets between the two bones as well as two strong ligaments, one proximal and one distal, that traverse the tarsal sinus. The talocalcaneal articulation does not have any external ligaments.

iii. Talar fractures can be managed with closed reduction and prolonged application of a transarticular external fixator. Alternatively, open reduction and placement of Kirschner wires as small crossed pins can be used to maintain the reduction, taking care not to penetrate the articular surface of the talus at the tibiotarsal joint. Internal fixation should be augmented by a prolonged period of external coaptation or application of a transarticular external fixator for a shorter duration of time (e.g. 4 weeks), as was done in this cat (79c).

80 i. Most dogs' carpi are positioned in a standing angle of 5–10° of extension. Some breeds, such as German shepherd dogs, normally have more hyperextension of the antebrachiocarpal joint.

ii. (1) Hyperextension can develop in young growing puppies. This condition is probably related to an imbalance in growth rate between the osseous and musculotendinous components of the musculoskeletal system. (2) Hyperextension can also be a sequela to external coaptation of the distal forelimb in young puppies and should not be mistaken for a carpal hyperextension injury due to traumatic rupture of the palmar carpal ligaments. Stress radiographs in a dog with carpal hyperextension secondary to coaptation will be normal.

iii. In most puppies, carpal hyperextension will improve with time. Owners should be advised regarding feeding a proper diet, screening for intestinal parasitism, and allowing appropriate exercise. Moderate controlled exercise and maintaining a low plane of nutrition to mitigate rapid growth spurts should be advocated. In some breeds a degree of carpal hyperextension is normal and should not cause any problems. The carpal hyperextension in this puppy resolved within 2 weeks once the dog's dietary intake had been reduced and intermittent short periods of exercise were implemented.

81 A dissection of a normal dog's stifle is shown (81).

i. Name the anatomic structure identified by the arrows.

ii. How could alterations in the dimensions of this structure contribute to the pathogenesis of CrCL disease?

iii. What additional conformational abnormalities of the stifle are purported to predispose dogs to develop CrCL insufficiency?

iv. Briefly describe how gait and stifle joint kinematics may play a role in the development of CrCL insufficiency.

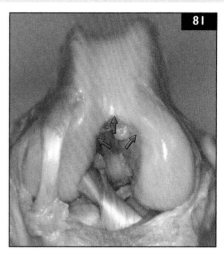

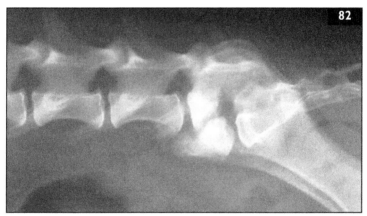

82 A 2-year-old male Yorkshire terrier hit by a car 3 days previously had been unable to ambulate since the accident. Abnormalities found during the physical examination suggested that the dog's inability to ambulate was the result of a neurologic injury. Radiographs of the vertebral column were obtained and a lateral view of the lumbosacral region is shown (82).

i. Describe the fracture.

ii. What type and severity of neurologic deficit could be expected with this fracture?

iii. Describe the treatment options for this fracture.

81 i. The intercondylar fossa of the femur.
ii. The intercondylar fossa in breeds at high risk for CrCL disease is narrow in comparison with breeds that rarely sustain CrCL disease. The narrowed fossa is associated with biochemical alterations, such as increased fibrocartilage content, in the portion of the CrCL subjected to impingement. These fibrocartilaginous alterations may lead to weakening and eventual rupture of the CrCL in breeds at high risk of developing CrCL insufficiency (e.g. Labrador retrievers), but may be adaptive to exercise in low-risk breeds (e.g. greyhounds). The intercondylar fossa can also become narrowed due to osteophyte development secondary to osteoarthritis, thereby impinging on the CrCL. The CrCL and CaCL have their origins on the femoral condyles and pass obliquely through the intercondylar fossa.
iii. Other conformational abnormalities include excessive tibial plateau angle, erect hindlimb posture, and excessive tibial torsion or internal rotation of the tibia as associated with medial patellar luxation or genu varum.
iv. Altered gait as demonstrated by stifle kinematics may contribute to abnormal loading of the CrCL in breeds at high risk of developing CrCL insufficiency. Greyhounds have a positive phase across the stifle, tarsus, and metatarsophalangeal joints at the end of the stance, indicating an active push-off, whereas the only positive phase evident in the hindlimbs of Labrador retrievers is across the tarsal joint and this is small.

82 i. There is an oblique fracture through the body of L7 with concurrent luxation of the articular facets of the lumbosacral joint. The fracture is displaced cranioventrally.
ii. Damage to the sciatic nerve roots or nerves (L6–S1 [S2]) results in lower motor neuron paresis or paralysis of the musculature innervated by the sciatic nerve and, possibly, loss of pain sensation in the sciatic dermatomes. Pudendal and pelvic nerve injury (S1–S3) can result in urinary and fecal incontinence. Clinically, these dogs will dribble urine, their bladders are easy to express, and they have poor or no anal tone. Damage to the caudal nerves (Cd1–Cd5) causes tail paralysis. The femoral nerve roots leave the spinal canal between L4 and L6. A normal to exaggerated (due to loss of sciatic antagonism) patellar reflex is therefore expected. Surprisingly, minor neurologic deficits are often observed in dogs with L7 fractures despite substantial fracture displacement, as seen in this dog; the spinal canal in the lumbosacral region is spacious and the nerves of the cauda equina are reasonably tolerant of compression.
iii. Decisions regarding treatment and prognosis depend on the severity of neurologic deficits, not the amount of radiographic fracture displacement. Conservative treatment with strict cage confinement and analgesics can be used to manage dogs with no or minor deficits, provided serial neurologic examinations are performed. Dogs with more severe deficits should undergo exploration, decompression, fracture reduction, and stabilization. Dogs that have lost deep pain perception have a grave prognosis, irrespective of whether or not surgery is done.

83 A 12-month-old male neutered Labrador retriever presented with a 4-week history of hindlimb lameness. There was no history of trauma and the lameness had an insidious onset. The dog was slightly overweight, but otherwise the remainder of the physical examination was unremarkable. Pain was elicited on manipulation of both coxofemoral joints, but was worse on the left. A ventrodorsal view radiograph of the pelvis is shown (83).

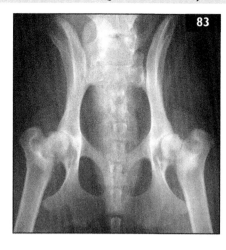

i. Describe the radiological abnormalities.
ii. What is the most likely diagnosis?
iii. What is the etiopathogenesis of this condition?
iv. What are the treatment options for this disease?

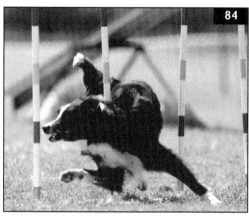

84 A 6-year-old spayed female Border collie with a 5-month history of intermittent weight-bearing right forelimb lameness is shown (84). The dog competes in agility events and has begun to pull out of weave poles and takes wide sweeping turns rather than the typically performed tight turns. During the orthopedic examination, the dog was uncomfortable on manipulation of the right shoulder. Spasm and discomfort of the surrounding musculature were noted when the right shoulder was abducted. The abduction angle of the right scapulohumeral joint was noted to be 60°.

i. What is the diagnosis?
ii. Briefly describe potential treatment options for this dog.

83 i. A linear radiolucent line traverses through the neck of the left femur extending from proximal to distal. There is a small amount of mineralization subjacent to the lateral margin of the femoral head. The contour of the right femoral head is distorted, with apparent shortening of the femoral neck.

ii. A slipped femoral capital physis (epiphysiolysis), given the radiographic appearance of a fracture of the subcapital femoral region in an overweight young dog with no traumatic event leading to the fracture. The pathologic appearance of the contralateral femoral head and neck region supports the diagnosis.

iii. The etiopathogenesis is uncertain. Biochemical and mechanical factors are theorized to be involved in the pathophysiology, resulting in weakening of the capital physis and, therefore, slippage of the femoral head. Histopathologic changes of affected canine femoral heads include bone necrosis and remodeling of the femoral head and osteochondrosis of the articular cartilage. The degree of slippage of the femoral head that occurs categorizes this condition into acute, chronic, or acute-on-chronic slippage.

iv. Appropriate treatment depends on the stage of disease. Acute cases should be treated as traumatic physeal fractures with anatomic reduction and internal fixation using either divergent Kirschner wires or lag screw fixation. Surgical stabilization can also be performed in dogs with chronic lesions in which the epiphysis is minimally displaced and when there is minimal neck resorption. Femoral head and neck excision or total hip replacement (may be challenging or not possible if there is extensive remodeling of the calcar region of the femur) is recommended for more advanced cases.

84 i. The dog has a high abduction angle that is strongly suggestive of medial shoulder instability. Medial shoulder instability is a common cause of unilateral forelimb lameness, especially in performance and sporting dogs. Instability develops as a result of repetitive activity and increased abnormal biomechanical loads on the medial compartment of the scapulohumeral joint. Consequently, repeated strain and sprain injuries occur.

ii. Treatment options for medial shoulder instability vary according to severity, and optimal treatment of this condition is still in question. Arthroscopy is warranted to characterize the pathology present and guide decisions regarding therapy. Treatment options include conservative management utilizing a DogLeggs® shoulder support system and rehabilitation therapy, which can be effective in managing many mildly and some moderately affected dogs. Radiofrequency treatment and/or arthroscopic imbrications can be used to address joint capsule and subscapularis muscle laxity or disruption if present. Primary stabilization using bone anchors and prosthetic ligaments or TightRope stabilization has been described to address marked instability of the medial compartment of the scapulohumeral joint. Postoperative shoulder support systems and rehabilitation therapy should also be used after these procedures have been done.

85 An 18-month-old male domestic shorthaired cat presented with a history of chronic, mild right hindlimb lameness and reluctance to jump. The lameness had suddenly become worse just prior to presentation for evaluation. Pain was elicited on manipulation of both coxofemoral joints. A pelvic radiograph was obtained (85).

i. What is the radiographic diagnosis?

ii. Discuss the pathogenesis of this condition in cats.

iii. Describe appropriate treatment for this cat.

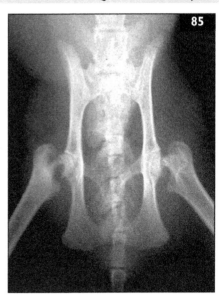

86 A 6-year-old male cat sustained right antebrachial fractures after unknown trauma. Craniocaudal and mediolateral radiographs were obtained (86a, b). There is a segmental diaphyseal fracture of the ulna and a transverse mildly comminuted proximal diaphyseal fracture of the radius. The fractures are closed and displaced proximolaterally.

i. At what level are antebrachial fractures most likely to occur in cats?

ii. What method of stabilization would be preferable to limit the potential for postoperative complications for this cat's fractures?

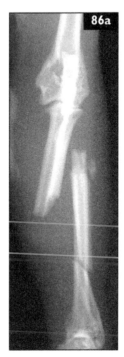
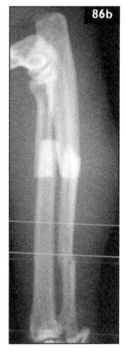

85 i. Bilateral spontaneous femoral capital physeal fracture. This condition is characterized radiographically by loss of bone within the femoral neck (indicating osseous necrosis), which may eventually lead to fracture. Over half of affected cats eventually develop bilateral disease. Clinically, these cats usually have a chronic mild hindlimb lameness that worsens acutely when fracture occurs.

ii. Spontaneous femoral capital physeal fractures predominately occur in young adult male cats neutered at a young age. The high incidence of this condition in neutered males between 12 and 24 months of age suggests that there is an association with delayed physeal closure ascribed to early neutering. The pathologic changes in affected cats are similar to those observed in dogs with metaphyseal osteopathy (also referred to as hypertrophic osteodystrophy or Barlow's disease). The terms spontaneous femoral capital physeal fracture, slipped capital femoral epiphysis, proximal femoral or femoral neck metaphyseal osteopathy, and femoral capital physeal dysplasia syndrome describe conditions with similar radiographic and clinical signs and may all be manifestations of the same condition.

iii. Femoral head and neck ostectomy. This may be performed on both hips in cats affected bilaterally. Total hip replacement is another salvage option that could be considered.

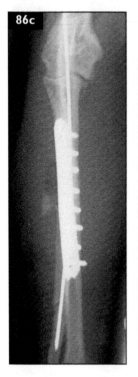

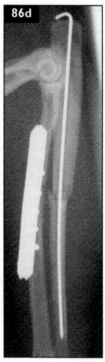

86 i. Radial fractures are located more commonly in the mid and proximal diaphyseal region in cats, while most antebrachial fractures involve the distal radius and ulna in dogs.

ii. Stabilization of both the radius and ulna has proved to be an effective repair strategy: in one study only 12.5% of fractures in which both bones were stabilized required revision compared with 27.8% of fractures in which only one bone was stabilized. In this cat the ulna fracture was stabilized with a 1.2 mm Kirschner wire and the radial fracture was repaired with a 2.0/1.5 mm veterinary cuttable plate with 2.0 mm screws (**86c, d**).

87 Surgery was performed on the dog in case 59. A post-operative radiograph is shown (87).
i. What are the spherical implants used in this dog?
ii. Describe the indications and properties of this therapeutic modality.
iii. Discuss the advantages and disadvantages associated with use of these implants.

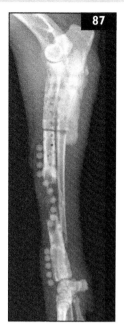

88 A 2-year-old male beagle presented with a history of walking on its 'tip-toes', which began when the dog was a young puppy. The dog walked with all joints in all four limbs rigidly extended, including its digits (88). Bilateral valgus deformity of the carpus was also evident. The dog 'bunny hopped' when running. When the dog sat, the hindlimbs were flexed at the hips with the remainder of both distal hindlimbs extended forward. The abaxial digits

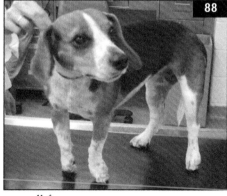

were noted to be disproportionally short on all four paws.
i. Abnormalities of which body systems should be considered?
ii. What specific syndromes could account for this clinical presentation?
iii. In addition to a complete orthopedic and radiographic evaluation, what other diagnostic tests would be indicated in this dog?
iv. In addition to limb stiffness, this dog's skin was noted to be thickened and its muscles were very firm on palpation, suggesting fibrosis. Abnormalities of which biochemical pathways play a major role in the etiopathogenesis of tissue fibrosis?

87 i. Antibiotic-impregnated PMMA beads.
ii. Indications for use of antibiotic-impregnated PMMA beads include chronic osteomyelitis, open fractures, soft tissue infections, septic arthritis, tenosynovitis, chronic rhinitis and/or sinusitis, and cellulitis. The beads are used as a local antibiotic delivery system. Bacteriocidal, heat-stable antibiotics (e.g. gentamicin, cefazolin, amikacin, tobramycin, vancomycin, clindamycin, or cephalothin) are typically used after obtaining a preoperative culture and sensitivity of the affected tissue. There is a rapid release of antibiotic from the beads in the first 24–48 hours, followed by a slow sustained release for weeks following implantation.
iii. Advantage: The beads afford a prolonged release of high local concentrations of antibiotics at the site of infection; initially the concentration can be 200 times as high as can be achieved through systemic antibiotic administration. Disadvantages: A number of potentially useful antibiotics cannot be incorporated into PMMA beads because they are not heat stable. The beads can promote a foreign body reaction, local toxicity, or even infection associated with prolonged implantation. A second surgery may be required to remove the beads.

88 i. The musculoskeletal system (bones and joints), the neuromuscular system (specifically muscle and peripheral nerve), and the skin.
ii. The differential diagnoses should include chronic myopathies and neuropathies associated with fibrosis, arthropathies associated with contractures, and generalized connective tissue diseases similar to Marfan's syndrome or scleroderma in humans.
iii. Appropriate diagnostics would include serum creatine kinase levels, electro-diagnostics, and biopsies of the muscle, nerve, and skin.
iv. Transforming growth factor-beta (TGF-β) and the extracellular matrix (ECM) play important roles in medical problems associated with fibrosis. TGF-β activity is regulated primarily in the ECM by tissue microfibrils, the glycoprotein fibrillin 1 and fibronectin. This dog was confirmed to have Musladin–Lueke syndrome, a TGF-β dysregulation syndrome identified in beagles and associated with a mutation in *ADAMTSL2*, a gene that encodes for a TGF-β regulating protein. This is a genetic disease with an autosomal recessive inheritance. Affected dogs should not be bred from and genetic testing of related dogs should be performed prior to breeding. The effectiveness of antifibrotic drugs has not been determined in this disease.

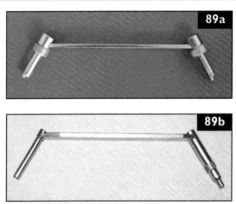

89 Two instruments are shown (89a, b).
i. Name the instruments.
ii. How much effective compression is achieved when placing a 2.0 mm, 2.7 mm, or 3.5 mm diameter screw using the end of the instrument with the gold collar in 89a?
iii. Does screw insertion order influence the amount of compression generated?
iv. Which plate – the locking compression plate (LCP) or the dynamic compression plate (DCP) – allows for greater compression of a fracture?
v. Which instrument will generate more compression when used with a DCP?

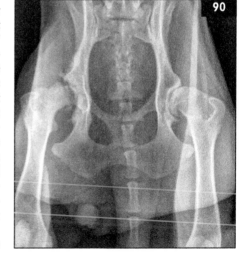

90 A 10-year-old female Labrador retriever presented with a right hindlimb lameness of 4 months' duration. During orthopedic examination pain was localized to the right coxofemoral joint. A pelvic radiograph is shown (90). The right coxofemoral joint is both osteolytic and productive, with diffuse periosteal reaction extending along the ilial wing and an area of smooth periosteal reaction on the medial ischium. There is severe destruction of the right femoral head. Differential diagnoses to consider include neoplasia and infection.
i. What is the most likely cause of the lameness in this dog?
ii. What are the most commonly recognized histologic subtypes of this lesion?
iii. Which histologic subtype has a worse prognosis?

89 i. A Synthes DCP drill positioning guide (**89a**) and a universal drill positioning guide (**89b**).

ii. The gold collar signifies that the end of the instrument is the compression drill guide and that the hole drilled in the bone will be positioned eccentrically within the hole in the plate, causing translation of the screw relative to the plate and, consequently, the engaged bone segment as the screw is tightened. The effective compression achieved when placing a 2.0 mm screw in this manner is 0.6 mm; when placing a 2.7 mm screw it is 0.8 mm; when placing a 3.5 mm screw it is 1.0 mm.

iii. A biomechanical study found that screw insertion order does influence the amount of compression generated. To maximize compression when using a load screw in a bone plate (after securing the opposite segment to the plate), the load screw should be placed before a neutral screw is placed. Another study found that more compression could be achieved when placing a third compression screw in a DCP if the third screw was placed on the opposite side to the fracture rather than placing all three screws in the same fracture segment.

iv. There is no significant difference in compression achieved between the first two compression screws in either a DCP or the combi-hole in the LCP.

v. The DCP drill positioning guide generates more compression than the universal drill positioning guide when placing screws in the plate holes of a DCP.

90 i. With this signalment, history, and radiographic abnormalities the most likely diagnosis is primary neoplasia involving the coxofemoral joint. Given that the osteolysis involves both the pelvis and the femur, the likely specific diagnosis is synovial cell sarcoma.

ii. Recently, synovial cell sarcoma and histiocytic sarcoma have emerged as the most common subtypes of joint tumors. Synovial cell sarcoma can be described as monophasic or biphasic. Biphasic synovial cell sarcomas are characterized by the presence of both phenotypically epithelioid and phenotypically mesenchymal cells within the tumor. When immunohistochemical staining is performed to further characterize these two cell populations, biphasic tumors are characterized by cells that express both vimentin (present in cells of mesenchymal origin) and cytokeratin (present in cells of epithelial origin). Synovial tumors containing solely one or the other type of cell are thus described as monophasic synovial cell sarcomas. Histiocytic sarcomas are characterized by CD18 positivity (present in cells of histiocytic origin). The distinction between histiocytic sarcomas of the synovium and synovial cell sarcoma is important because there is a marked difference in prognosis.

iii. Histiocytic tumors of the synovium have a worse prognosis than synovial cell sarcoma. In one study the mean survival time for dogs with histiocytic tumors was 5.3 months. Dogs with synovial cell sarcomas had a reported mean survival time of 31.8 months.

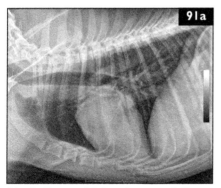

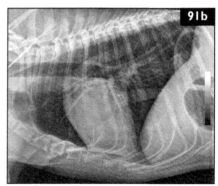

91 A 5-year-old female spayed German shepherd dog has a poor appetite and has lost a considerable amount of weight over the past month. The owner has noted that the dog has difficulty rising after lying down, is reluctant to ambulate, and perceives that the dog has back pain. On physical examination the dog has a kyphotic posture and hyperpathia is elicited when pressure is applied to the thoracic vertebral column. Radiographs of the thorax are obtained (**91a, b**).
i. Describe the radiographic abnormalities.
ii. What is the diagnosis?
iii. What particular etiology should be considered when this disease occurs in a German shepherd dog?

92 The radiation treatment plan superimposed on a CT sagittal image for a proximal humeral osteosarcoma in a large-breed dog is shown (**92**).
i. What type of radiation procedure is being planned for in this image?
ii. What is the name of the colored lines?
iii. Briefly discuss the underlying concept of this type of radiation therapy; in particular, state how high doses of radiation can be delivered in a single setting.

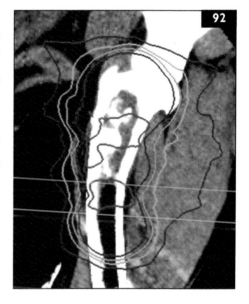

91 i. There are focal areas of lysis along the cranial and caudal vertebral end-plates at multiple intervertebral disc spaces. The vertebral bodies of T1 and T2 are lytic. In addition, there is ill-defined osseous proliferation associated with the T4–T5 and T7–T8 vertebral body end-plates.

ii. Discospondylitis, an infection of the intervertebral disc and adjacent vertebrae.

iii. Discospondylitis can be either bacterial or fungal, and German shepherd dogs have a breed predilection for developing discospondylitis secondary to systemic *Aspergillus* spp. infections. The breed is believed to have an hereditary immune defect that predisposes young and middle-aged female dogs to systemic aspergillosis. The primary species involved are *A. deflectus* and *A. terreus*. Dogs usually present with non-specific clinical signs. Typical radiographic abnormalities of aspergillosis include discospondylitis; however, polyostotic osseous lesions of multiple long bones and enlargement of the tracheobronchial lymph nodes may also be seen. Radiographs of the thorax and the appendicular skeleton are warranted to accurately stage the disease. Other organ systems that may be involved include the central nervous system, retina, spleen, and kidneys. Fungi can be present in the urine sediment. Abdominal ultrasound may reveal abnormalities of the liver, kidneys, and spleen including changes in the size, margin, and echogenicity of these organs.

92 i. A stereotactic radiosurgery (SRS) procedure.

ii. Isodose lines. The lines represent the dose of radiation within each outlined topographic anatomic location. In this example the radiation doses that the lines represent are as follows: red – 50 Gy, blue – 40 Gy, salmon – 30 Gy, turquoise – 20 Gy, purple – 10 Gy.

iii. Conventional radiation therapy is performed via a limited number of simulated, static fields and relies on the use of fractionation schemes to minimize damage to surrounding normal tissue. For example, a dose of radiation greater than 4–5 Gy given in a single fraction will result in greater damage to late-responding normal tissues than the same dose divided into two smaller fractions. In contrast, SRS minimizes collateral damage to normal tissues adjacent to the tumor by relying on extreme accuracy of radiation delivery to a tumor target and a steep dose gradient between the tumor target and the adjacent normal tissues. With SRS the entire radiation treatment is delivered as a single, large dose via multiple, non-coplanar beams or, in some instances, arcs of radiation that are stereotactically focused on the target. Stereotactic delivery results in a summation effect of the radiation dose where the beams intersect beneath the skin in the center of the tumor.

93 An 18-week-old female Newfoundland is positioned in dorsal recumbency on the operating table in preparation for juvenile pubic symphysiodesis (JPS) surgery (**93a**).

i. Explain the mechanism by which JPS alters pelvic development in dogs affected with hip dysplasia.

ii. Why is concurrent or subsequent neutering mandatory in dogs undergoing JPS?

iii. What is the age range that has been recommended for performing JPS in dogs?

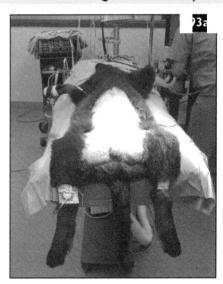

94 A 6-year-old, 27 kg female mixed-breed dog sustained a comminuted right tibial fracture, which was stabilized with a plate-rod fixation and cerclage wires. Nine weeks following surgery the dog presented with a mild weight-bearing lameness and an open draining wound on the medial side of the crus, over the mid-diaphysis of the tibia. On palpation, the area was warm, swollen, and painful. Radiographs of the crus were obtained (**94a, b**).

i. Evaluate the repair and assess the progression of fracture healing on these radiographs.

ii. What is the diagnosis?

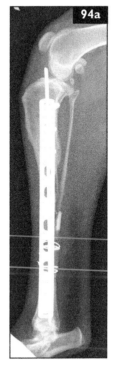
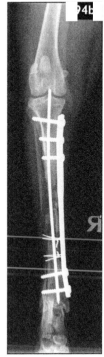

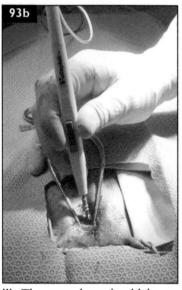

93 i. During JPS an electrosurgical device (cautery pen with needle tip) is used to thermally ablate the cranial two-thirds of the pubic symphysis (**93b**). The thermal cytotoxic effects on the pubic symphysis cause cessation of ventral acetabular growth (pubic rami), thereby resulting in relative overgrowth of the dorsal acetabulum (triradiate physis). This growth pattern results in bilateral acetabular ventroversion, which improves dorsal acetabular coverage of the femoral heads.

ii. JPS changes a dog's phenotype without changing the dog's genotype. Therefore, a dog with a genetic predisposition for hip dysplasia could potentially be promoted as a normal dog and unethically used for breeding. In addition, female dogs will develop a smaller-diameter pelvic canal, which could potentiate dystocia if allowed to breed.

iii. The procedure should be performed in dogs between 12 and 20 weeks of age. Studies in large-breed dogs have shown that performing JPS during this time frame is associated with clinically relevant changes in acetabular angle and relative acetabular ventroversion, as well as improvements in coxofemoral joint conformation and clinical function. This is also the earliest time frame for reliably determining the extent of hip laxity (distraction index) in puppies if this assessment is to be used as a criterion for JPS treatment.

94 i. The fracture alignment is good with the proximal and distal tibial segments correctly orientated with respect to each other. The plate, screws, and intramedullary pin are in place without evidence of loosening; however, the cerclage wires appear to be loose. There is little evidence of callus formation or fracture healing. There are large areas of lucency mid diaphysis indicative of substantial bone resorption in the comminuted fracture zone, with the remaining fragments being displaced and sclerotic.

ii. These radiographic findings together with the open draining wound are typical of an infected, necrotic non-union. The intermediate bone fragments are very likely sequestra. This adverse outcome is usually associated with poor local vascularity secondary to the trauma causing the fracture, as well as excessive iatrogenic trauma incurred during the attempted reduction and improper application of cerclage wires.

95 An 18-month-old female Italian greyhound sustained a fracture of the right radius and ulna after jumping off a bed. The fracture was managed sequentially by external coaptation, then intramedullary pinning and thirdly with an external fixator. The fixator was removed 12 weeks after application and the dog was referred 3 weeks later for further evaluation. The radiograph shown (**95**) was obtained at this time.

i. Elaborate on the categorization of non-union fractures based on the classification scheme described by Weber and Cech.

ii. How would this dog's fracture be classified according to Weber and Cech's classification scheme?

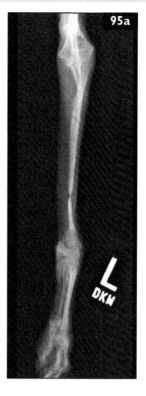

96 A 10-month-old male brindle Great Dane (**96a**) was presented with progressive exercise intolerance, muscle wastage, and body tremors. Exercise and excitement exacerbated the clinical presentation, resulting in collapse, but the dog could resume physical activity following a period of rest.

i. What is the most likely diagnosis given this dog's signalment, history, and clinical abnormalities?

ii. What diagnostic tests should be done to substantiate the diagnosis?

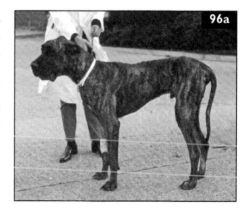

iii. What is the prognosis for dogs affected with this condition?

95 i. Non-union fractures are classified into two major groups (vascular or biologically active, and avascular or biologically inactive) based on the viability of the ends of the bone segments adjacent to the fracture. Biologically active (vascular) non-unions (subclassified as hypertrophic [elephant's foot], slightly hypertrophic {horse's foot}, or oligotrophic), must be differentiated from biologically inactive non-unions because active fractures have a much better prognosis based on the viability of the fracture site. There are four subclassifications of biologically inactive (avascular) non-unions: dystrophic and necrotic non-unions, which develop in comminuted diaphyseal fractures and in which there is a devascularized butterfly fragment or fragments; defect or gap non-unions, which are the result of bone loss at the fracture site; and atrophic non-unions, which are particularly difficult to treat because vascularity is compromised, a gap is often present, and bone quality is often poor, the result of predominating osteoclastic resorption of the involved bone segments. In a dystrophic non-union the fragment(s) heals to one of the major fracture segments and is subsequently partially revascularized. In necrotic non-unions the comminuted fragment(s) remains devitalized.

ii. The radiographic appearance of this dog's fracture is compatible with an atrophic non-union. A gap has developed at the fracture site. There has been progressive loss of bone without appreciable callus formation. The ends of the bone segments are conical with closure of the medullary canal.

96 i. Inherited myopathy of Great Danes, formerly described as central core myopathy of Great Danes. This condition has been most commonly reported in fawn and brindle dogs of both sexes.

ii. Routine hematology is generally normal. Serum biochemistry in most affected dogs will reveal a significant increase, up to 26-fold, in creatine kinase. In one study, electromyography was shown to be the most useful electrophysiological test, with 16 of 18 affected dogs having generalized fibrillation potentials and positive sharp waves. Histopathologic examination of affected muscle biopsies revealed abnormal basophilic central areas in 10–50% of the myofibers demarcated by a distinct basophilic ring (**96b**). Histochemistry showed these central basophilic areas

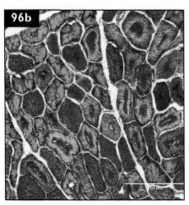

to be strongly reactive to the mitochondrial oxidative enzymes cytochrome c oxidase and succinate dehydrogenase, suggestive of increased mitochondrial accumulations. This is the primary difference of inherited myopathy of Great Danes to central core disease in humans, in which the cores are devoid of mitochondrial activity. Both type I and II myofibers are affected by these changes, but there appears to be a predominance of type I myofibers in affected muscles.

iii. Generally poor as there is no effective treatment for this condition.

97 A 2-year-old racing greyhound sustained a fracture of the calcaneus. Mediolateral and plantarodorsal radiographs of the tarsus were obtained; the mediolateral view is shown (**97**).
i. What soft tissue structures would be compromised as a result of this fracture?
ii. What are the possible consequences if this fracture is managed conservatively without surgery?
iii. Which other tarsal bones are fractured in the so called 'triad of the tarsus' in racing greyhounds?

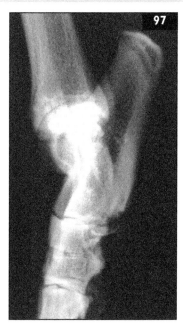

98 i. What are the orthopedic implants shown in **98a**?
ii. Describe the unique functional property of this implant.
iii. What is the most common clinical application for this implant in dogs?

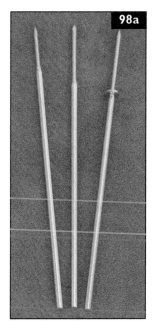

97 i. This dog has an avulsion fracture of the base of the calcaneus, which has also been described as a small oblique plantar distal chip fracture. This is an intra-articular fracture. The fracture will result in loss of function of the plantar ligament. The long plantar ligament originates from the base of the calcaneus and inserts on the plantar process of tarsal bone IV as well as on the plantar processes of metatarsal bones IV and V. This ligament, together with the plantar fibrocartilage, is one of the major stabilizers of the tarsal joint.

ii. As there is an avulsion component to this fracture, osseous union is unlikely without surgical intervention. If left untreated, this fracture will likely become a fibrous non-union with proximal plantar intertarsal instability.

iii. Fracture of the central tarsal bone and a compression fracture of tarsal bone IV.

98 i. Orthofix self-compressing pins (Orthofix Magic Pin). The smooth shaft has a larger diameter than the threaded segment of the pin, with a tapered chamfer located at the smooth shaft–thread interface. Pins are available in small (1.2 mm thread diameter, 1.5 mm shaft diameter), medium (1.6 mm/2.0 mm), and large (2.2 mm/3.0 mm) sizes. All are 120 mm in length with variable thread lengths. The two larger diameter pins also have compatible washers (**98a**).

ii. The ability to generate interfragmentary compression without the normally obligatory step of overdrilling the *cis*-fragment to prepare a glide hole. The implant is designed such that when the chamfer (or washer) contacts the cortex of the *cis*-fragment, further advancement of the pin preferentially strips the threads cut in the bone of the *cis*-fragment. The threads continue to maintain purchase in the *trans*-fragment and advancing the pin creates interfragmentary compression.

iii. This implant has been used to repair articular fractures of the humeral condyle, especially Salter–Harris type IV fractures in smaller, skeletally immature dogs (**98b**). A Kirschner wire is generally placed from the condylar segment proximally through the epicondylar crest to provide adjunctive stability. A report reviewing the results in 23 dogs that had humeral condylar fractures stabilized with Orthofix self-compressing pins concluded that the implant was convenient and simple to use, and complications were infrequent. On long-term follow-up dogs had good clinical outcomes with little or no osteoarthritic changes in the repaired elbow.

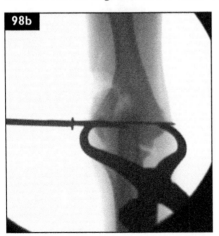

98b

99 Briefly describe two methods of surgical treatment for the fracture shown in case 97.

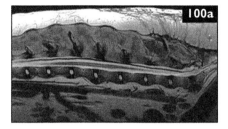
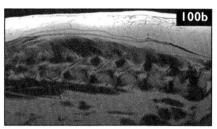

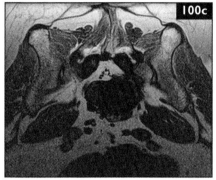

100 A 6-year-old castrated male mastiff presents for a 4-week history of difficulty rising. On physical examination the dog is overweight and has hindlimb weakness, which is more severe in the left hindlimb. The dog intermittently holds the left hindlimb in a flexed non-weight-bearing position and has marked low-lumbar hyperpathia. MRI was performed, focused on the caudal lumbar spine and lumbosacral junction. Shown are T2-weighted images including sagittal (**100a**) and left parasagittal (**100b**) images of the caudal lumbosacral region as well as an axial image (**100c**) obtained at the level of the L7–S1 intervertebral disc space.
i. Describe the finding of the MRI examination.
ii. What is the diagnosis?
iii. What is the pathophysiology of this disease?

99 (1) The fragments can be reduced and stabilized with one or two Kirschner wires and a figure-of-eight tension band. In the presence of mild comminution, it may be necessary to stabilize additional small fragments with lag screws. In this case two Kirschner wires, a lag screw, and a tension band wire were used (99a, b). While technically

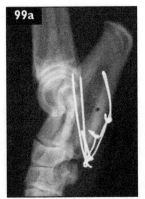 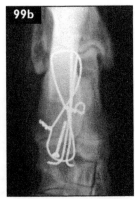

demanding, this option offers the best prognosis for return to racing performance. (2) In fractures with severe comminution, in which the fracture is deemed unreconstructable, the best solution would be a proximal intertarsal arthrodesis stabilized using either a Steinmann pin and a tension band wire or by application of a lateral plate. Unfortunately, the prognosis for return to competitive performance following application of a plate is poor because of fusion of the calcaneoquartal joint.

100 i. At the lumbosacral junction, there is moderate low-signal intensity material bridging the intervertebral disc space, with absence of the normal, high-signal intensity associated with the nucleus pulposus of the L7–S1 intervertebral disc. On the axial image, there is a large volume of low-signal intensity material causing complete attenuation of the left L7–S1 intervertebral foramen, with compression of the left L7 nerve root. On the parasagittal image there is also a region of low-signal intensity at the level of the L7–S1 intervertebral foramen.
ii. The MRI findings are compatible with intervertebral disc degeneration at L7–S1, characterized by dessication of the intervertebral disc, bridging spondylosis deformans, protrusion, and possible extrusion of the annulus fibrosis. This dog has left-sided foramenal stenosis with resultant compression of the L7 nerve root.
iii. Degenerative lumbosacral stenosis is the most common cause of cauda equina compression in dogs and results from various degenerative changes in the osseous and soft tissue structures surrounding the nerve roots. CT and MRI offer non-invasive means of characterizing nerve root compression and identification of involved structures. While agreement between the CT and MRI findings is high, correlation between the MRI abnormalities, surgical findings, and clinical signs is often low. Surgical outcome is correlated with the severity of clinical signs; specifically, the presence of urinary or fecal incontinence correlates with poor outcomes.

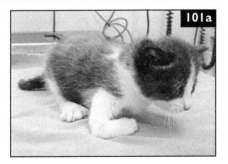

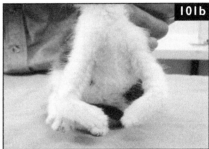

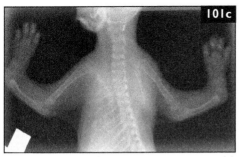

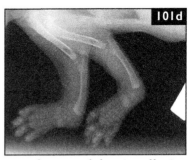

101 A 3-week-old female kitten presented because of a varus deformity affecting both forelimbs (**101a, b**). The kitten behaved and played normally, but the deformity caused a markedly abnormal forelimb gait. There was only one other littermate, which was similarly affected. Physical examination of the forelimbs did not elicit any pain response on manipulation of any joint or when direct pressure was applied to any of the appendicular long bones. Radiographs of both forelimbs were obtained (**101c, d**).

i. What is the diagnosis?
ii. What other conditions have been reported as co-existing with this problem in cats?
iii. What are the implications for further growth and development of the forelimbs of this kitten?
iv. What treatment should be advised for this kitten?

102 What considerations should be made before including any NSAID in the preoperative protocol for a dog undergoing elective orthopedic surgery?

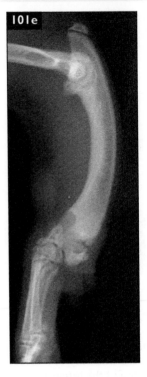

101 i. Bilateral radial agenesis (also referred to as 'intercalary hemimelia'). Both radii appear to be completely absent in this kitten. The ulnae appear fully formed. Using the classification system for similar developmental deformities in humans, the complete absence of the radius suggests this is a type IV deformity, which is the most commonly reported variant of radial agenesis in dogs and cats.
ii. Cardiomegaly and hindlimb polydactyly.
iii. The ulnae in response to the applied forces will remodel as predicted by Wolff's law. The distal diaphysis and metaphysis will enlarge and the articulation between the ulnar styloid process and the ulnar carpal bone will remodel to enable better dispersion of the forces of weight bearing. The humeroulnar joint will remodel, with enlargement of the coronoid processes to accommodate the humeral condyle. These adaptive changes are seen in the radiograph of a 15-week-old kitten with type IV radial agenesis (**101e**).
iv. Cats affected with type IV hemimelia function well without surgical intervention and treatment was not advised for this kitten. Despite shortening and varus deformity of the forelimbs, cats learn to compensate for their disability and behave and play normally.

102 Dogs should be screened with respect to renal and hepatic function as well as for a history of NSAID gastrointestinal tolerance. As a class of drug, NSAIDs are most commonly associated with adverse reactions affecting the gastrointestinal tract (64%), kidneys (21%), and liver (14%). Hepatic and/or renal compromise may not necessitate withholding administration of an NSAID; however, justification should be made. The dog should not have recently been administered corticosteroids or a different NSAID. Aspirin administration within the prior 7–10 days would be a contraindication for administration of an NSAID because of complications associated with aspirin-triggered lipoxin. Additionally, to minimize the potential for acute renal failure, the dog must be sufficiently hydrated prior to anesthesia and surgery.

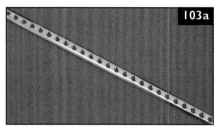

103a

103 A plate commonly used in small animal orthopedics is shown (**103a**).
i. Name the implant.
ii. Describe the properties and advantages of this implant.
iii. How does the stiffness of the 2.0/2.7 mm version of this plate compare with the stiffness of a 2.7 mm dynamic compression plate (DCP)?

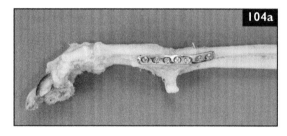

104a

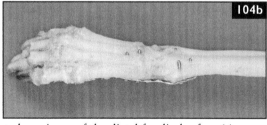

104b

104 The macerated specimen of the distal forelimb of an 11-year-old male Boston terrier that had undergone a pancarpal arthrodesis to address an antebrachiocarpal hyperextension injury is shown (**104a, b**). The dog functioned well on the limb for 3 years after surgery before dying of congestive heart failure.
i. How was the plate applied to stabilize this dog's pancarpal arthrodesis?
ii. What are the reported advantages of positioning the plate in this position to stabilize a pancarpal arthrodesis?

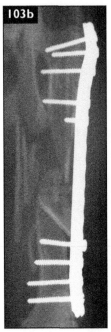

103b

103 i. A veterinary cuttable plate. These plates are available in two sizes: 1.5/2.0 mm plates and 2.0/2.7 mm plates. The plates are designed to accommodate two different diameter screws (smaller plate: 1.5/2.0 mm screws; larger plate: 2.0/2.7 mm screws), as implied by each plate's name.
ii. The plates can be cut to the desired length, which negates the need to maintain a large inventory of different length plates. The holes in the plates are evenly spaced, so two plates of the same size or different sizes can be used together (sandwiched or stacked) to increase construct stiffness, as illustrated in **103b**, where two 2.0/2.7 mm plates were used in a stacked fashion to stabilize a comminuted femoral fracture in a cat.
iii. The 2.0/2.7 mm plate is only about a third as stiff as a 2.7 mm DCP (578 N/mm compared with 1,507 N/mm). Stacking two 2.0/2.7 mm plates effectively doubles the construct stiffness to 1,066 N/mm, but it is still not as stiff as a single 2.7 mm DCP.

104 i. A seven-hole 2.0 mm LC-DCP bone plate contoured to provide 10° of carpal extension was applied to the caudomedial aspect of the distal radius, carpus, and proximal second metacarpal bone. Seven 2.0 mm cortical screws were used to stabilize the construct with the distal screws engaging multiple metacarpal bones.
ii. The surgical approach to the medial aspect of the distal forelimb is straightforward and the arthrodesis can be performed faster and with less associated surgical morbidity than with previously reported techniques. A small amount of valgus is normally present in dog carpi and applying the plate to the medial surface of the carpus positions the plate along the tension surface of the joint. The medial technique also results in the bone plate being loaded on edge, which provides a greater area moment of inertia and makes the plate highly resistant to bending forces. Screws placed medial-to-lateral through the radius have greater purchase than screws placed cranial-to-caudal. Compared with dorsal plating techniques, in which the distal screws are typically placed in only a single metacarpal bone, medial application results in screws engaging multiple metacarpal bones, which potentially provides more stable distal fixation.

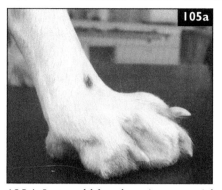
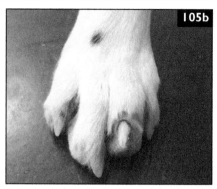

105 A 5-year-old female springer spaniel was presented with a history of developing an acute right forelimb lameness while running in a field 2 weeks previously. The dog's lameness was transient, lasting only a couple of days, but the owner was concerned about the appearance of one of the dog's digits (**105a, b**).

i. Describe the appearance of digit III.

ii. What is the most likely cause of this abnormality?

iii. What treatment would be appropriate for this dog?

106 A 6 year old springer spaniel that has had surgical stabilization of a fracture of the lateral aspect of the humeral condyle is shown (**106a**). The dog had a nerve block performed prior to surgery.

i. Which peripheral nerve blocks provide analgesia during forelimb surgery?

ii. How can the chances of performing a successful nerve block be increased?

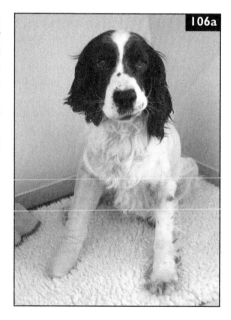

105 i. The third phalanx and nail of the third digit of the right fore paw are deviated dorsally. The digital pad is only partially in contact with the ground. This abnormality is colloquially referred to as a 'kicked up' or 'knocked up' toe.
ii. An isolated rupture of the deep digital flexor tendon to the affected digit.
iii. If rupture of the deep digital flexor tendon occurs in a pet dog, surgical intervention is probably not warranted as the deformity should not produce any adverse functional consequences. Surgery is often recommended for show or athletic dogs; however, owners should be warned that the tenorrhaphy often stretches or fails with the affected digit resuming some degree of hyperextension. If the injury is left untreated, the abnormal contact of the digital pad with the ground can result in the formation of a corn. This dog's injury was already 2 weeks old and the dog was not lame, so treatment was not advocated.

106 i. A 'traditional' brachial plexus block may be performed, although this is unlikely to provide analgesia proximal to the elbow. For surgery involving the humerus and shoulder, a cervical paravertebral block may be used, although this is technically more difficult and carries an increased risk of complications. For surgery involving structures distal to the elbow, a radial, ulnar, median, and musculocutaneous (often abbreviated RUMM) block may be performed, which carries less risk of morbidity than brachial plexus blockade.
ii. Success can be dramatically improved by identifying accurately the location of the nerves using either an electrical nerve stimulator or ultrasound guidance. Electrical location is more commonly done in dogs, but requires a dedicated nerve stimulator (**106b**) and special needles. These needles have a shaft that is electrically insulated, with only the metal of the bevel remaining exposed (**106c**). Consequently, lower current strengths are required to locate nerves. The non-cutting tip of these needles also reduces the risk of nerve damage.

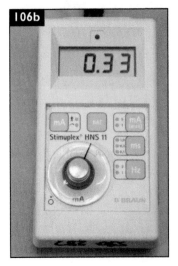

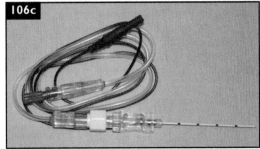

107 A 7-year-old male crossbreed dog jumped from a first floor window. The dog suffered an acute-onset left forelimb lameness. Orthopedic examination revealed a swollen effusive left carpus, which was painful on palpation. Treatment was instigated with bandaging and NSAID administration. The dog was referred for definitive treatment 6 weeks later. A mediolateral radiograph was obtained at this time, with the carpus in a hyperextended stressed position (107a).
i. What is the diagnosis?
ii. Describe appropriate treatment options for this dog and the advantages and disadvantages of each of these treatment options.

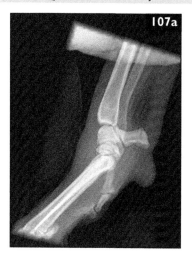

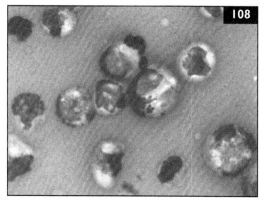

108 A 5-year-old, neutered female Old English sheepdog presented with a 3-week history of a right hindlimb lameness that had progressively increased in severity. The picture shows a 100x magnified photograph of Wright–Giemsa-stained cytologic preparations of synovial fluid aspirated from the right stifle (108).
i. What is the most likely diagnosis?
ii. What specific diagnostic technique would have the greatest potential to yield an etiologic agent in this dog?
iii. What general mechanisms are responsible for the development of this condition?

Answers: 107, 108

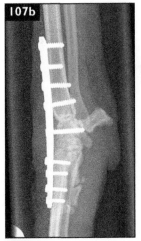
107b

107 i. This dog has sustained a carpal hyperextension injury with palmar instability of the carpometacarpal joint, implying that there is disruption of the palmar carpal fibrocartilage attachment to the metacarpal bones as well as the accessoriometacarpal ligaments.

ii. Conservative treatment utilizing coaptation is an ineffective means of managing carpal hyperextension injuries. Healing of the palmar fibrocartilage and palmar ligamentous structures is typically insufficient to support weight bearing, even following prolonged coaptation in flexion. Two surgical options are partial carpal arthrodesis or pancarpal arthrodesis. Pancarpal arthrodesis fuses the antebrachiocarpal, middle carpal and metacarpal joints (**107b**) and has an excellent outcome with a low complication rate. As the entire carpus is fused, motion in the antebrachiocarpal joint is eliminated. The aim of a partial carpal arthrodesis is to achieve fusion of the middle carpal and carpometacarpal joints, while preserving normal motion in the antebrachiocarpal joint. Retaining motion at the antebrachiocarpal joint should allow the dog the possibility of returning to full athletic function. Partial carpal arthrodesis is reported to have a good outcome with a low complication rate. Additional surgery is occasionally required due to subclinical ligament damage affecting the antebrachiocarpal articulation, resulting in development of degenerative joint disease, pain, and lameness.

108 i. The nucleated cell population consists primarily of neutrophils, many of which are degenerate. Phagocytized cocci are present within one neutrophil (right of center) suggesting that the dog has septic arthritis.

ii. Although the presence of large numbers of neutrophils in the synovial fluid is suggestive of septic arthritis, immune-mediated arthropathies must also be considered, particularly if the neutrophils are non-degenerate. Identifying intracellular bacteria in this dog substantiates the diagnosis of septic arthritis; however, bacteria are not observed cytologically in most dogs with septic arthritis. While culture of the synovial fluid is critical to establishing a diagnosis of septic arthritis, <50% of synovial fluid cultures from infected joints will initially yield positive bacterial growth. Inoculating synovial fluid into blood culture medium and an aerobic culturette, then incubating for 24 hours, followed by inoculation onto blood agar, significantly increases the possibility of obtaining positive culture results.

iii. Joint infections can be initiated by hematogenous spread of bacterial organisms from a remote site of infection, extension of local (juxta-articular) infection into the joint, or by traumatic penetration of the joint. Joints may also be infected iatrogenically as a result of surgery or intra-articular injections. The most common organisms isolated from infected joints in dogs and cats include *Staphylococcus* spp., *Streptococcus* spp., *Corynebacterium* spp., *Escherichia coli*, and other coliforms.

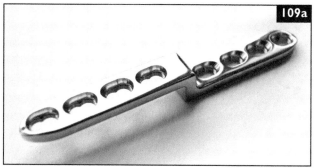

109 A picture of an implant is shown (**109a**).
i. For what procedure was this implant developed?
ii. What are the recommended selection criteria for deciding to apply this implant?
iii. What possible complications might be anticipated after implant application?

110 A craniocaudal radiograph of the left femur of a 10-month-old spayed female Labrador retriever with an obvious weight-bearing left hindlimb lameness of 6 weeks' duration is shown (**110**). The yellow line represents the anatomic proximal femoral longitudinal axis (aPFLA) drawn between center points identified at the proximal third and mid-point of the femur. The white line represents the joint reference line (JRL) drawn along the distal-most articular surface of the medial and lateral portions of the femoral condyle.

i. Describe the radiographic abnormalities.
ii. What term has been applied to denote the obtuse angle formed by the intersection of the yellow and white lines?
iii. What does a large angle indicate?
iv. List the characteristics of a properly positioned radiograph that would allow accurate determination of this measurement and discuss how inappropriate positioning can affect accuracy when making this measurement.
v. What surgical procedure could be done to improve this dog's femoral conformation?

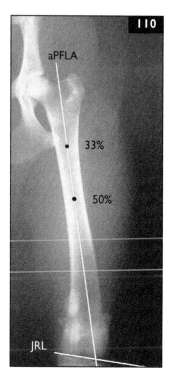

Answers: 109, 110

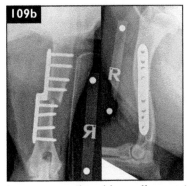

109 i. To stabilize the humerus when performing a sliding humeral osteotomy. The plate features combination locking/non-locking screw holes and has a centrally-located 7.5 or 10 mm step. The plate is applied to the medial surface of the humerus such that the distal humeral segment is translated medially (109b). ii. Sliding humeral osteotomy acts to transfer the weight-bearing load towards the normal lateral joint compartment in dogs with medial compartment disease of the elbow. Clinical selection criteria include: marked or persistent lameness attributable to elbow pain refractory to medical or conventional surgical treatment; medial compartment disease, which is characterized by full-thickness cartilage erosion of all or part of the medial articular surface of the elbow; absence of significant cartilage pathology affecting the lateral compartment of the elbow.

iii. Major complications include humeral fracture, catastrophic multiple screw failure, and delayed osteotomy union. Minor complications include incidental screw breakage, wound dehiscence, and hematoma or seroma formation. Possible complications (e.g. implant-associated infection, iatrogenic intraoperative neurologic or vascular injury, lateral compartment disease) have not been documented. Refinement of implant design and surgical technique have reduced the complication rate from 35% to 5%.

110 i. This dog has a left medial patellar luxation and there appears to be mild varus of the distal femur.

ii. The anatomic lateral distal femoral angle (aLDFA), which is a measure of frontal plane femoral conformation.

iii. Varus conformation is reflected by a positive aLDFA value, whereas a negative value indicates valgus conformation. A large aLDFA reflects an increase in femoral varus conformation. This dog's aLDFA was 107°.

iv. The femur is a three-dimensional object. Accurate measurement of frontal plane conformation from a two-dimensional radiograph requires a well-positioned craniocaudal (or caudocranial) image. With proper positioning: both fabellae are bisected by the ipsilateral femoral cortex; the apex of the lesser trochanter protrudes from the medial femoral cortex; and there is (often but not always) an end-on view of the nutrient foramen. Slight obliquity of the radiographic image will reveal normal sagittal plane procurvatum as artifactual angular deviation in the frontal plane. Subtle external rotation of the femur, a common positioning error, is detected by excessive protrusion of the lesser trochanter, superimposition of the lateral fabella on the distal femur, and isolation of the medial fabella. Such a positioning error would artifactually increase the radiographic measurement of an aLDFA.

v. A distal femoral corrective osteotomy could be done to reduce this dog's femoral varus. The osteotomy can be performed as a laterally-based closing wedge ostectomy, a medially-based opening wedge osteotomy, or a radial or dome osteotomy.

111 A 5-year-old female spayed Jack Russell terrier presented for evaluation of an intermittent non-weight-bearing lameness of the right forelimb of several weeks' duration. After examining the dog, the lameness was determined to be neurologic in origin with a suspected nerve root signature (**111**).

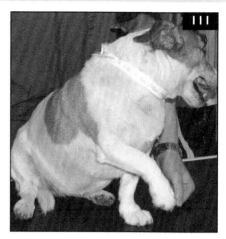

i. What is the most likely location of this dog's lesion?
ii. What differential diagnoses should be considered in this dog?

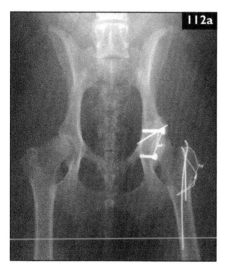

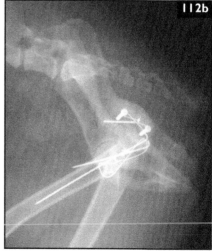

112 Two-year follow-up radiographs of a 3-year-old female spayed Labrador retriever that underwent open reduction and stabilization of an acetabular fracture are shown (**112a, b**).
i. What fixation method was used to stabilize this fracture?
ii. Describe how this fixation is applied.

Answers: 111, 112

111 i. Dogs that intermittently hold a forelimb off the ground in a partially flexed position due to neurogenic pain are described as having a 'root signature'. This posture is most commonly associated with C6–T2 spinal segment lesions, but can also be associated with C1–T2 nerve root entrapment. Important considerations when formulating a list of differential diagnoses and developing a diagnostic plan are that the responsible lesion must be lateralized or asymmetric.

ii. The most common cause of a root signature is extrusion of intervertebral disc material that has lateralized toward the vertebral foramen. Cervical disc disease in dogs, which accounts for up to 25% of intervertebral disc disorders in this species, is usually a consequence of disc extrusion rather than protrusion. The predominant clinical abnormality observed in dogs with cervical disc disease is cervical pain: approximately 60% of affected dogs have pain, but no neurologic deficits. Studies have reported the incidence of root signature to be anywhere from 22–50% in dogs with cervical disc disease. Other important differential diagnoses include traumatic nerve injury such as a brachial plexus trauma, nerve root tumors, discospondylitis, and, rarely, nerve root entrapment associated with degenerative spondylosis.

112 i. The screw/wire/PMMA composite fixation technique.

ii. The fracture is exposed using a dorsal approach via a greater trochanteric osteotomy combined with a tenotomy of the tendons of insertion of the gemelli and obturator muscles to improve exposure. A second approach is made to apply bone reduction forceps to the tuber ischii in order to manipulate the caudal acetabular segment to obtain reduction. Once the fracture is reduced anatomically, one or more interfragmentary Kirschner wires are placed to maintain the reduction. A bone screw is placed in both the cranial and caudal acetabular segments, 5–10 mm from the fracture. A line drawn between the two screws should intersect the fracture at a right angle. The screws should be approximately 4 mm longer than the measured depth of the drill holes so that the shank and one or two revolutions of thread remain exposed. Stainless steel orthopedic wire is then placed around the exposed shank in a figure-of-eight pattern. The free ends of the wire are tightened using a wire tightener. When the wire is tight, the braided strands are cut, leaving at least three twists. The exposed implants are then covered with a small aliquot of methyl methacrylate, which, after polymerizing *in situ*, will prevent cyclic fatigue of the wire while the fracture is healing. Strict asepsis must be maintained to prevent contamination of the PMMA and the sciatic nerve must be retracted to avoid thermal damage as the PMMA is polymerizing.

113 With regard to the dog in case **111**, what further diagnostic evaluations would be most helpful to establish a diagnosis?

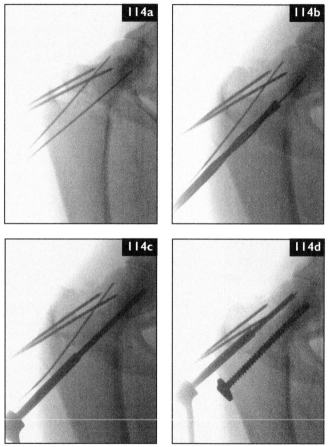

114 Intraoperative fluoroscopic images of a femoral neck fracture being stabilized via a limited open reduction in a 20-month-old male castrated Great Dane are shown (**114a–d**). The fracture was sustained when the dog was hit by a car.
i. How would this dog's femoral neck fracture be categorized?
ii. What is the unique characteristic of the drill bits used during repair of this fracture?

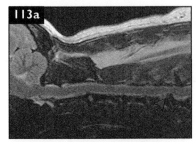

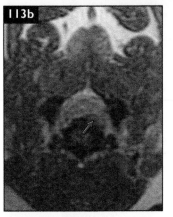

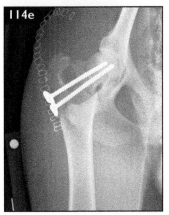

113 Some form of cross-sectional imaging is necessary to determine the causative lesion for lateralized cervical spinal cord signs. CT with myelography or MRI should be considered. MRI is advantageous if the lesion extends beyond the foramen into soft tissues. If the lesion is not mineralized, identification on a CT scan would be difficult without administration of intrathecal contrast. The sagittal MR scan of this dog revealed a ventral compressive lesion at the C5–C6 intervertebral disc space (arrowhead) (**113a**) with right-sided lateralization (arrow) (**113b**). Electrophysiological tests (needle electromyography and nerve conduction testing) can assist in substantiating the localization of the lesion if the disease process has been present for more than 5 days. Electrodiagnostic tests, however, do not provide information that allows characterization of the underlying disease process.

114 i. Fractures can be classified as intracapsular (subcapital or transcervical) or extracapsular (basilar or intertrochanteric). This is an extracapsular basilar fracture, which could be exposed by reflecting the origin of the vastus lateralis muscle at the base of the femoral neck without entering the joint capsule.
ii. The drill bits are cannulated, having a central longitudinal hole that runs the length of the drill bit, which accepts a small diameter wire. This facilitates accurate drilling in preparation for screw placement. Once this dog's fracture was reduced, multiple Kirschner wires were placed to maintain reduction (**114a**). One mm (smaller diameter wires) Kirschner wires were placed and imaged fluoroscopically to ensure that alignment and depth was optimal. The trochanteric fracture segment was overdrilled with a 4.5 mm cannulated drill bit (**114b**). A centering drill sleeve was placed in this hole and the hole in the femoral neck and head was made with a 3.2 mm cannulated drill bit (**114c**). Fluoroscopy was utilized to ensure the holes in both fracture segments were made to the proper depth. The more proximal 1.0 mm Kirschner wire was replaced at a more appropriate angle once the first screw had been placed (**114d**), as seen on the immediate postoperative craniocaudal radiograph (**114e**).

115 Linear fixator constructs have been applied to two tibiae (115a, b).

i. How would the two constructs illustrated in these photographs be classified according to conventional nomenclature established to describe linear fixators?

ii. In order to maximize a linear fixator's stiffness and limit implant complications, what relationship should be maintained with respect to fixation pin diameter and the diameter of the stabilized bone segment?

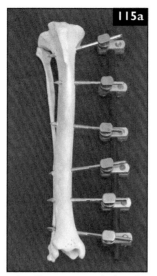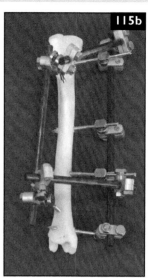

iii. Describe the relative mechanical and clinical advantages of using the construct in **115a** compared with the construct in **115b** for stabilization of a diaphyseal tibial fracture.

116 This diagram (116) is of a craniodorsal approach to the coxofemoral joint, which is used for open reduction and stabilization of an acetabular fracture in a dog. An osteotomy of the greater trochanter of the femur has been done to expose the acetabulum.

i. What muscle inserts on the third trochanter?

ii. What two muscles insert on the greater trochanter?

iii. What muscles insert in the trochanteric fossa of the femur?

iv. What type of fixation should be used when reattaching the greater trochanter to the femur?

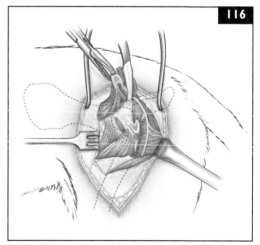

115 i. Both are type I constructs. The pins engage both the *cis-* and *trans*-cortices of the bone, but only protrude from the soft tissues on one side of the limb (half-pins), therefore both constructs are unilateral. The construct in **115a** is also uniplanar, as all the pins are in the same longitudinal plane and attached to a single connecting rod. These unilateral, uniplanar fixators are known as type Ia constructs. The construct in **115b** is biplanar, as the pins have been placed in orthogonal planes. Two connecting rods, one medial and one cranial, form the external frame. Unilateral, biplanar fixators are referred to as type Ib constructs.

ii. The pin diameter should not exceed 25–30% of the bone's diameter. The stiffness of a pin is proportional to the diameter to the fourth power: larger diameter pins increase stiffness; however, fixation pins that exceed 30% of the bone's diameter potentiate the risk of fracture through the pin hole.

iii. Type Ib fixators offer greater resistance to axial, bending, and torsional loading than type Ia constructs. Torsional stiffness can be further enhanced by articulating the two connecting rods, creating a diagonal strut. Type Ib fixators are more resistant to shear loads than type II constructs, therefore a type Ib construct offers substantial biomechanical stability without the potential soft tissue morbidity associated with placement of full-pin splintage pins in the proximal tibia when applying a type II construct.

116 i. The superficial gluteal muscle inserts on the third trochanter. This muscle's tendon of insertion is incised and the muscle is reflected dorsally prior to performing the trochanteric osteotomy.

ii. The middle and deep gluteal muscles insert on the greater trochanter. These muscles are reflected with the greater trochanter to expose the dorsal aspect of the acetabulum during this approach.

iii. The gemelli as well as the internal and external obturator muscles insert on the trochanter fossa. These muscles are reflected to expose the caudal aspect of the acetabulum. After pre-placing a stay suture through these muscles, tenotomies are performed near the fossa. Traction can be applied to the stay suture, pulling the muscles caudally. The muscles can be used as a physiological retractor, protecting the sciatic nerve, while affording the surgeon greater exposure of the caudal aspect of the acetabulum.

iv. Following anatomic reduction, the greater trochanter should be stabilized using either pin-and-tension band fixation or screws placed in a lag fashion. In a study that assessed healing and complications associated with greater trochanteric osteotomies performed in 24 dogs, only one dog (4% of all cases) developed a pertinent clinical complication despite the observation that the osteotomies had achieved normal radiographic union in only 38% of the dogs at 6 weeks following surgery. The authors concluded that the method of stabilization did not influence radiographic healing and that despite the high incidence of abnormal radiographic findings, trochanteric osteotomy was associated with a low incidence of postoperative morbidity.

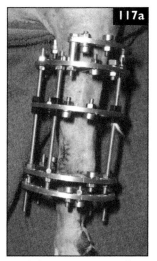
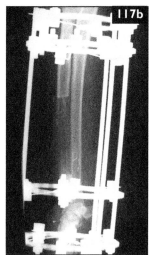

117 A 6-year-old female bullmastiff pre-sented for treatment of an osteosarcoma of the distal right radius and underwent a limb salvage procedure (117a). A radiograph taken 16 weeks after surgery is shown (117b).

i. What limb salvage technique was used in this dog?

ii. What are the advantages of using this limb salvage technique in comparison to other more traditional surgical techniques?

iii. What are the disadvantages associated with using this method of limb salvage?

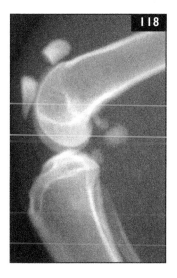

118 A 2-year-old male neutered Russian blue cat that was kept indoors presented with an acute-onset right hindlimb lameness. Pain was localized to the right stifle. Radiographs of the stifle were obtained and the mediolateral view is shown (118). The cat had suffered a similar fracture in the contralateral stifle 3 months previously. No traumatic incident had been observed with either injury.

i. Describe the fracture.

ii. What is the likely etiology of this cat's fracture?

iii. What is the likelihood of a cat sustaining bilateral fractures?

iv. What is the recommended method of treatment for these types of fracture?

v. What dental abnormalities have also been noted in cats with this particular fracture?

117 i. Bone transport osteogenesis. In this technique the segment of diseased bone is excised. A circular external skeletal fixator is applied to the limb. A transport segment of bone is created in the bone immediately proximal to the defect and is secured by a transport ring. The ring is translated along the threaded rods by turning nylon nuts placed on either side of the ring. The nylon nuts can be turned simultaneously using a special double wrench, moving the transport ring and the secured transport segment distally toward the carpus. This process is used to initiate distraction osteogenesis in the distraction gap that develops between the transport and the proximal radial segment.

ii. Advantages include: creation of autologous viable bone in the defect; residual implants do not remain in the limb at the completion of the procedure; and the incidence of catastrophic infection is much lower when using this technique compared with placement of an allograft or an endoprosthesis.

iii. Disadvantages include: the bone segment is transported at a rate of 1 mm/per day – because a large segment of the bone typically needs to be removed in most dogs, the fixator needs to be maintained for a very long period of time (mean of 205 days in one case series); the technique requires a high level of owner compliance and daily care for the procedure to be successful; and the technique is technically demanding to perform and requires experience.

118 i. There is a transverse fracture of the right patella, with wide displacement of the fracture fragments and sclerosis of the patella.

ii. Transverse patellar fractures in cats are suspected to be stress fractures. There is evidence of pre-existing sclerosis in the patella prior to acute fracture and often an absence of identifiable causative trauma. There may be underlying metabolic bone disease, as many cats with patellar fracture develop additional stress fractures at other locations. Atraumatic fractures of the proximal tibia, acetabula, ischial tuberosity, and humeral condyle have been seen in cats with pre-existing or subsequent transverse patellar fractures.

iii. Both patellae will fracture in at least 50% of affected cats. The median time interval between fractures is 3 months.

iv. Pin and tension band wire fixation has a very high failure rate, often resulting in additional fracture of the patella because the bone is sclerotic and brittle and liable to further fragmentation. The optimal treatment method is unknown, but placing a wire that encircles the patella or treating these fractures conservatively may be a preferable approach, as the likelihood of these fractures healing, regardless of the fixation method, is low.

v. Retained deciduous teeth, a rare finding in the normal cat population, is frequently reported in cats with patellar fractures.

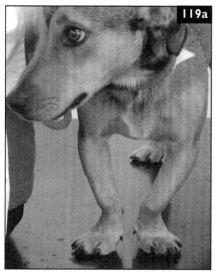

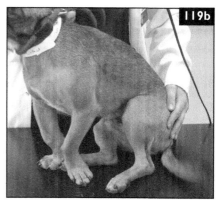

119 This 9-month-old crossbred dog was presented because of the owner's concerns regarding the appearance of its forelimbs (**119a, b**). The dog had moderate forelimb gait abnormalities and mild pain was elicited on manipulation of the forelimb joints during an orthopedic examination.

i. What disorder is responsible for this dog's conformational abnormalities?

ii. Describe the etiopathogenesis of this disorder.

120 A 3-year-old male castrated Australian shepherd dog developed an acute non-weight-bearing lameness of the left hindlimb after jumping to catch a ball. Dorsoplantar (**120a**) and lateral (**120b**) radiographs were taken of the left tibiotarsus.

i. Describe the radiographic abnormalities. What is the radiographic diagnosis?

ii. What anatomic structures must sustain damage for this condition to occur?

iii. What treatment options exist for this condition?

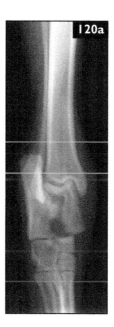

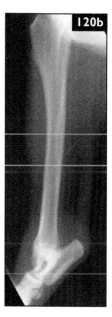

119 i. Osteochondrodysplastic dwarfism.
ii. The general term osteochondrodysplasia embraces a group of genetic skeletal anomalies. These anomalies are due to defects in growth and development of cartilage and bone and are usually characterized by various dwarfish features. While the underlying cause is complex and poorly understood, the condition is known to arise from defective chondroblast activity during endochondral ossification. This results in premature physeal closure or retarded physeal growth. The distal ulnar physis is particularly affected, which results in features characteristic of radius curvus syndrome, as seen in this dog. Some breeds (e.g. Pekingese, shih tzus) are bred to be achondroplastic dwarfs and have dwarfish features of both their skulls and limbs. Other breeds (e.g. corgis, bassett hounds) have dwarf features of the limbs but normal or dolichocephalic skulls and these breeds are known as hypochondroplastic dwarfs. Osteochondrodysplastic dwarfism occurs sporadically in non-chondrodystrophic breeds including the Alaskan malamute, Scottish deerhound, Norwegian elk hound, Maremmano–Abruzzese shepherd dog, Great Pyrenees, German shepherd dog, miniature poodle, Labrador retriever, beagle, and cocker spaniel. Most of the alterations in these dogs result from a *de novo* mutation, but in some dogs the abnormalities appear to be due to autosomal recessive inheritance. This dog had mild humeroulnar subluxation, which was the cause of the elbow pain.

120 i. There is an increased talocalcaneal joint space with medial displacement of the distal aspect of the talus relative to the central tarsal bone. This is a talocalcaneal luxation with associated talocentral luxation.
ii. The proximal and distal talocalcaneal ligaments must be disrupted to allow for talocalcaneal luxation. The talocalcaneal ligaments span the tarsal sinus and

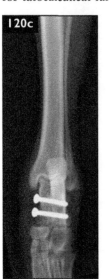

attach to each bone at a position between the proximal and middle articular facets (proximal talocalcaneal ligament) and near the distal articular facets (distal talocalcaneal ligament). **iii.** Talocalcaneal luxations have been managed conservatively with external coaptation after open or closed reduction, although internal fixation is recommended to reduce chronic instability and the development of degenerative joint disease. Placement of screws in a lag fashion from talus to calcaneus is the most commonly reported method of internal fixation (**120c**). The joint is not arthrodesed in these cases due to the difficulty of accessing and debriding the articular cartilage, but debridement, grafting, and eventual osseous union do not seem necessary for obtaining a good functional outcome.

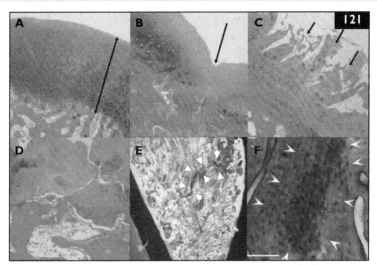

121 These images are of toluidine blue/basic fuchsin-stained photomicrographs taken at ×100 magnification (**121A–D**) and basic fuchsin-stained photomicrographs taken at ×200 (**121E**) or ×40 magnification (**121F**) of sections through the medial aspect of the coronoid process (CP).

i. Describe the articular cartilage histopathologic abnormalities associated with medial CP disease in the dog.

ii. Describe the subchondral bone histopathology associated with medial CP disease in the dog.

iii. What is the likely etiopathogenesis responsible for these histopathologic abnormalities?

122 A cat's distal humerus is shown (**122**).

i. Name the anatomic structure centered in the red box.

ii. What neurovascular structures pass through this structure?

iii. Is it preferable to place an intramedullary pin in a normograde or retrograde fashion when stabilizing a supracondylar humeral fracture in a cat?

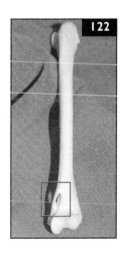

121 i. A wide spectrum of abnormalities can be present, ranging from thickening of cartilage (**121A**) to healed or non-healed full-thickness fissures (**121B**), superficial fibrillation (**121C**), mixed pathology including fissuring and fragmentation (**121D**), or complete abrasional loss of cartilage.

ii. Gross pathology of subchondral bone may vary from intact to fissuring or fragmentation of the lateral aspect of the CP. Subchondral microfracture is a consistent histopathologic finding. There may be large microcracks (**121E**) or more diffuse microdamage (**121F**). Microfracture may be associated with variable degrees of necrosis, microcrack healing (by fibrous, cartilaginous, or osseous infilling), or penetration of microcracks into the articular cartilage. This variation is largely dependent on chronology and severity of disease. Importantly, microfracture can be identified throughout the entire medial aspect of the CP, and is not limited to the areas of visible gross pathology.

iii. Mechanical overload of the medial aspect of the CP during load bearing, resulting in 'stress' microfracture, is the most probable explanation. A range of scenarios for this mechanical overload has been postulated, including static or dynamic radial–ulnar length incongruity, ulnar trochlear notch shape-associated joint incongruity, primary humeral–antebrachial rotational instability, and osseous–soft tissue mismatch (including excessive supination forces asserted on the medial aspect of the CP by the biceps brachii and brachialis musculotendinous units), but remain unproven.

122 i. The supracondylar foramen, which is a distinguishing anatomic feature of the cat's humerus.

ii. The brachial artery and median nerve.

iii. Intramedullary pinning of the humerus is arguably more difficult in cats than in dogs. The pin should optimally be seated distally in the condyle; however, care must be taken to avoid iatrogenic damage to the brachial artery, the median nerve, and the articular cartilage of the humeral condyle. While cats do not have a supratrochlear foramen, the cat's trochlea is situated more medial to the anatomic axis of the humerus than in dogs, which complicates effective seating of a pin distally. In addition, an appreciable medullary canal is only present in approximately 50% of cat humeri distal to the supracondylar foramen. In one study using cat cadavers, pins introduced from a simulated fracture into the condylar segment in retrograde fashion were much more likely to inflict damage to the articular cartilage and periarticular vital structures than pins placed in normograde fashion. Thus, normograde pin placement via a limited approach to the trochlea was advocated when utilizing an intramedullary pin to stabilize supracondylar fractures in cats.

123 A 4-year-old, 20 kg female Border collie dog injured its left hind paw jumping a fence. The dog presented with a non-weight-bearing lameness of the left hindlimb, with swelling, pain, and crepitus of the paw on that limb. A dorsoplantar radiograph of the left hind paw is shown (**123a**). The dog's fractures were stabilized with external skeletal fixation.
i. Describe this dog's fractures.
ii. List the advantages and disadvantages of the stabilization technique used for the fractures in this dog.

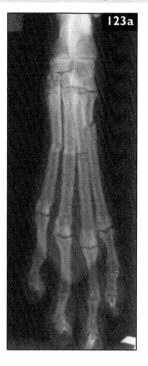

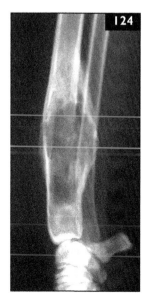

124 A 6-year-old male castrated greyhound presented with progressive forelimb lameness. The dog had recently developed a painful swelling centered at the distal antebrachium. A radiograph of the affected antebrachium (**124**) revealed an aggressive lesion that was confirmed cytologically to be an osteosarcoma.
i. What treatment options exist for this dog?
ii. What survival times might these options offer?

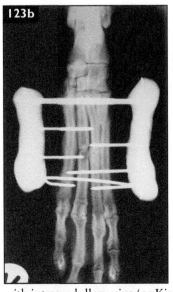
123b

123 i. This dog has transverse mid-diaphyseal fractures of the second, third, and fourth metatarsal bones and a proximal diaphyseal fracture of the fifth metatarsal bone.

ii. External skeletal fixation, as used in this dog, is suitable for stabilizing a variety of fracture configurations. External fixators can be applied via closed reduction, thereby limiting the amount of iatrogenic trauma associated with surgery. In addition, postoperative external coaptation is not required. The main disadvantages of stabilizing metatarsal fractures with an external fixator are that pin placement in small dogs can be challenging and fracture reduction may not be anatomic, although as long as paw alignment is maintained, the functional results are not affected by individual bone alignment. Individual bone alignment is easier to achieve by using external skeletal fixation in conjunction with intramedullary pins (or Kirschner wires), which can be articulated or 'tied-in' to the fixator. Pin placement, unfortunately, requires an open approach and the pins may need to be placed through the metatarsophalangeal joints, which can lead to degenerative joint disease. In this dog, epoxy putty was used to form the connecting columns. The fixator was removed 6 weeks after application when healing had progressed satisfactorily (123b).

124 i. Palliative options include administration of analgesic medications such as NSAIDs, tramadol, gabapentin, amantadine, and/or bisphosphonates (e.g. pamidronate) and coarse fractions of external beam radiation. Curative-intent options include amputation or limb-sparing procedures, including surgical excision of the involved bone segment and implantation of an allograft or endoprosthesis, or high-dose radiation (single fraction stereotactic radiosurgery, stereotactic radiotherapy, fractionated radiotherapy). Systemic chemotherapy administration is indicated to treat the micrometastatic disease presumably present in all dogs diagnosed with appendicular osteosarcoma.

ii. Palliative options are likely to provide 2–6 months of effective relief before the pain becomes unremitting or the limb fractures. Amputation alone is associated with a median survival time of 3–4 months, but the median survival time can be increased to 10–12 months with administration of adjunctive chemotherapy, typically carboplatin or doxorubicin, alone or in combination. Surgical or radiation therapy limb-sparing techniques do not extend overall survival compared with amputation unless the surgical site becomes infected, which has been shown to increase the median survival time to 480 days.

125 A 5-month-old female kitten presented because it was reluctant to exercise, had a poor appetite, and was not growing at an appropriate rate. The kitten was significantly smaller than its littermates. During the physical examination the kitten walked with a stiff, stilted gait and there was swelling of the metaphyseal regions of the appendicular long bones. The following results were noted on the serum chemistry analysis:

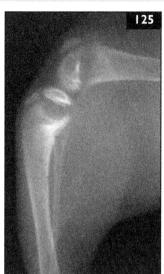

Alkaline phosphatase	955 U/L (normal range: 14–192U/L)
Ionized calcium	1.14 mmol/l (normal range: 1.2–1.8 mmol/l)
Parathyroid hormone	448 pg/ml (normal: <23 pg/ml)
25(OH)D (vitamin D)	11.7 ng/ml (normal range: 5–30 ng/ml)
1,25(OH)$_2$D (calcitriol)	590 pg/ml (normal range: 20–50 pg/ml)

Radiographs of the appendicular skeleton were obtained and a representative radiograph of the right stifle is shown (125).
i. What is the diagnosis?
ii. Explain the abnormal laboratory results.

126 An anatomic dissection of the medial aspect of a cat's carpal joint is shown (126a).
i. Name the two anatomic structures identified by the arrowhead and arrow in this photograph.
ii. Describe the origin and insertion of each of these structures.
iii. Describe the clinical abnormalities that would be expected in a cat when the structure that the large arrow is pointing to is ruptured.

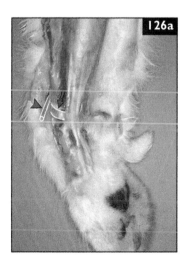

125 i. This kitten has vitamin D-dependent rickets (VDDR) type 2 (VDDR-2) (calcitriol resistant). Four main forms of rickets have been identified. The first is nutritional rickets resulting from a dietary vitamin D or phosphorus deficiency; the second is hereditary X-linked hypophosphatemic rickets; the third is VDDR-1; and the fourth is VDDR-2. VDDR-1 is attributable to a defect in calcitriol production; type 2 is attributable to impaired responsiveness of target organs to calcitriol because of defects in the vitamin D receptors.

ii. Levels of 25(OH)D are within normal ranges, reflecting normal levels of vitamin D nutrition; levels of 1,25(OH)$_2$D (calcitriol) are markedly elevated. Ionized calcium levels are below the normal range and parathyroid hormone levels are elevated. VDDR-2 was originally described as 'vitamin D or calcitriol resistant rickets', as affected individuals have high levels of vitamin D, but a lack of, or deficiency in binding to, vitamin D receptors. Calcitriol is therefore unable to affect target organs (primarily intestine and bone) due to this receptor dysfunction. This results in hypocalcemia, which leads to a secondary hyperparathyroidism. Both calcitonin (release stimulated by hypocalcemia) and hyperparathyroidism activate 1-α-hydroxylase in the kidney, increasing calcitriol production from vitamin D, hence the extremely high levels of calcitriol in cases of VDDR-2. Normally, calcitriol itself decreases 1-α-hydroxylase activity, but this negative feedback pathway fails in VDDR-2 as the pathway requires a functional vitamin D receptor.

126 i. The arrowhead is pointing to the tendon of the abductor pollicis longus muscle. The large arrow is pointing to the medial collateral ligament of the antebrachiocarpal joint.

ii. The medial collateral ligament of the carpus runs obliquely from dorsoproximal on the radius to insert palmarodistal on the radial carpal bone. The abductor pollicis longus muscle has a broad origin, arising from the lateral surface of the radius, the ulna, and the interosseous membrane. The tendon of the abductor pollicis longus muscle courses superficial to the medial collateral ligament and inserts at the base of the first metacarpal bone.

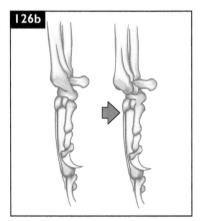

126b

iii. The oblique course of the medial collateral ligament provides medial stability for the antebrachiocarpal joint and restricts palmar displacement of the radial carpal bone. Rupture of the medial collateral ligament in cats does not just result in a pure medial instability (as is the situation in dogs), but also causes palmar subluxation or, potentially, complete luxation of the radiocarpal joint. The instability created by medial collateral ligament rupture in cats is similar to a positive drawer test, as illustrated in **126b**.

127 A ventrodorsal radiograph of the pelvis of a 36-month-old, 33 kg female Labrador retriever that was submitted for evaluation for abnormalities consistent with hip dysplasia is shown (**127**). The owners were unaware of the dog having any clinical lameness or dysfunction.

i. How would this dog's radiograph be assessed by the Orthopedic Foundation for Animals (OFA) and the British Veterinary Association/Kennel Club (BVA/KC)?

ii. What eponym is given to the curvilinear line of enthesophyte seen at the base of each of this dog's femoral necks?

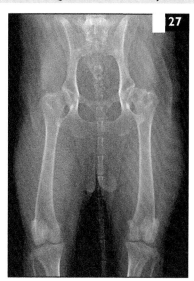

128 A 7-month-old-female boxer dog sustained a comminuted proximal diaphyseal radial fracture and a simple transverse ulna fracture while playing with another dog. The fractures were stabilized by placing an intramedullary pin in the ulna and an external fixator on the radius (**128**).

i. Describe the type of external fixator connecting column that was used in this dog.

ii. List the advantages inherent to using this type of connecting column.

iii. List the disadvantages inherent to using this type of connecting column.

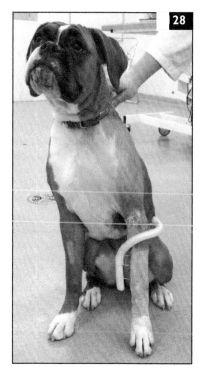

127 i. The OFA evaluates the radiographs for coxofemoral joint subluxation, assessment of acetabular coverage of the femoral heads, assessment of the acetabular margins, and detection of osseous remodeling of both the acetabula and the femoral heads, as well as for the presence of secondary degenerative osteoarthritic changes. Both of this dog's coxofemoral joints are incongruent with <50% acetabular coverage of the physeal scar of either femoral head and marked remodeling and exostosis of both femoral heads. There is also early, bilateral remodeling of the cranial acetabular margin and acetabular fossa. This dog would be considered to have severe bilateral hip dysplasia according to the OFA's grading criteria. BVA/KC scoring is based on different criteria. Nine specific points are evaluated for each hip: (1) subluxation, (2) cranial acetabular margin, (3) dorsal acetabular edge, (4) cranial effective acetabular rim, (5) a Norberg angle of 105° or greater, (6) femoral head and neck exostosis, (7) caudal acetabular edge, (8) femoral head recontouring, and (9) acetabular fossa. Each criterion is scored on a scale from 0–6, except for the caudal acetabular edge, which is scored on a scale from 0–5. The individual scores of the right and left coxofemoral joints are summed, giving a minimum total score of 0 and a maximum of 106 (53 for each hip). The higher the score, the greater the pathology. This dog's radiographs would receive a BVA/KC score of 50 (24/26).

ii. A 'Morgan line'. The line of enthesophytes, which can be indistinct or well-defined, has been suggested as being an early indicator of hip dysplasia in dogs as young as 24 weeks of age.

128 i. This dog's antebrachium has been stabilized with a linear fixator employing an acrylic connecting column. These constructs are sometimes referred to as free-form external skeletal fixation systems. While free-form systems have traditionally utilized acrylic, specifically PMMA, for the connecting column, the use of epoxy resin is becoming increasingly popular.

ii. Advantages of the free-form external fixator include the fact that fixation pin diameter and alignment are not restricted by the size of clamp or the conformation of a connecting rod. The column can be molded to conform to the regional anatomy, which is one reason this type of connecting column was used to stabilize this dog's antebrachial fractures. The constructs are economical, relatively easy to apply, as there is no need for construct preassembly or complex planning, and light in weight.

iii. There are several disadvantages associated with the use of a free-form external skeletal fixation system. A relatively large diameter acrylic or epoxy column must be used to provide comparable strength and stiffness to that of commercially available rigid connecting rods. A 2 cm diameter acrylic connecting column is able to withstand greater shear and compressive loads than unilateral fixators with medium Kirschner–Ehmer clamps and a 4.8 mm connecting bar. Making adjustments with regard to fracture reduction or fixation pin placement is difficult once the material has polymerized.

129 An 18-week-old male neutered chihuahua became acutely non-weight-bearing lame in the right forelimb after jumping from a chair. On physical examination the right elbow was swollen and crepitus and a pain response were elicited on manipulation of the joint. A radiograph of the right elbow was obtained (**129a**).

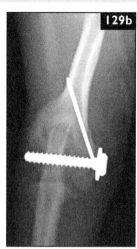

i. What are the correct anatomic terms used to describe the two articulating regions of the humeral condyle?

ii. How would this dog's fracture be described with respect to the Salter–Harris classification scheme?

iii. What is atypical about this dog's fracture?

iv. A transcondylar screw, placed in lag fashion, and an anti-rotational Kirschner wire were used to stabilize this fracture (**129b**). The screw was placed at the level of the physis. What effect will this screw have on subsequent longitudinal bone growth?

v. What concurrent orthopedic injury is evident on this dog's postoperative radiograph?

130 A transverse CT scan of a 9-year-old mixed-breed dog with a 6-week history of mild right forelimb lameness and soft tissue swelling distal to the elbow joint is shown (**130a**).

i. Describe the CT findings.

ii. What is the most likely diagnosis?

iii. Discuss the treatment options.

iv. What is the prognosis?

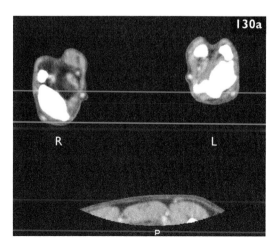

129 i. The lateral portion of the humeral condyle, which articulates with the radial head, is the capitulum. The medial portion of the condyle, which articulates primarily with the ulna, is the trochlea.

ii. This dog has sustained a Salter–Harris type IV fracture.

iii. The fracture is medial, involving the trochlea. The majority of unicondylar fractures involve the capitulum. Approximately one in six unicondylar humeral fractures involves the trochlea. The medial portion of the humeral condyle is more resistant to fracture than the capitulum because the trochlea is directly in line with and buttressed by the metaphysis and is not subjected to eccentric loading (i.e. shear forces) by the radial head. Indirect forces transmitted via the radial head subject the capitulum to shear loads. Bone is weakest when loaded in shear, explaining why unicondylar fractures typically involve the capitulum and are often the result of minor trauma.

iv. A study evaluating humeral length in adult dogs that had undergone stabilization of humeral condylar fractures when the dogs were skeletally immature demonstrated that placement of a transcondylar screw did not impair humeral growth. Fractured humeri were actually found to be longer when compared with the normal contralateral humeri in these dogs.

v. Fracture or fragmentation of the medial coronoid process. This frequently occurs in dogs with unicondylar humeral fractures.

130 i. There is an expansile fat density mass that is displacing the antebrachial musculature and in some areas there is evidence of invasion of the fatty tissue into the muscle. There is no evidence of osseous involvement.

ii. This mass is an infiltrative lipoma.

iii. Due to the invasive nature of infiltrative lipomas, complete surgical excision would only be possible with amputation. Alternatively, local control of the tumor could be achieved via radiation therapy. Ideally, radiation is given in the postoperative setting. This dog's tumor was surgically debulked (**130b**). Fractionated radiation therapy was administered following surgery and local tumor control was achieved.

iv. There is a high chance for recurrence or regrowth of infiltrative lipomas. In one report, single or multiple recurrences followed surgical removal in 4/8 dogs:

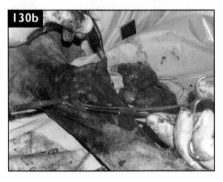
130b

no follow-up was possible in the other four dogs. In a retrospective study of 16 dogs, the lesion had previously been excised in 8 dogs prior to referral. Two dogs were euthanized immediately after surgery because the tumor could not be completely excised. Five (36%) of the remaining 14 tumors recurred. Median time to recurrence for these five tumors was 239 days (range, 96–487 days). The percentage of dogs disease-free 1 year after surgery was 67%.

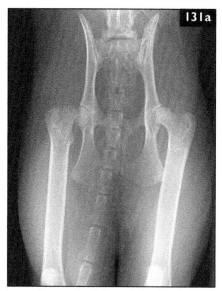

131 A ventrodorsal view radiograph of the pelvis of a 6-month-old female domestic shorthaired cat that presented for acute hindlimb lameness is shown (**131a**).
i. What is the radiographic diagnosis?
ii. Discuss the pathogenesis of this cat's injury.
iii. Describe appropriate treatment for this cat.

132 This 3-year-old, 28 kg male mixed-breed dog is being evaluated 4 months following surgical stabilization of a femoral fracture (**132a**). The dog has undergone extensive physical rehabilitation three times a week, which was initiated 2 weeks after surgery.
i. Name the instrument being used to assess this dog.
ii. Describe the use and value of this particular instrument.

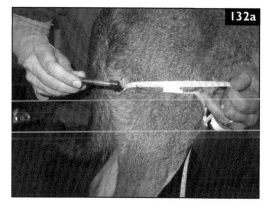

131 i. Femoral capital physeal fracture. Separation of the proximal femoral growth plate occurs in skeletally immature cats: most are Salter–Harris type I fractures with separation through the physis. Typically, the epiphysis (femoral capitus) remains in the acetabulum while the femoral neck is displaced craniodorsally. Occasionally, displacement at the physis is minimal and careful examination of the radiographs or additional frog-leg and extended view radiographs are required to confirm the diagnosis.

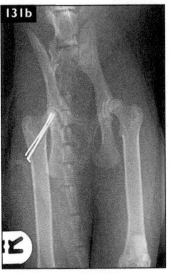

ii. This condition is usually a result of trauma in immature cats. Spontaneous femoral capital physeal fractures have been described in heavier, neutered male cats between 12 and 24 months of age with delayed physeal closure, ascribed to being neutered at a young age.

iii. This cat's fracture was anatomically reduced and stabilized with multiple Kirschner wires (**131b**). Alternatively, screw fixation can be performed in large cats. Femoral head and neck excision can be done in cats with chronic fractures with extensive remodeling of the femoral neck or if complications arise during or after surgery. Conservative therapy (cage confinement followed by limited activity) can be attempted if the epiphysis is minimally displaced; however, the efficacy of this approach is unknown. Surgical intervention is generally warranted, especially if the epiphysis is markedly displaced.

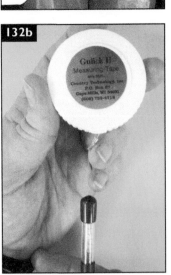

132 i. A Gulick tape measure.

ii. This instrument is used to measure limb or body circumference. The device at the end of the tape measure ensures that a consistent amount of tension (4 ounces) has been applied when one red ball can be seen in the window (**132b**). This device improves the accuracy and consistency of measurements within and between individual animals. If an ordinary tape measure is used, variation in the measurement is influenced by the amount of tension the observer applies.

133 A 5-year-old female neutered pit bull dog developed an acute non-weight-bearing left forelimb lameness after the dog got caught in a railing during a fall off a deck. The dog sustained a lateral scapulohumeral joint luxation. Closed reduction of the luxation was performed and an external coaptation device was applied to the limb (133).

i. Name the coaptation device used to stabilize this dog's reduction.

ii. List indications for use of this coaptation device.

iii. What open reduction and stabilization technique can be employed if the closed reduction fails?

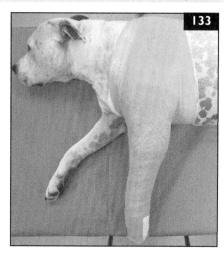

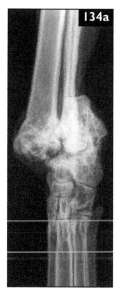

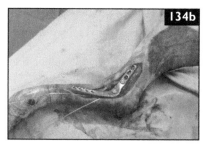

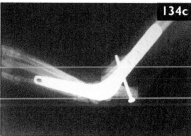

134 A 5-year-old male cat presented with a severe right hindlimb lameness and a painful swollen hock. A craniocaudal radiograph of the tarsal joint is shown (134a). The cat had a chronic dislocation of the right tibiotarsal joint and a decision was made to perform an arthrodesis of the affected joint (134b, c).

i. What type of arthrodesis should be performed in this cat?

ii. If the arthrodesis is stabilized with a plate and screws, discuss the advantages of dorsal versus medial plate application.

133 i. A Spica splint.

ii. Spica splints are used to immobilize the forelimb to treat injuries involving or proximal to the elbow such as fractures of the scapula or the humerus and avulsion of the triceps tendon. Spica splints are more commonly used following closed or open reduction of shoulder and elbow luxations. In this dog the Spica splint was used after closed reduction of a lateral shoulder luxation. The splint was maintained for 14 days, which resulted in a successful outcome.

iii. Surgical stabilization of a lateral scapulohumeral luxation can be accomplished by a variety of different techniques. One technique involves lateral transposition of the tendon of origin of the biceps brachii muscle. Transposition of the tendon creates a 'bowstring' effect and exerts a medially directed force on the humeral head. Imbrication of the joint capsule is concurrently performed and the forelimb typically is placed in a Spica splint for 2 weeks following surgery with exercise restriction imposed for an additional 4 weeks. A prosthetic ligament reconstruction with a screws and suture technique can be used to replicate the lateral glenohumeral ligament.

134 i. Although only the talocrural joint is affected, a pantarsal arthrodesis rather than a partial tarsal arthrodesis was recommended. Selective fusion of the talocrural joint alone will place excessive stress on the adjacent intertarsal and tarsometatarsal joints and can result in development of subsequent degenerative joint disease. This is particularly true for the calcaneal (calcaneoquartal and calcaneotalar) joints. The talocrural joint is the high motion joint of the hock, but substantial motion also occurs at the level of the calcaneal joints.

ii. Medial plating offers the advantages of a simpler surgical approach, better implant biomechanics, and thus more stable fixation. Postoperative coaptation may not be necessary. Medial plate application is performed using customized plates; a medial tarsal arthrodesis plate with an angle of 120° is available for cats. Medial plating is less suitable in animals with medial shearing injuries. Dorsal plate placement is biomechanically inferior and requires adjunctive fixation using either talocrural screws or a transarticular pin. Postoperative coaptation is advisable for the initial 4–6 weeks following surgery. Advantages of dorsal plating are that standard plates can be used and the angle of fusion can be customized to the individual cat. Dorsal plating can be an effective technique in cats.

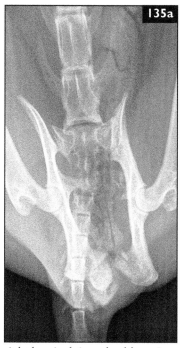

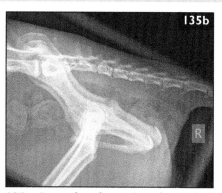

135 A male domestic shorthaired cat, injured in a road traffic accident, was reluctant to ambulate on either hindlimb. On physical examination the cat was painful on manipulation of the pelvic region. On neurologic assessment, proprioceptive reflexes were considered to be slow in the right hindlimb and there was also a reduced withdrawal reflex in that limb. Ventrodorsal and lateral radiographs of the cat's pelvis were obtained (135a, b). There is cranial displacement of the right hemipelvis and subluxation of the right sacroiliac joint. There are fractures of the pubic and ischial rami resulting in an unstable pelvic floor, but these fractures are minimally displaced on the mediolateral radiograph. The sacroiliac joint is part of the hindlimb's weight-bearing axis and this cat's sacroiliac luxation would benefit from reduction and stabilization. The majority of sacroiliac luxations are stabilized with a screw placed in lag fashion. How can correct sacroiliac screw placement be optimized in this cat?

136 Two plates designed for specific applications in dogs are shown (136).
i. Name the two implants.
ii. Describe the intended use for each of these plates.

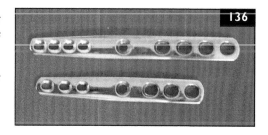

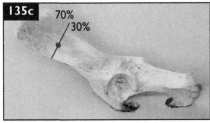

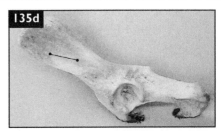

135 The hole for the sacral screw is drilled at a 90° angle to the articular surface of the sacrum. The drill hole in the sacrum should be placed in the center of the craniocaudal axis of the wing of the sacrum slightly dorsal to the midpoint of the dorsoventral axis. To find the correct craniocaudal position on the ilium, align the ilial and sacral wings, visualize the drill hole in the sacrum, and then position the drill bit on the corresponding spot on the lateral ilium. The craniocaudal location of the screw hole on the ilium lies at a distance of about 70% of the sacral tuber length, measured from the craniodorsal to caudodorsal iliac spine. The dorsoventral location on the ilium lies just slightly ventral to the center of the ilial wing height (135c). The ventral gluteal line, a thin bony crest between the insertion area of the middle and deep gluteal muscles, serves as an additional landmark for positioning the ilial screw hole (135d). Following reduction, a 2.7 or 2.0 mm screw is placed in lag fashion across the articulation. The screw should traverse at least 60% of the width of the sacrum to reduce the potential for the screw to pull out.

136 i. The longer plate is a hybrid carpal arthrodesis plate; the shorter plate is a hybrid intertarsal plate.
ii. The carpal arthrodesis plate is designed for stabilization of pancarpal arthrodeses. The dimensions of the hybrid plate taper distally, reducing the stress riser effect at the distal end of the plate. The plate is also designed to accept small diameter screws to stabilize the metacarpal bone, reducing the incidence of postoperative metacarpal bone fractures. It is recommended that the plate extends distally at least 50% of the length of the third metacarpal bone when performing pancarpal arthrodesis with dorsal plate application. Hybrid carpal arthrodesis plates come in a variety of lengths, so this recommendation can be met. The intertarsal plate is similar to the carpal arthrodesis plate, but has fewer screw holes, primarily to accommodate the shorter length of the calcaneus. The 2.7/2.0 mm plate is specifically designed for use in Shetland sheepdogs, a breed predisposed to proximal intertarsal subluxation, which usually requires treatment by proximal intertarsal arthrodesis.

137 An 8-year-old male mastiff presented with a right forelimb lameness of 2 months' duration. The lameness was noted initially after the dog was playing in deep snow. The lameness did not respond to 4 weeks of empirical treatment consisting of administration of an NSAID and rest. Abnormalities on the physical examination were confined to the right proximal humerus. A radiograph of the right humerus is shown (**137**). Given the age, breed, and radiographic abnormalities, the dog most likely has a primary osteosarcoma of the right proximal humerus.

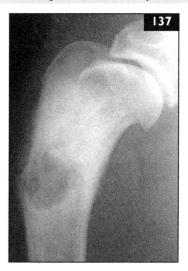

i. What additional diagnostic imaging tests would be indicated in this dog?

ii. What would be the recommended method for obtaining a definitive diagnosis?

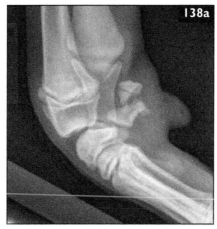

138 A radiographic image of the right carpus of a 6-month-old, 22 kg male greyhound that apparently sustained a right forelimb injury while turned out in an exercise pen is shown (**138a**). The dog was not observed to be lame until the following day and even then the lameness was subtle. On physical examination there was mild swelling and pain isolated to the region of the accessory carpal bone (ACB) and a mild pain response was elicited on flexion of the right carpus.

i. Describe the fracture.

ii. Discuss the probable etiology of this injury.

iii. Describe potential methods of managing this dog's fracture.

137 i. A whole body nuclear bone scan and three-view (ventrodorsal, right lateral, left lateral) thoracic radiographs should be considered to determine the systemic extent of disease. Osteosarcoma most commonly metastasizes to the lungs and less commonly to other bone. Skeletal sites may have subclinical (occult) metastases. If metastasis to either the lungs or skeleton is documented, the prognosis is significantly poorer than for dogs without detectable metastasis. The presence or absence of metastasis may influence the owners' decision regarding treatment options.

ii. A bone biopsy using a Jamshidi bone marrow biopsy needle. This method provides a small cylindrical core of bone and does not require the surgeon to penetrate both the *cis*- and *trans*-cortices. The advantage of penetrating only the *cis*-cortex is that the risk of fracture is decreased. An alternative method involves using a standard surgical trephine. This method provides a larger core sample and requires penetration of both cortices, increasing the potential for a post-biopsy fracture. Regardless of the method used to obtain the specimen, owners must be warned that a histologic diagnosis of 'reactive bone' is not uncommon. To avoid this possibility, the biopsy should be obtained from the center of the lesion and not the periphery, where there is often reactive bone surrounding the neoplasm.

138 i. ACB fractures have been classified based on fracture morphology: type 1, distal basilar fracture; type II, proximal basilar fracture; type III, distal apical fracture; type IV, proximal apical fracture; and type V, comminuted body fracture. This is a comminuted extra-articular Salter–Harris type IV fracture with fragmentation of the avulsed apical component, and this would be classified as a type V ACB fracture.

ii. ACB fractures occur mostly commonly in racing greyhounds and are usually physiologically-induced avulsion injuries. This fracture has two primary components. The distal apical fragment is characteristic of a type III injury (avulsion fracture of the origin of the accessoriometacarpal ligament, which inserts on the fourth and fifth metacarpal bones). The proximal apical fragment is characteristic of a type IV injury (avulsion fracture of the insertion of the flexor carpi ulnaris muscle).

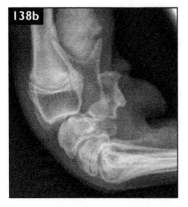

138b

iii. One or both of the major fragments could be stabilized using divergent Kirschner wires, pin and tension band fixation, or screws; however, repair of comminuted fractures is rarely feasible. The fracture could be allowed to heal or articular fragments excised. Regardless of the method of treatment, the carpus is immobilized at 20° of flexion in a splint or cast for a month, followed by gradual return to activity. This dog was managed with a splint and obtained union by 6 weeks (**138b**). The dog made a functional pet.

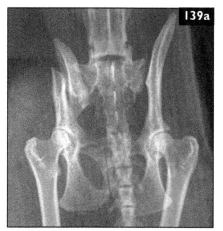

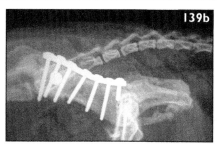

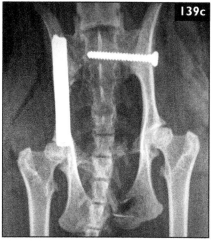

139 A 3-year-old male cat sustained multiple pelvic fractures in a road traffic accident. The cat was not ambulatory at presentation. Voluntary movement and deep pain sensation were present in both hindlimbs, but there were proprioceptive deficits. A ventrodorsal radiograph of the pelvis is shown (139a). The cat was taken to surgery and the ilial fracture was stabilized with a plate and screws (139b, c).

i. What are the general indications for surgical stabilization of pelvic fractures in cats?
ii. What advantages are ascribed to positioning the plate dorsally, as was done in this cat?
iii. What important neuroanatomic structures would need to be protected during surgical stabilization of this cat's pelvis?

140 i. Name the surgical instrument shown (140a).
ii. What specific orthopedic application is this instrument most commonly used for in dogs?

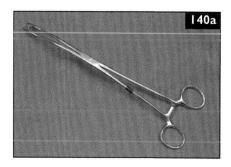

139 i. There are no absolute indications for surgical stabilization, but general considerations include: acetabular fractures; fractures of the ilial body with concurrent fractures that result in an unstable acetabular segment; sacroiliac fracture-separation (especially if subluxation exceeds 50%); pelvic canal narrowing (especially if the narrowing is greater than 40% and has the potential to result in constipation and megacolon); extreme pain; and neurologic deficits. Stabilization should also be considered with widely displaced pelvic floor fractures and for avulsion fractures of the ischial tuberosity that may result in substantial lameness or pain.

ii. Lateral plating of ilial fractures in cats has been associated with a high incidence of screw loosening and narrowing of the pelvic canal. Implant failure has been ascribed to the ilium having thin cortices, providing limited purchase for screws. Dorsal plate application results in greater screw purchase and has been shown to significantly decrease postoperative pelvic canal narrowing. Dorsal plating allows placement of longer plates with more screws, as the plate can be extended caudally, dorsomedial to the acetabulum. In addition, if there is a concurrent sacroiliac luxation, there is no need to reposition the cat to approach and stabilize the ilial fracture after the sacroiliac screw has been placed.

iii. The caudal ilial fracture segment can impinge on the sciatic nerve if it is displaced craniomedially. The nerve may be damaged due to this impingement either from manipulation of the fracture during surgery or during placement of implants such as screws or wires.

140 i. A pair of vulsellum forceps, sometimes referred to as Schroeder vulsellum forceps.

ii. Vulsellum forceps are long scissor-type forceps with ratchet handles. The long thin curved blades are somewhat elastic and have opposing double-pointed hooks or claws. This intrument was designed for grasping the uterus, but the elasticity of the blades and the double-pointed claws make vulsellum forceps particularly useful for temporary fracture stabilization when performing closed or open reduction and stabilization of humeral condylar fractures in dogs (**140b**).

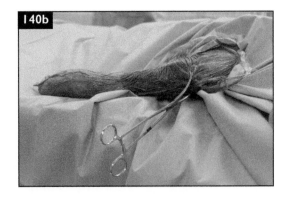

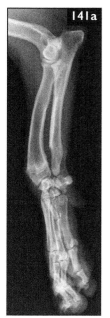

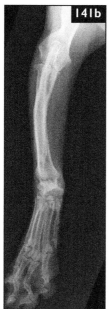

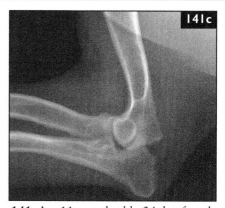

141 An 11-month-old, 24 kg female pit bull dog presented for evaluation of a right antebrachial deformity. On physical examination the dog had an obvious weight-bearing right fore-limb lameness. There was valgus, procurvatum, and external rotation. The medial aspect of the right fore paw contacted the ground when the dog placed weight on the right forelimb and a moderate pain response was elicited when the right elbow was extended. Radiographs of the right distal forelimb (141a, b) and elbow (141c) are shown.

i. What is the most likely etiology of this dog's deformity?

ii. What are the clinical implications associated with the radiographic abnormalities affecting this dog's right elbow?

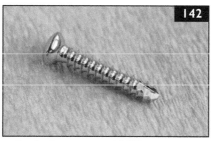

142 This is a photograph of a bone screw (142).

i. What is the function of the longitudinal channels located at the end of the screw?

ii. What are the advantages of using this type of screw?

iii. What are possible disadvantages of this type of screw?

141 i. This dog's deformity is likely secondary to premature closure of the distal ulnar physis, which is responsible for 85% of the longitudinal growth of the ulna. The conical shape of the dog's distal ulnar physis predisposes the physis to traumatic closure following even minor trauma. This dog has developed valgus, procurvatum, and external rotation of the radius, which typically result from the restricted ulnar growth subsequent to distal ulnar physeal closure.

ii. This dog has elbow incongruency, specifically the radial head is positioned proximal to the coronoid processes, causing elbow subluxation. One study evaluated the prognostic significance of various factors in dogs with antebrachial deformities that underwent lengthening procedures using circular fixator constructs. Factors that correlated with poorer long-term functional outcomes included marked lameness prior to surgery, the degree of pre-existing radiographic evidence of osteoarthritis, and larger discrepancies in the relative radial and ulnar length. This dog had a prominent lameness at the time of evaluation, mild degenerative changes in the elbow on the preoperative radiographs, and the radial head was positioned 5 mm proximal to the distal aspect of the semilunar notch of the elbow and was laterally subluxated. Therefore, the prognosis for a full return to soundness in the short and long term was guarded.

142 i. These are cutting flutes, which indicate that this is a self-tapping screw.

ii. Self-tapping screws are inserted immediately after drilling. The step of using a specific instrument (a tap) to cut threads in the bone is omitted, shortening screw insertion and surgical time, which can be particularly advantageous when working in areas where visualization is limited, maintaining fracture reduction is difficult, or in animals that are high anesthetic risks.

iii. Self-tapping screws are more difficult and costly to manufacture than screws that require tapping. If the treads of a self-tapping screw do not fully engage the *trans*-cortex, axial pullout of the screw will be reduced by approximately 20%, so the surgeon should add an additional 2 mm after measuring the depth of the pilot hole to account for the deficiencies inherent to the cutting tip. The exposed cutting tip has the potential to irritate the adjacent soft tissues. If a self-tapping screw is placed, removed, and reinserted, the screw may cut a new thread in the bone and destroy the original thread. Self-tapping screws may generate more heat during insertion, although the clinical relevance of this is unclear. Self-tapping screws are not as sharp or as efficient in clearing debris as a proper tap, therefore the threads can become obstructed with debris during insertion.

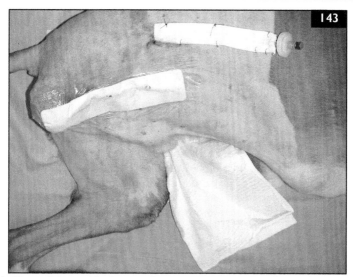

143 This Pharaoh hound had severe lameness associated with a pathologic fracture of a hemangiosarcoma lesion affecting the right proximal femur. Hemipelvectomy was performed and a 'soaker' catheter was placed for postoperative analgesia (**143**).

i. What are the reported intravenous doses of lidocaine and bupivacaine that have been shown to result in acute central nervous system toxicity?

ii. Why are soaker catheters used in dogs and cats undergoing amputation?

iii. In a study published by Abelson *et al.* (2009) that evaluated the use of soaker catheters in 56 dogs, what percentage of the dogs developed incisional infections?

144 Describe appropriate surgical treatment to address the deformity of the dog in case **141**.

143 i. The neurotoxic dose for intravenous lidocaine is 16 mg/kg. For intravenous bupivacaine it is 4 mg/kg.

ii. The brachial and hindlimb nerves are easily accessible in the surgical field, allowing the catheter to be placed in close proximity to severed nerves. This maximizes the effects of the local anesthesia and facilitates blockade of the incised nerves and muscles in the surgical wound.

iii. Incisional infection developed in approximately 5% of dogs.

144 This dog would benefit from surgical correction of the angular and rotational components of the dog's antebrachial deformity as well as correction of the elbow incongruency. Correction could be done acutely at the time of surgery or sequentially in the postoperative convalescent period using distraction osteogenesis. In this dog an acute correctional ostectomy was done to address the angular and rotational deformity: a segmental distal ulnar ostectomy and a cuneiform distal radial ostectomy were performed and a hybrid construct applied to stabilize the realigned radius and ulna. The elbow incongruency was addressed by postoperative distraction of the ulna through a second oblique, proximal osteotomy. An intramedullary pin was placed in the ulna and a partial ring and one fixation wire were placed to secure the proximal ulnar segment. Distraction (1 mm/day) was initiated the day after surgery and performed for 7 days to translate the proximal ulnar segment proximally until the elbow was congruent (**144a, b**). This invoked regenerate bone formation in the developing distraction gap. The fixator was removed 48 days following surgery. The dog was ambulating with nominal lameness when examined 5 months after surgery and radiographs obtained at that time showed that elbow congruency and limb alignment were substantially improved. The residual valgus deformity was similar to the natural valgus deviation present in the contralateral forelimb (**144c, d**).

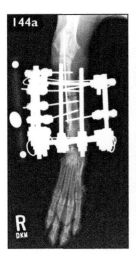 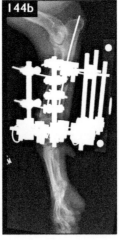 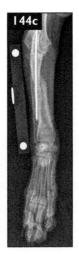 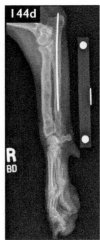

145 A 7-year-old female spayed domestic shorthaired cat was presented for an open left femoral fracture sustained the previous day when attacked by a dog. The fracture was stabilized using a 2.4 mm limited contact dynamic compression plate (**145a**). A substantial amount

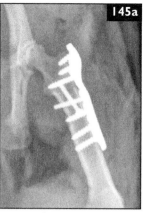

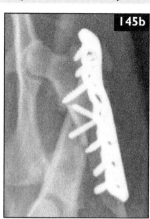

of soft tissue trauma, in particular avulsion of the majority of the adductor magnus muscle from the caudal aspect of the femur, was noted at surgery. *Enterococcus* and *Enterobacter* were grown from cultures obtained at the time of surgery. Six weeks after the original surgery, the cat presented with recurrent lameness. The cat had sustained a new fracture originating distal to the plate on the femur after jumping off a counter (**145b**). The fracture was re-plated and grafted, using a combination of cancellous autograft, collected from the ipsilateral proximal humerus, and 0.5 ml aliquot mixture of feline cancellous bone allograft and demineralized bone matrix (Veterinary Transplant Services, Kent, WA, USA) (**145c**).

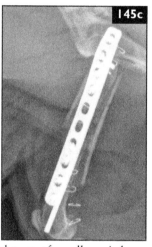

i. List the properties of an autogenous cancellous bone graft that promote bone healing.

ii. List advantages and disadvantages associated with the use of an allogenic bone graft.

146 A tibial plateau leveling osteotomy is being performed in a dog (**146a**).

i. What type of plate is being used to stabilize this dog's osteotomy?

ii. Describe the features that make this plating system unique compared with other locking plate systems.

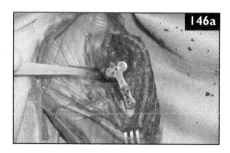

145 i. An autogenous cancellous bone graft provides viable osteoblasts that begin synthesizing new bone at the recipient site within days of transplantation (direct osteogenic effect). The trabecular structure of cancellous bone is conducive to rapid ingrowth of capillaries and subsequent new bone formation (osteoconduction). As the transplanted bone is resorbed, bone morphogenic proteins and other growth factors are released, inducing nearby mesenchymal cells to differentiate into osteoblasts, promoting further bone growth (osteoinduction).

ii. Use of allograft bone decreases the length of surgery and anesthesia associated with autograft collection and eliminates any potential morbidity associated with the harvest site. Possible detriments of allograft use include expense, lack of any viable cells and thus direct osteogenesis, and risk of infectious disease (bacterial contamination from harvesting or storage or direct transmission of disease from the donor to the recipient [e.g. feline leukemia virus or feline immunodeficiency virus in cats]). Occasionally, an allogenic bone graft will resorb, probably an immunogenic response, rather than promote new bone formation.

146 i. A Fixin plate.

ii. Fixin plates have been used successfully for the stabilization of arthrodeses, osteotomies, and fractures. This is a locking plate system with several technical novelties. The locking mechanism, which secures the screws in the plate, consists of a conical coupling mechanism between the screw head and the intermediary bushing-insert (**146b, c**), affording the unique advantage that each individual plate can accommodate two different diameter screws. Another advantage is that the presence of the intermediate inserts allows for easy implant removal either by uncoupling of the screws from the inserts or unthreading the inserts from the plate. This feature eliminates concerns associated with cold welding and difficult screw removal reported with other locking plate systems. An additional advantage of incorporating an intermediate bushing is that the thickness required for an adequate surface area of conical coupling between the plate and the screws is not dependent on the actual thickness of the plate.

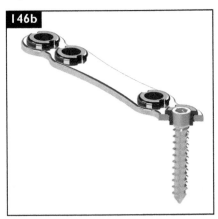

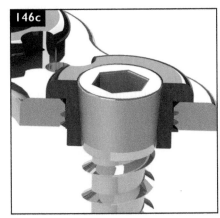

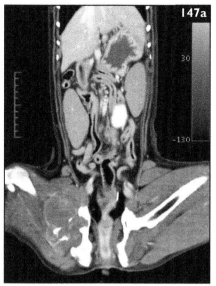

147a

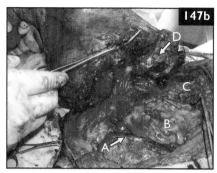

147b

147 A 3-year-old female German shepherd dog presented with a non-weight-bearing lameness of the right hindlimb. The dog had a large, firm palpable mass in the region of the right proximal femur. Manipulation of the right coxofemoral joint elicited a marked pain response. Contrast CT of the pelvis was performed (**147a**). The dog underwent a right hemipelvectomy surgery (**147b**).

i. Describe the abnormalities present on the CT scan.
ii. Provide a list of differential diagnoses.
iii. List the anatomic structures labeled A, B, C, and D.
iv. List indications for performing hemipelvectomy?
v. What possible complications should be anticipated after performing a hemipelvectomy?

148 An 11-month-old male English bulldog was presented with a history of hindlimb stiffness. On orthopedic examination pain was elicited on extension of both coxofemoral joints. A radiograph of the pelvis is shown (**148**).

i. Describe the radiographic abnormalities and state the most likely diagnosis.
ii. What hematologic effects can result from this dog's osseous abnormalities?

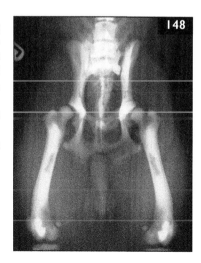

148

147 i. There is a large soft tissue mass in the region of the proximal right femur. The mass is displacing normal soft tissue structures and is enhanced by contrast administration. The extensive destruction of the proximal femur and the regions of mineralization within the mass suggest it may be a tumor of bone origin. The right femoral head is absent. The mass is in contact with and invading the ilium and acetabulum.

ii. Differentials would include osteosarcoma, chondrosarcoma, fibrosarcoma, soft tissue sarcoma, hemangiosarcoma.

iii. A, the incised pubic symphysis; B, omentum as the prepubic tendon and caudal abdominal wall separated from the pubic brim, effectively exposing the caudal abdomen; C, the articular surface of the sacrum, which has been exposed via sacroiliac disarticulation; D, the medial surface of the ilium.

iv. Soft tissue neoplasia involving the coxofemoral joint or thigh; bone tumors involving the proximal femur or ilium, ischium or pubis; severe pelvic trauma; infection; malunion.

v. Complications include iatrogenic trauma to the urethra and rectum; inadequate planning of the position of the skin incision leading to insufficient skin for closure; overzealous muscle resection leading to poor muscle reconstruction of the pelvic diaphragm; poor adherence of surgical oncology principles with consequent exposure or penetration of the tumor capsule and contamination of the surgical field with tumor cells; hematoma and seroma formation; decubital ulcers, especially over the ischium if an osseous protuberance is prominent and painful.

148 i. There is bilateral subluxation of both coxofemoral joints, with early degenerative and dysplastic changes characteristic of hip dysplasia. There is increased radiodensity of all bones. The medullary cavities of the bones are nearly obliterated by abnormal intramedullary bone, with only small remnants of medullary canal remaining in the ilial bodies and femora. These changes are compatible with a diagnosis of osteopetrosis.

ii. The osteopetroses are a heterogenous collection of skeletal disorders in which abnormal osteoclast function results in decreased bone resorption and increased bone deposition. The reduction in active medullary bone can result in a reduced production of red blood cells, leading to a severe non-regenerative anemia. One case report described a 1-year-old male Australian shepherd dog that developed a severe non-regenerative anemia associated with osteopetrosis. The dog's anemia was attributed to aplastic marrow development as well as failure to develop effective compensatory extramedullary erythropoiesis. Blood transfusions sustained the dog's life for 15 months, but the dog ultimately died of a hemolytic transfusion reaction. The owners of the English bulldog described in this question declined further diagnostic evaluation or treatment of the condition and follow-up information was not available.

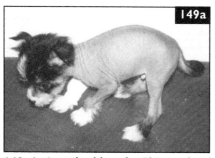
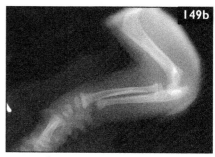

149 A 4-week-old male Chinese hairless crested puppy (**149a**) was presented by the breeder for evaluation. A problem had been noted with the puppy's left forelimb from approximately 2 weeks of age. A mediolateral radiograph of the dog's antebrachium is shown (**149b**).
i. What is the diagnosis?
ii. What is the typical signalment for dogs affected with this condition?
iii. Describe appropriate treatment options for this condition.

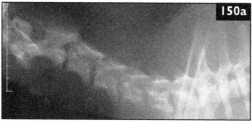
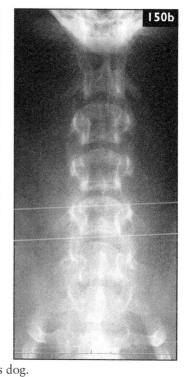

150 Radiographs of the cervical vertebral column of a 4-year-old male neutered Beagle are shown (**150a, b**). The dog had a history of progressive weakness and reluctance to ambulate. On physical examination the dog was bradycardic, had a dull hair coat, and was tetraparetic. A pain response was elicited on manipulation of the dog's neck.
i. Describe the radiographic abnormalities.
ii. List potential differential diagnoses.
iii. Results of a complete blood count, serum biochemistry analysis, and hormonal assay were normal aside from a resting thyroid level of 0.10 μg/dl. Provocative testing using thyroid stimulating hormone resulted in a post-stimulation test of 0.12 μg/dl. Discuss the pathogenesis of the disease process affecting this dog.

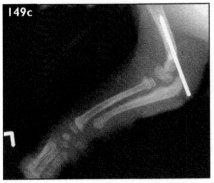

149 i. This puppy has a congenital type II elbow luxation. The luxation involves the humeroulnar articulation, with the ulna displaced lateral to the humeral condyle.

ii. Humeroulnar luxation occurs most commonly in small breeds and is generally first recognized when affected dogs are 3–6 weeks of age.

iii. Treatment involves closed or open reduction of the luxation. Transarticular pinning and/or a modified transarticular fixator with pins and elastic bands have been employed to maintain the reduction if performed in a closed manner. If an open reduction is necessary, transposition and fixation of the olecranon, medial imbrication and placement of support sutures, transarticular pinning, and reconstruction of the trochlear notch and trochlea are procedures that have been used to maintain reduction. Reduction is most effective if performed at a young age. Arthrodesis can be performed in older dogs. Surgical intervention may not be warranted in older dogs with acceptable limb function. In this dog the luxation was successfully reduced in a closed fashion. A percutaneous transarticular Kirschner wire was placed from the caudal aspect of the olecranon and into the humerus (149c). The Kirschner wire was removed after 10 days and the reduction was successfully maintained.

150 i. The vertebral bodies are stunted with irregular margins and epiphyseal fragmentation. All vertebral physes are open. There is narrowing of the vertebral canal over the cervical intervertebral disc spaces, especially C4–C5 and C5–C6, with rounded mineralized structures protruding into the vertebral canal over C2–C3 to C5–C6. Similar but less severe changes are noted at C6–C7.

ii. This dog has polyostotic axial delayed physeal closure. Differential diagnoses include congenital hypothyroidism, panhypopituitarism (lacking normal thyroid and growth hormonal interactions) and mucopolysaccharidosis I or VI.

iii. This dog has a thyroid hormone deficiency, which is likely congenital. Clinical abnormalities associated with congenital hypothyroidism include decreased mental cognition and skeletal developmental abnormalities characterized in this dog by a failure of normal physeal closure. Causes of congenital hypothyroidism can range from a lack of responsiveness to thyroid-releasing hormone or thyroid-stimulating hormone, as well as thyroid dysgenesis or hypoplasia. Thyroid hormones are essential for normal bone growth, including the normal stimulation of cartilage growth, as well for influencing bone resorption. Normal thyroid hormone has an indirect effect on skeletal growth through the stimulation and release of growth hormone. Growth hormone then has a direct anabolic effect on osteoblasts. This dog's tetraparesis was the result of spinal cord compression caused by dorsal displacement of epiphyseal fracture fragments in the caudal cervical region.

151 Initial postoperative radiographs of a dog that underwent correction of an antebrachial deformity performed using an external fixator are shown (**151a, b**).

i. What type of fixator was used in this dog?

ii. What are the advantageous properties inherent to this type of fixator system?

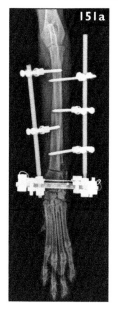
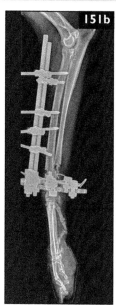

152 A 14-month-old male rottweiler presented with a history of the dog developing an acute left forelimb lameness 2 weeks prior to examination. The lameness was initially subtle and intermittent, but had subsequently become somewhat more pronounced and consistent. On examination the dog had a moderate weight-bearing left forelimb lameness and resented flexion and extension of the metacarpophalangeal joint of the fifth digit of the left fore paw. A radiograph of the left fore paw is shown (**152**).

i. What is the diagnosis?

ii. At what age is this disease most commonly diagnosed?

iii. How should this dog be treated?

iv. Describe the most likely pathogenesis of this condition.

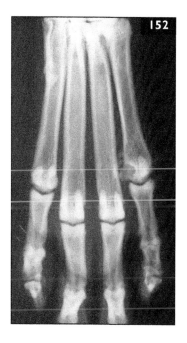

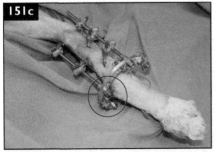

151 i. A hybrid linear-circular construct. The limb is shown when the bandage was changed 3 days after surgery (151c). The construct utilizes half-pin splintage fixation pins and two hybrid connecting rods (referred to as a type Ia hybrid construct).

ii. Hybrid constructs confer the advantageous properties of both linear and circular systems. The ring component is particularly useful for stabilizing short, juxta-articular fracture or osteotomy segments. Divergent, small diameter wires have been used as fixation elements on the ring component and provide stable, multiplanar fixation of the short distal radial and ulnar segments. The use of wires as fixation elements, as opposed to larger diameter more rigid fixation pins, allows for some degree of axial micromotion, which potentiates callus formation and osseous union. The linear hybrid rods and half-pin splintage fixation pins afford stable fixation of the proximal radial segment, but are associated with less morbidity during the postoperative convalescent period in comparison with traditional circular fixators. Half-pins can be placed through defined safe corridors, minimizing impingement of large muscle masses as well as major vital neurovascular structures. In addition, hybrid constructs are much simpler to apply than traditional circular fixators, particular hinged circular constructs.

152 i. There is fragmentation of the seventh metacarpophalangeal sesamoid bone. The bone is disrupted into at least three fragments, which are slightly displaced into the interosseous space. Paired sesamoid bones are located at the head of the second, third, fourth, and fifth metacarpal bones and numbered (from medial to lateral) I–VIII. The second and seventh sesamoid bones are involved in more than 90% of affected dogs.

ii. Clinical lameness commonly develops in dogs at 6–9 months of age. Lameness is usually acute in onset and transient, persisting for approximately 2 weeks in most dogs. Some affected dogs will remain chronically lame, with pain and synovial effusion of the adjacent metacarpophalangeal joint evident on physical examination.

iii. Strict rest is indicated when lameness has been present for less than 4 weeks and administration of an NSAID should be considered. This dog's prognosis for a return to soundness is good. If lameness persists beyond 6 weeks and the lameness can be clearly ascribed to the metacarpophalangeal joint, excision of the smaller fracture fragments or the whole sesamoid bone often resolves the lameness, although excision may predispose the joint to the development of osteoarthritis.

iv. Mechanical stress has been strongly implicated in the pathogenesis of sesamoid disease. Due to anatomic peculiarities of the second and fifth digits, the flexor tendons reportedly place greater loads on the second and seventh sesamoid bones. In addition, sesamoids II and VII appear to have a poor blood supply and may be susceptible to avascular necrosis, which would alter the physical properties of these two sesamoid bones and therefore make the bones more likely to fail under mechanical load.

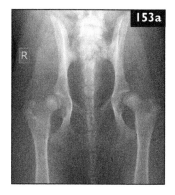

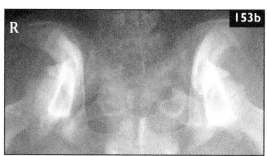

153 A 7-month-old female golden
retriever presented with hindlimb weakness and intermittent right hindlimb
lameness. On physical examination the
dog was resistant to manipulation of
both coxofemoral joints. Under sedation
a positive Ortolani sign was elicited in
both hips. The angle of reduction was
45° for the right hip and the angle of
subluxation 25°. The angle of reduction
was 35° for the left hip and the angle of

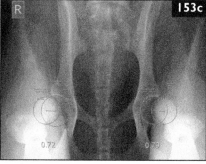

subluxation 15°. Crepitus was elicited while performing the Ortolani test on the right
hip. A standard ventrodorsal radiographic view of the pelvis (153a) showed bilateral
hip dysplasia with marked subluxation, but no degenerative changes. A ventrodorsal
frog-leg view indicated right acetabular filling, while congruency was restored in the
left coxofemoral joint. On the dorsal acetabular rim view radiograph (153b) there was
less than 50% femoral head coverage by the right acetabulum, while approximately
half of the left femoral head was covered by the acetabulum. Erosion of the lateral
margin of the right acetabulum and slight rounding of the left acetabular margin were
also evident on the dorsal acetabular view radiographs. The right acetabular slope was
25° and the left acetabular slope was 18°. A distraction view radiograph was obtained
(153c) and the right distraction index (DI) was calculated as 0.72 while the left DI was
calculated as 0.79.

i. What surgical procedure would be most appropriate to treat this dog's right hip?
ii. What surgical procedure would be most appropriate to treat this dog's left hip?
iii. What additional diagnostic evaluation could be done to establish which surgical
treatment option is appropriate?

154 Name the assembly components circled in 151c (page 152), and describe the
utility of using these components when securing a hybrid rod in a ring.

153 i. The right hip has advanced dysplasia with erosion of the lateral border of the dorsal acetabular rim. The DI reveals that there is less laxity in the right hip attributable to capsular fibrosis, consistent with more advanced degenerative joint disease. Corrective osteotomy would not arrest or effectively mitigate subsequent degeneration of this hip and a total hip replacement would be the most appropriate surgical option. Alternatively, femoral head and neck excision could be considered if surgical intervention is warranted.

ii. Cartilage erosion is not evident in the left hip and the joint is congruent on the frog-leg view. The subluxation observed on the standard view and the high DI suggest that further progression of the disease will occur if this hip is managed conservatively. Corrective pelvic osteotomy is indicated to modify the biomechanics of the joint and resolve the subluxation of the femoral head. Degeneration of the left coxofemoral joint can rapidly progress, so surgery should be performed as soon as possible.

iii. Arthroscopy of the hip could be done to assess the integrity of the acetabular labrum as well as to confirm whether or not there is extensive articular cartilage damage of the acetabulum or femoral head.

154 Hemispherical washers and nuts. One surface of the washer has a concave contour, which accommodates the conical surface of the hemispherical nut. Interdigitation of these two surfaces allows the threaded portion of the hybrid rod to be secured in one of the holes in the ring at an oblique angle (**154**, outlined in red). If standard nuts are used to secure a hybrid rod in the ring, the rod will be orientated perpendicular to the surface of the ring (**154**, outlined in yellow). The degree of obliquity is limited by the thickness of the ring. An 84 mm diameter ring was used in this dog, allowing approximately 10° of angulation. Hemispherical washers and nuts function as universal joints and afford the surgeon considerable latitude in adjusting the alignment of the stabilized limb segment during deformity correction or when performing fracture reduction.

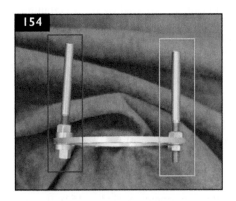

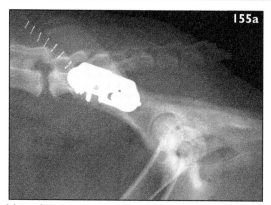

155 A left double pelvic osteotomy using a 25° plate was performed on the 7-month-old golden retriever with hindlimb weakness in case 153. A postoperative radiograph is shown (155a). What are the advantages of performing a double, rather than a triple, pelvic osteotomy?

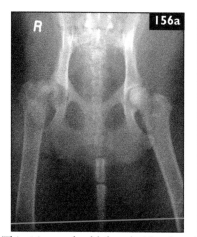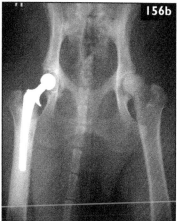

156 This 11-month-old female Newfoundland dog slipped on the kitchen floor 2 weeks previously and became acutely lame on the right hindlimb. The dog had a severe right hindlimb lameness at presentation and pain was elicited on extension of the right hip. A ventrodorsal radiograph of the pelvis is shown (156a). A right cemented total hip replacement (BioMedtrix CFX) was performed to address this dog's injury. A postoperative ventrodorsal radiograph is shown (156b).
i. What is the preoperative diagnosis?
ii. What substance is added to the PMMA to make the cement radiopaque?
iii. Describe improvements that have been instituted in cementing techniques for total hip surgery.

Answers: 155, 156

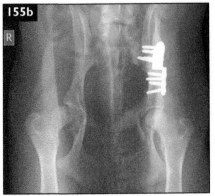

155 Double pelvic osteotomy reduces joint laxity and improves joint congruity by creating ventroversion of the acetabulum, similar to triple pelvic osteotomy. With a triple pelvic osteotomy, the ilium, pubis, and ischium are all osteotomized to create a fully mobile acetabular segment. With a double pelvic osteotomy, the ischial osteotomy is omitted. The effective acetabular rotation obtained with a double pelvic osteotomy is 5° less than that obtained after triple pelvic osteotomy, using the same pre-angled plate, and this difference must be accounted for when selecting which plate to use during surgery. Screw loosening and narrowing of the pelvic canal are common complications following triple pelvic osteotomy. By leaving the ischium intact during a double pelvic osteotomy, the hemipelvis is much more stable during the early postoperative convalescent period. Healing of the ilial and pubic osteotomies occurs rapidly, restoring the anatomic integrity of the pelvis (155b is a radiograph obtained 2 months following a left double pelvic osteotomy). Double pelvic osteotomy is much more effective in preserving pelvic geometry than triple pelvic osteotomy and, when combined with restoration of coxofemoral joint congruity, results in a more normal gait and improved limb function.

156 i. The dog has a fracture of the right capital femoral epiphysis, also known as a slipped capital femoral epiphysis. The sclerosis in the femoral neck is compatible with the chronic nature of the injury.
ii. Barium sulfate is added to make the PMMA radiopaque.
iii. A key determinant of a cement mantle's longevity is the technique of cementing. Third-generation cementing techniques involve procedural improvements now commonly used during cemented total hip replacement. Vacuum mixing of cement improves blending of the liquid and powder components of the cement, resulting in decreased porosity and a stronger cement. Improvements in bone preparation include placement of a plug, which allows for compression of cement, and pulsatile lavage of the femoral canal after reaming to remove loose cancellous bone and blood and improve interdigitation of cement with the bone. Cement delivery has also been improved with the use of a cement gun to provide consistent retrograde filling of the canal followed by pressurization of the cement mantle during polymerization. Centralization of the femoral stem increases the likelihood of long-term success on the cemented femur. Both proximal and distal centralizers, now considered part of the third-generation cement technique, are widely used as these have been shown to increase the probability of maintaining a more uniform circumferential cement mantle around the stem.

157 A 2-year-old male neutered cat underwent an open reduction of an acute traumatic right coxofemoral luxation that had occurred after unknown trauma. An initial postoperative radiograph is shown (157).

i. What technique has been utilized to maintain the reduction in this cat?

ii. What diameter implant should be used when performing this procedure in an average sized adult cat?

iii. What is the most commonly reported complication associated with the technique utilized in this cat?

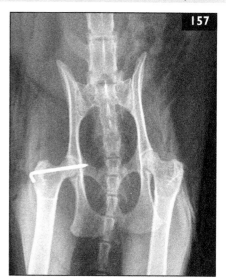

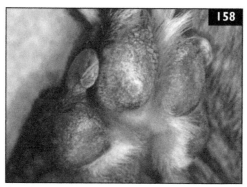

158 A 7-year-old female retired racing greyhound presented for evaluation of a chronic progressive right forelimb lameness. The owner noted that the dog had an obvious weight-bearing lameness, which was accentuated when the dog walked on hard surfaces such as gravel, concrete, or tile. While examining the right fore paw, the dog was found to have a circular, non-pigmented nodule on the pad of the fourth digit (158). A marked pain response was elicited when pressure was applied to the affected pad.

i. What is the lesion affecting this dog's pad?

ii. What are the purported etiologies for this condition?

iii. Describe the anatomic distribution where these lesions most commonly occur.

iv. Discuss potential treatment options for this dog.

157 i. A temporary transarticular pin has been placed to stabilize the reduced coxofemoral luxation.

ii. A 1.6 mm Kirschner wire. Use of a smaller diameter Kirschner wire is likely to result in implant breakage.

iii. In a study of 20 cats with coxofemoral luxations, reluxation of the femoral head occurred in 2/13 cats with available long-term follow-up evaluations. One of these cats had bilateral coxofemoral luxation, and immediate postoperative radiographs with the transarticular pin in place showed subluxation of the right hip. The hip was still reduced when the pin was removed, but at radiographic evaluation 6 months after surgery, the right hip was reluxated. Other rare complications include pin loosening with reluxation of the hip, aseptic necrosis of the femoral head, osteoarthritis, and femoral head fracture.

158 i. A pad keratoma, commonly referred to as a corn.

ii. Pad keratomas have been ascribed to repetitive, chronic, low impact mechanical overloading of the digital pads. Corns occur most often in racing or retired greyhounds, whippets, and lurchers. The digital pads in these breeds have a small relative surface area with a lower adipose tissue content compared with other breeds of dogs, resulting in larger ground reaction forces being transmitted through the digital pads with less cushioning. One report stated that 40% of affected dogs also had concurrent paw deformities, which potentially could cause abnormal weight bearing on the affected digital pad. Foreign body penetration resulting in the introduction of small particles of epithelium into the subcutis has also been postulated, although this is considered a less likely etiology. There is no tangible evidence to support previous suggestions that corns are associated with papilloma virus infection.

iii. Ninety percent of corns develop on digits III and IV, with 90% of the lesions occurring in the fore paws.

iv. Surgical intervention by either excision or distal digital ostectomy has been recommended; however, in one report the 3-month recurrence rate exceeded 50%. Physical extrusion or hulling out of the corn via curettage are other suggested treatments. Specific recurrence rates have not been reported with these techniques, but recurrence is anecdotally comparable to, or higher than, following surgical excision. The use of padded boots may decrease the rate of recurrence following interventional therapies.

159 Initial postoperative radiographs from an 8-year-old, 30 kg spayed female Labrador retriever that underwent total knee replacement to address lameness ascribed to severe chronic degenerative joint disease of the left stifle are shown (**159a, b**).

i. What is the composition of each of the components of this total joint replacement system?

ii. Describe the design configuration of this total knee joint replacement system.

iii. List some major potential complications of this procedure.

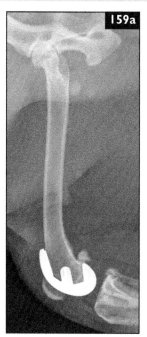
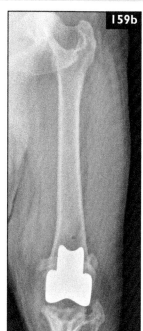

160 A 6-month-old male intact Staffordshire bull terrier is shown (**160**). The dog was presented collapsed, distressed, and unable to walk. All four limbs were held rigidly extended caudally. The dog had a history of lacerating a digital pad 10 days prior to presentation.

i. What is wrong with this dog?

ii. List the facial abnormalities typically seen in dogs with this condition.

iii. Describe the underlying pathogenesis of this condition.

iv. What physiological process is required for recovery from this condition?

v. What is the recommended treatment for dogs affected with this condition?

vi. What two forms of the disease are recognized in small animals?

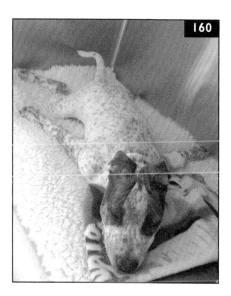

159 i. The femoral component is made of cobalt-chromium alloy (ASTM-F75). The fixation surface is covered with three layers of sintered cobalt-chromium beads for macrosurface roughness. This roughened surface is manufactured to promote osseointegration of the component with the femur, with the aim of long-term stability of the femoral component being achieved via cementless fixation. The tibial component is machined entirely from highly cross-linked ultra-high molecular weight polyethylene. This implant is cemented into place with PMMA.
ii. It is a condylar-style prosthesis that is semi-constrained and designed to mimic the natural motion and stability of a normal dog's femorotibial articulation. The concave surfaces of the tibial component match the convex surfaces of the femoral component in the sagittal and coronal planes. Thus, craniocaudal and mediolateral translation are mitigated by maximizing contact between the prosthetic articular surfaces. Most of the joint's normal axial rotation and flexion–extension range of motion is maintained following surgery.
iii. Potential intraoperative complications include: iatrogenic damage to the collateral ligaments, popliteal tendon, long digital extensor tendon, or patellar tendon; malpositioning of the implants; hemorrhage; and fracture. Potential post-operative complications include: infection; aseptic loosening; fracture; luxation; and collateral ligament injury.

160 i. This dog has tetanus, caused by infection of the pad wound with the bacterium *Clostridium tetani*.
ii. Facial changes include third eye-lid protrusion, abnormal ocular position, trismus, erect ear carriage, and an abnormal facial expression known as *ricus sardonicus*.
iii. *C. tetani* is a gram-positive anaerobic spore-forming bacillus widely distributed in the environment. Following infection, and in an anaerobic environment, the spores vegetate and release toxins: tetanolysin and tetanospasmin. Tetanospasmin enters the peripheral nerves distally at the neuromuscular end-plate and then moves in a retroaxonal manner to the central nervous system, where the toxin binds irreversibly to presynaptic sites on inhibitory neurons and inhibits the release of glycine and gamma-aminobutyric acid, leading to sustained muscle spasms.
iv. Recovery requires synthesis of new presynaptic components, which must be transported to the distal axon. A 2-week delay is typical before improvement becomes evident.
v. Supportive therapy including nursing, nutrition, sedation, and muscle relaxation, together with antibiosis (penicillin G or metronidazole) to prevent clostridial growth and toxin production. Administration of tetanus antitoxin is usually too late to be effective by the time tetanus is diagnosed. Similarly, wound debridement will usually not alter the course of the disease unless performed early.
vi. A local form in which the signs are limited to a specific body region, for example a limb, and a generalized form in which the entire body is affected, as was the case in this dog.

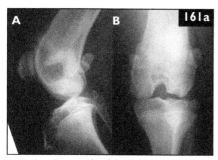

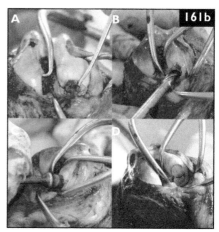

161 An 8-month-old male Great Dane is presented with a 2-week history of a left hindlimb lameness that had an insidious onset, but progressed in severity such that the dog placed only nominal weight on the limb. On examination the dog was uncomfortable when the left stifle was manipulated and there was a palpable stifle effusion. The dog has an osteochondrosis lesion, visible as an articular subchondral bone defect on the radiographs of the left stifle (**161a**) affecting the lateral femoral condyle.

i. What surgical procedure is being performed to treat this condition in the series of intraoperative photographs (**161b**)?
ii. What factors might contribute to the uniformly poor clinical outcomes following traditional surgical treatment of this condition?
iii. What are the postulated benefits of the treatment modality being performed in **161b** over traditional surgical treatment?

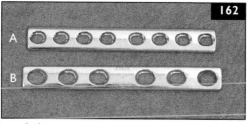

162 A 3.5 mm broad dynamic compression plate (A) and a 4.5 mm dynamic compression plate (B) are shown (**162**).
i. What is the definition of area moment of inertia (AMI)?
ii. What is the equation for the AMI of a rectangular object such as a bone plate?
iii. Which of the two plates has a greater AMI?

161 i. An osteochondral autograft transfer (OAT) procedure. 'A' shows the loose flap being removed. 'B' shows creation of a recipient socket using the OATS™ Cannulated Recipient Site Drill Bit in preparation for insertion of a donor osteochondral core. 'C' shows an autogenous osteochondral core being inserted into the prepared socket. 'D' shows the final appearance of the lesion with two donor cores *in situ* as well as the empty donor sockets from osteochondral core harvesting on the abaxial aspect of the medial trochlear ridge.
ii. Traditional surgical treatment typically involves removal of diseased cartilage and subchondral bone, followed by curettage or osteostixis of the underlying subchondral bone plate to stimulate defect infilling with fibrocartilaginous repair tissue. Poor clinical outcomes might be associated with: the poor biomechanical properties of fibrocartilaginous repair tissue by comparison with hyaline cartilage; failure of restoration of articular and subchondral bone contour, resulting in effective joint incongruity and 'rim stress concentration' during weight bearing; exposure of subchondral bone to synovial fluid allowing exchange of inflammatory mediators precipitating osteoarthritis.
iii. OAT procedures can achieve: joint resurfacing with hyaline-type cartilage; accurate reconstruction of articular and subchondral bone contour; and provide an immediate barrier to exchange of inflammatory mediators. OAT procedures result in superior outcomes compared with microfracture for treatment of articular cartilage defects in the knee of human athletes.

162 i. AMI is a mathematical representation of the distribution of mass about a defined central axis through an object's cross-section. This expression takes into account both the cross-sectional area of the object and the cross-sectional shape of the object. The AMI, along with the modulus of elasticity (material stiffness) of the material composing the object, are parameters that determine bending stiffness.
ii. AMI = $bh^3/12$. In this equation, b is the dimension defined as being directed parallel to the AMI that is being calculated and h is the dimension defined as being directed parallel to the applied load. Thus, small differences in the thickness (h) of a plate have a profound effect on the implant's bending stiffness because the AMI is proportional to the plate's thickness (h) to the third power.
iii. The width (b) of a 3.5 mm broad dynamic compression plate is 12 mm and the plate is 3.8 mm thick (h). Thus, the calculated AMI of a 3.5 mm broad dynamic compression plate is 54.9 mm^4. The width (b) of a 4.5 mm dynamic compression plate is 12 mm and the plate is 3.6 mm thick (h). Thus, the calculated AMI of a 4.5 mm dynamic compression plate is 46.7 mm^4 (i.e. slightly less than that of a 3.5 mm broad dynamic compression plate).

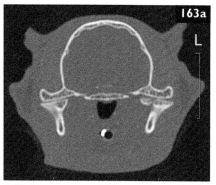

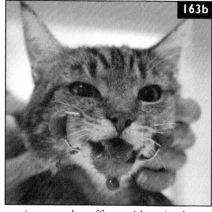

163 A transverse CT scan through the skull of a 2-year-old male domestic shorthaired cat that sustained facial trauma in a road traffic accident is shown (163a). The cat has malocclusion. Attempts to perform an oral examination prior to being anesthetized elicited a pain response. A photograph of the cat following surgery is shown (163b).

i. Describe the abnormalities present on the CT scan.

ii. Describe the stabilization technique used to manage this cat's injury and the potential advantages of managing this cat's injury in this manner.

iii. To what degree should the mouth be left open when applying this stabilization technique?

164 A radiograph of the elbow of an 8-month-old male French bulldog that had a humeral condylar fracture surgically repaired 2 weeks ago is shown (164).

i. Describe the complication that has occurred.

ii. Is this complication more likely to be the result of acute overloading or cyclic loading?

iii. How should this complication be addressed?

iv. How is a screw's stiffness related to the implant's diameter?

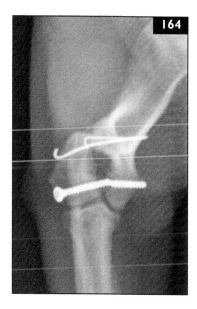

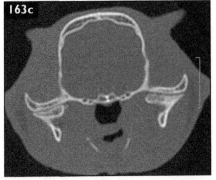

163 i. There is a minimally-displaced articular fracture through the medial aspect of the condylar process of the left hemimandible.

ii. Direct reduction and internal stabilization of this fracture were not deemed feasible. Indirect stabilization of caudal mandibular fractures can be achieved by immobilizing the jaw in either a closed or a slightly open position. In this cat a maxillomandibular external fixator was used to stabilize the mouth in a slightly open position. Alternatively, interdental bonding of the ipsilateral upper and lower canine teeth with acrylic columns could have been used. Open mouth stabilization techniques allow the animal to eat and drink during the convalescent period and decrease the potential for aspiration pneumonia. This fracture had healed and the fixator was removed 4 weeks after surgery (163c).

iii. The cusps of the upper and lower canine teeth should overlap slightly, leaving a 10–12 mm gap between the upper and lower incisors, to assure functional occlusion. This allows the cat to lap water and soft food while the fixator is in place, although placing an esophagostomy tube soon after injury is prudent. The tube can be used to provide nutritional support prior to and after surgery, until the cat is able maintain a normal calorie intake orally.

164 i. The transcondylar screw placed in lag fashion to stabilize the fracture has broken. In addition, the fracture has displaced and is no longer anatomically reduced.

ii. Implant failure in this dog is most likely due to cyclic loading. The screw has broken, but there is no apparent gross deformation (bending). This mode of failure is due to repetitive cyclic loading within the elastic region of the implant, which fatigues the metal and will eventually result in the implant breaking. Failure produced by acute mechanical overloading is more typically characterized by bone failure or bending of the implant.

iii. The broken screw should be removed. The fracture should again be anatomically reduced and restabilized with a larger diameter, transcondylar screw placed in lag fashion. The transcondylar hole from placement of the original screw can probably be used again once the hole is enlarged to the appropriate diameter for placement of the new screw.

iv. A cylindrical implant's bending stiffness is directly proportional to the implant's core diameter to the fourth power. Therefore, if a screw that has twice the core diameter of the original screw is placed, the bending stiffness of the implant would be increased 16-fold.

165 A 7-month-old male Bernese mountain dog was presented with a complaint of an irregular gait affecting both hindlimbs. The dog circumducted both hindlimbs during the swing phase of the stride. The medial aspect of both hind paws contacted the ground first at the end of the swing phase and there was pronounced external rotation of both hindlimbs during the propulsive phase of the stride. When the dog was placed in lateral recumbency and the hindlimbs extended, a bilateral deformity causing external rotation of the pes was evident as the plantar surfaces of the hind paws were positioned parallel to each other. Orthogonal radio-

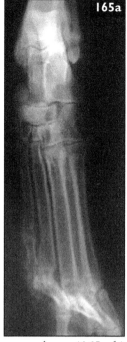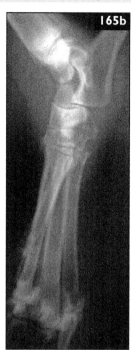

graphs of one of the affected paws are shown (165a, b).
i. What is the diagnosis?
ii. On this dog's radiographs, what anatomic abnormality is present in association with this deformity?
iii. List five other breeds in which this deformity has been reported.
iv. What treatment should be recommended for this dog?

166 A 2-year-old male golden retriever with a forelimb lameness ascribed to fragmentation of the medial coronoid process is scheduled for elbow arthroscopy. Postoperatively, intra-articular analgesia is planned as part of a balanced analgesia protocol.
i. At what stage should the intra-articular analgesia be given?
ii. Which local anesthetics are suitable for use as intra-articular analgesic agents?
iii. Which additional drug is often administered intra-articularly to provide local analgesia?

165 i. This deformity has been described as metatarsal rotation or external rotation of the pes. This condition is often bilateral, originating at the level of the proximal intertarsal joint, and resulting in an external rotation of the pes. These dogs are sometimes referred to 'seal puppies' or 'clapper puppies' because the plantar surfaces of the paws appose each other, resembling the fins of a seal or a person clapping.

ii. There is evidence of a fully developed first metatarsal bone resulting in polydactylia.

iii. Great Pyrenees, Saint Bernards, rottweilers, Abruzzese shepherd dogs, greyhounds.

iv. If the deformity does not produce a marked lameness, treatment is not warranted. In dogs with pronounced lameness, the metatarsal rotational deformity can be corrected by performing an intertarsal or tarsometatarsal arthrodesis. The articular cartilage of the intertarsal (and likely the tarsometatarsal) joints is debrided and a cancellous bone graft implanted in the debrided joint spaces. The alignment of the pes is corrected and the arthrodesis stabilized with an external fixator or a bone plate. Realignment of the pes can result in substantial improvement in limb function. This dog had a corrective arthrodesis stabilized by a fixator. The dog's gait improved markedly, although mild hyperextension of the hock persisted during ambulation.

166 i. Intra-articular analgesics are typically injected into the joint at the end of surgery, but analgesics can be infused pre-emptively when the joint is distended in preparation for arthroscopy (**166**).

ii. Lidocaine, bupivacaine, and ropivacaine; the shorter duration of action of lidocaine makes this agent less useful. Several clinical studies have suggested that

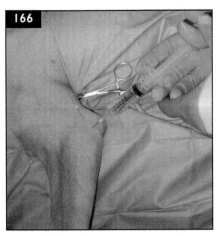

bupivacaine is associated with significant chondrotoxicity and its use is therefore not recommended. Ropivacaine appears to be much less chondrotoxic and is currently advocated for intra-articular administration. The maximum dose is 1.5 mg/kg.

iii. Opioid receptors are present in the synovial membrane and intra-articular morphine has been shown to have significant analgesic and anti-inflammatory effects in both human patients and horses. Morphine is given at a dose of 0.1–0.2 mg/kg and preservative-free morphine should be used when administered by this route.

167 A 4-year-old male springer spaniel presented with a history of moderate right forelimb lameness of 6-weeks' duration. During the orthopedic examination the dog showed no pain on full neutral flexion and extension of the elbow. However, pain was elicited when the elbow was fully flexed while pronating the right carpus. Orthogonal radiographs of the right elbow and shoulder did not reveal any abnormalities. Scintigraphy was performed (**167a**).

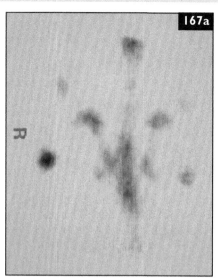

i. What substance is commonly used to perform scintigraphy in dogs?
ii. What additional imaging modality would be most useful for establishing a diagnosis in this dog?

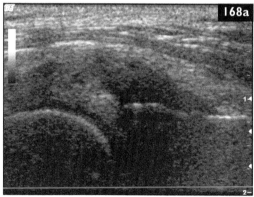

168 A 5-year-old male Labrador retriever had a left tibial plateau leveling osteotomy 7-months ago to address CrCL insufficiency. The dog's lameness had initially improved following surgery, but recently the dog had become intermittently non-weight bearing on the left hindlimb. An ultrasonographic image of the medial compartment of this dog's left stifle was obtained (**168a**).

i. Describe the pertinent ultrasonographic abnormalities.
ii. Based on the ultrasonic evaluation, what is the precise morphology of this dog's lesion?
iii. What is the risk and purported pathophysiology of this dog's lesion?

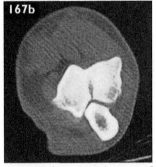

167 i. Intravenous technetium-99m-methylene diphosphonate, which is incorporated into bone mineral and accurately reflects tissue perfusion and the status of osseous remodeling.

ii. Fragmented coronoid process or incomplete ossification of the humeral condyle or a humeral condylar fissure would be differential diagnoses for a springer spaniel with chronic forelimb lameness and increased radiopharmaceutical uptake in the elbow region. Fragmented coronoid processes are infrequently identified on radiographs. In dogs with incomplete ossification of the humeral condyle, if the fissure is not complete or the radiographic beam is not aligned parallel to the fracture line, the lesion may be missed on radiographs. Additional lesion-oriented projection radiographs, CT, or arthroscopy can be used to investigate further. CT (**167b**) revealed that this dog had an incomplete fissure of the right humeral condyle. The dog was managed by placement of a transcondylar screw and the lameness resolved 3 days following surgery.

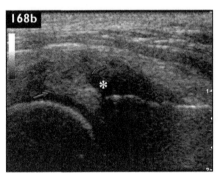

168 i. There is hypoechoic fluid (asterisk, **168b**) indicative of synovial effusion surrounding the medial meniscus, which is hyperechoic, abnormally shaped, with loss of the normal triangular appearance and flattening along the tibial margin of the meniscus (arrows, **168b**). There is abaxial displacement of the meniscus and remodeling along the margins of the femoral condyle (curvilinear structure in lower left-hand corner) and tibial plateau consistent with osteophytosis and thickening of the medial soft tissue structures.

ii. The abaxial displacement of the meniscus is consistent with the dog having a displaced bucket-handle tear of the caudal horn of the medial meniscus.

iii. This dog's medial meniscal tear is either a postoperative lesion that developed in a normal meniscus or a latent meniscal tear, which is the progression of meniscal pathology that was not recognized at the initial surgery. In one study, latent meniscal tears were diagnosed in 6.3% of dogs that had a tibial plateau leveling osteotomy (TPLO). Subsequent meniscal tears were 3.8 times more likely to occur in dogs that had an arthrotomy than in dogs that had arthroscopy at the time of TPLO. These findings raise questions regarding whether or not there was unrecognized pathology at the time of initial surgery.

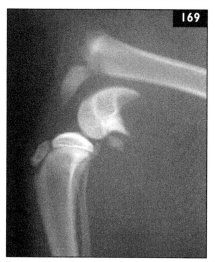

169 A distal femoral fracture in an 8-month-old male cat is shown (169).
i. What type of physeal fracture is shown?
ii. What eponym is used to describe the caudal metaphyseal fragment attached to the condylar fracture segment?

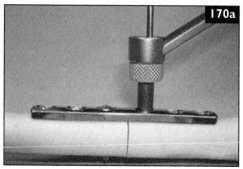

170 This image shows a load drill guide being used to drill a hole for insertion of a load screw in a dynamic compression plate (170a).
i. How much screw angulation does the dynamic compression plate hole allow in a longitudinal plane?
ii. How does angling a screw placed with the load drill guide, such that the tip of the screw is directed away from the fracture, affect the amount of interfragmentary compression achieved?
iii. How does angling a screw placed with the load drill guide, such that the tip of the screw is directed toward the fracture, affect the amount of interfragmentary compression achieved?

169 i. A Salter–Harris type II fracture.

ii. In Salter–Harris type II fractures, the line of separation extends through the physis for a variable distance and then extends through a portion of the metaphysis, thus producing the familiar triangular-shaped metaphyseal fragment, sometimes referred to as the 'corner' or Thurston Holland sign.

170 i. The oval hole in the plate allows the screw to be angled by up to 25° in either direction of the perpendicular position in the longitudinal plane.

ii. Angulation of a load screw directed away from the fracture line by 10° or more can double the amount of interfragmentary compression achieved compared with that achieved with a load screw placed perpendicular to the surface of the plate (**170b**). The graph represents the force created by screws placed at different angles to the bone and plate. For a screw placed at 89–91° there is approximately 50–70 kPa of force (interfragmentary compression) created. For a screw placed at 104–107°, with the screw angled away from the fracture, the compression created increases to over 125 kPa.

iii. For a screw placed at 70° to the perpendicular (angled towards the fracture line), the graph (**170b**) illustrates that the force created ranges from 25 kPa to neglible.

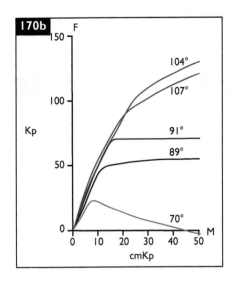

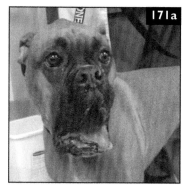

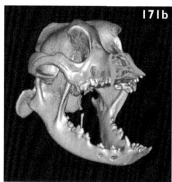

171 An 18-month-old male neutered boxer dog presented because the dog was unable to close its mouth (**171a**). The dog had four prior episodes over the past 3 months during which this had occurred but spontaneously resolved. On physical examination the dog appeared uncomfortable and the jaw could not be closed even when considerable pressure was applied to the rostral mandible. CT of the dog's skull was performed with the dog heavily sedated and two oblique cranial view images of the three-dimensional reconstructed images are shown (**171b, c**).

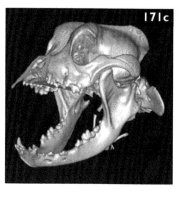

i. What is the likely etiology of this dog's problem?
ii. Describe how this dog's mandible should be manipulated to allow closure of this dog's mouth.
iii. Describe appropriate treatment for this dog.

172 A 2-year-old male Cairn terrier is being administered analgesic drugs in preparation for surgery to correct patellar luxation (**172a**).
i. What method is being used to provide regional analgesia in this dog?
ii. Describe how this technique is performed.

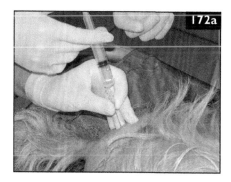

171 i. This dog is affected with a condition known as intermittent open-mouth (lower jaw) locking. The condition is typically the result of unilateral impingement of the coronoid process of the mandible on the ventrolateral zygomatic arch, as is evident on the CT image. Intermittent open-mouth locking has been associated with temporomandibular joint laxity and dysplasia. Bilateral temporomandibular joint incongruity is evident on the image with widening of the left temporomandibular joint. This laxity allows for abnormal lateral movement of the vertical ramus of the mandible and if sufficient laxity exists, the coronoid process becomes entrapped on the zygomatic arch. Dental malocclusion secondary to brachygnathism, as present in this dog, may have also contributed to the open-mouth locking. Other proposed underlying causes include flattening of the zygomatic arch and pterygoid muscle contracture.

ii. Opening the mouth further and applying rostral traction to the mandible, as this maneuver allows the apex of the coronoid process to move ventral to the zygomatic arch. The coronoid process is then pushed medially, allowing the mouth to be closed.

iii. Surgical intervention is warranted as locking was recurrent. Partial resection of the left zygomatic arch will relieve impingement. Locking is induced during surgery to identify the site of impingement and the rostroventral two-thirds of the zygomatic arch is excised with a pneumatic burr. Excision is continued until impingement can no longer be induced. Complete segmental ostectomy of the involved zygomatic arch and/or resection of the proximal portion of the coronoid process have been described in animals with severe impingement.

172 i. Epidural analgesia is being administered as part of a balanced anesthetic protocol.

ii. The dog is placed in lateral recumbency. The cranial borders of the wings of the ilium and the dorsal spinous process of the seventh lumbar vertebra are identified. The lumbosacral space may be palpated as a depression just caudal to the dorsal spinous process of L7 (**172b**, arrow). A 22G 38 mm Quincke point spinal needle is inserted in the midline at the lumbosacral space, with the long axis

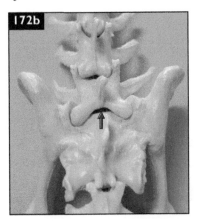

of the needle oriented perpendicular to the skin. A 'pop' may be detected as the needle passes through the ligamentum flavum into the epidural space. The hub of the needle is observed carefully for blood or cerebrospinal fluid. Correct positioning is confirmed by the 'loss of resistance' technique. Resistance to a test injection of a small volume of sterile saline is assessed – the saline should flow freely. Once correct placement is confirmed, the analgesic (local anesthetics and morphine are commonly used) is injected over 60–90 seconds.

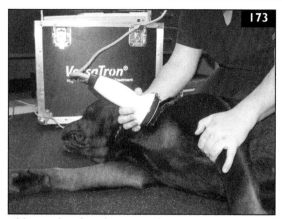

173 A 6-year-old, 39 kg female rottweiler receiving treatment for bicipital tendinopathy is shown (**173**).
i. Name the treatment modality being used on this dog.
ii. What form of energy is delivered to the tissues using this device?
iii. List three indications for the use of this therapeutic modality.
iv. List three anatomic locations where the use of this treatment modality is contraindicated.

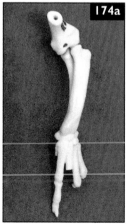 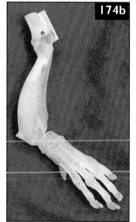

174 Models of the distal forelimb of two different dogs are shown (**174a, b**). Both dogs had an antebrachial deformity.
i. How are these models useful when considering correction of complex limb deformities?
ii. Describe the process by which models such as these are made.

173 i. This dog is receiving extra-corporeal shockwave therapy (ECST).

ii. ECST is an acoustic energy modality. Shockwaves can be created by electrohydraulic, electromagnetic, and piezoelectric mechanisms. The initiation of a wave that rapidly rises in pressure, typically reaching a peak pressure of around 50 Mpa within 10 nanoseconds, followed by a period of negative pressure, is characteristic of electrohydraulic shockwave therapy, the most common form of shockwave therapy used in veterinary medicine. Energy is released when a wave meets an area of high acoustic impedance such as a bone–tendon interface. Compressive and tensile forces result in cavitation and mechanical microstress to cells and tissue. The mechanical stimulation of cells is hypothesized to increase expression of cytokines and growth factors. ECST applied to an area of chronic inflammation signals the release of acute inflammatory mediators, facilitating appropriate progression of healing.

iii. (1) In conditions of delayed or disturbed healing, such as stimulating osseous union of delayed or non-union fractures. (2) To stimulate healing of soft tissue injuries such as Achilles, patellar, and bicipital tendinopathies, as well as chronic, non-healing wounds. (3) To provide analgesia in the multimodal approach to management of osteoarthritis. The analgesic effects are thought to be mediated through increased serotonin activity in the dorsal horn and descending inhibition of pain signals.

iv. Over the thorax or abdomen, over large nerves, or over blood vessels, particularly vessels with thrombi or vascular anomalies. ECST should not be used to treat neoplastic conditions because this modality enhances neovascularization.

174 i. The fabricated models allow for more accurate definition of the deformity, in particular characterizing its rotational component in addition to angular and length discrepancy when planning surgical correction of complex deformities. Identification of the anatomic axes and determination of the appropriate location and configuration of osteotomies or ostectomies can be done directly on the models. A sham procedure can be performed using the model to determine the efficacy of the planned correction prior to surgery.

ii. Precise morphologic models can be fabricated from CT scans. **174a** was fabricated using three-dimensional printing, a rapid prototyping process. A computer model is generated from the data acquired in the CT scan of the deformed limb segment by image segmentation, then converted into stereolithography file format, which is sent to the three-dimensional printer for fabrication. This rapid processing technology guides a printer head over a thin layer of powder, releasing a liquid powder binder in the pattern of the specimen's cross-sectional morphology. Successive layers of plaster are added at 0.2–0.3 mm increments to produce a model of the specimen. The model is then infiltrated with cyanoacrylate solution, which hardens the surface. Unfortunately, the three-dimensional printer model is brittle and not particularly compatible with the placement of implants or creation of osteotomies to emulate an *in-vivo* procedure. **174b** was fabricated using stereolithography. Stereolithography is a slower and more expensive process that produces a more detailed epoxy model of the deformed limb segment. Epoxy models have the advantages of being easier to cut and are more accepting of implant placement, allowing the surgeon to perform rehearsal surgery more easily.

175 A 9-year-old, 35 kg male crossbred dog presented for a left forelimb lameness of 3 weeks' duration. On physical examination there was a large, painful palpable mass in the region of the proximal scapula. A radiograph of the left scapula was obtained (**175a**).

i. Describe the radiographic abnormalities present.

ii. List the differential diagnoses.

iii. What surgical options might be applicable for treating this dog, assuming the disease is confined to the affected scapula?

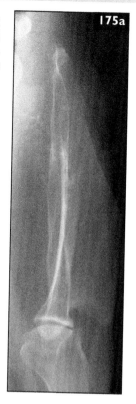

175a

176 A proximal humeral segment that has been stabilized with a linear external fixator is shown (**176**).

i. Describe the thread design of each of the fixation pins shown.

ii. Compare the respective mechanical properties of these fixation pins.

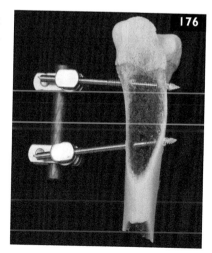

176

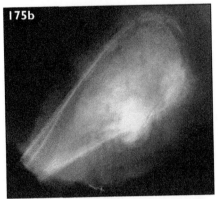

175 i. There is a destructive lytic lesion involving the proximal scapula. The proximal third of the scapula spine has been destroyed and replaced by an expansile mass containing areas of wispy mineralization, mostly concentrated medial to the scapula. There is minimal soft tissue mass effect.

ii. Differentials include osteosarcoma, chondrosarcoma, fibrosarcoma, soft tissue sarcoma, hemangiosarcoma.

iii. Curative-intent options include radical forequarter limb amputation or, alternatively, partial scapulectomy. A substantial portion of the scapula can be excised *en bloc* including the tumor capsule and surrounding soft tissues. The excised portion of scapula should be radiographed to assess if the excision was complete (175b). If necessary, the entire scapula proximal to the neck and the glenoid can be excised, but this can result in marked postoperative lameness. Removing 50% or less of the scapula can result in the dog having little observable lameness. The remaining portion of scapula should be anchored to the body wall with large non-absorbable sutures. These sutures function as a dorsal sling, allowing the dog to bear weight on the limb. Active physical therapy including range of movement exercises and non-weight-bearing activity (e.g. swimming) are encouraged during the postoperative convalescent period.

176 i. The proximal pin is a positive-profile, partially-threaded fixation pin. The distal pin is a negative-profile, partially-threaded fixation pin. Both pins are end threaded and intended for use as half-pins.

ii. The use of threaded pins is advocated to enhance the biomechanical properties of the pin–bone interface, resulting in greater resistance to axial extraction. Utilization of threaded fixation pins has been shown to decrease morbidity in dogs that had fractures managed with external fixators. The interface between the thread and smooth shaft of any pin serves as a stress concentrator and can predispose the pin to breakage at the thread–smooth shaft junction. Positive-profile, partially-threaded pins have threads that are raised above the pin's core diameter: the uniform core diameter minimizes the stress riser effect at the thread–smooth shaft interface. The threads of a negative-profile, partially-threaded pin are scored into the pin, which decreases the core diameter of the threaded portion of the pin. The positive-profile pin has threads that engage both the *cis-* and *trans-*cortices, which improves the pin's resistance to axial extraction. The threads of the negative-profile pin only engage the *trans-*cortex. Having a short thread length positions the thread–smooth shaft junction within the medullary cavity and protects the junction from axial forces during weight bearing, decreasing the potential for pin failure.

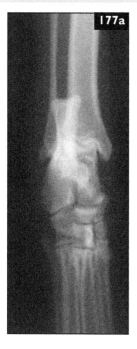

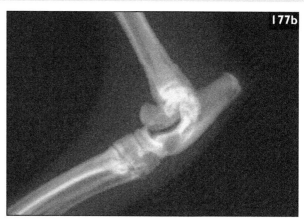

177 An overweight 4-year-old female neutered cat presented with an acute left hindlimb lameness sustained as the result of suspected trauma. Pain was localized to the tarsal region, but a detailed examination was not possible due to the cat's temperament. Radiographs of the cat's left tarsus were obtained after sedation (177a, b).
i. What is the diagnosis?
ii. How should this cat's injury be treated?

178 A 5-year-old, 33 kg male German shepherd dog was presented with a weight-bearing lameness of the left hindlimb of at least 3 months' duration. The lameness had an insidious onset, had become progressively more severe, and was characterized by a shortened stride with a rapid, elastic internal rotation of the paw, hock, and stifle, and external rotation of the tuber calcanei during the mid-to-late swing phase of the stride (178).
i. What is the tentative diagnosis?
ii. What specific physical examination abnormalities are typically present with this condition?
iii. Describe appropriate treatment for this condition.

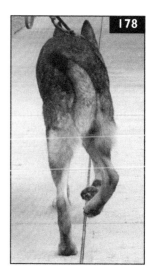

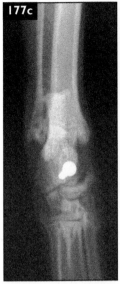

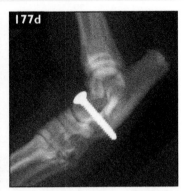

177 i. This cat has a subluxation of the talar body from the central tarsal bone (talocentral joint) and a concurrent subluxation from the talocalcaneal joint. This is often referred to as dorsal displacement of the talus.

ii. Displacement of the talus causes medial collapse of the tarsus, so reduction and stabilization are required. The talus can usually be reduced by digital pressure and reduction maintained by placement of a pair of small pointed reduction forceps. A 2.0 mm positional screw is placed to maintain the reduction between the talus and calcaneus, as was done in this cat (**177c, d**). External coaptation is not necessary, but the cat should be confined for 3–4 weeks. Small short locking plates placed to engage both the talus and central tarsal bone have also been used to stabilize the reduction transiently while the dorsal ligaments heal.

178 i. This lameness is associated with fibrotic myopathy of the gracilis or, less frequently, the semitendinosus muscle. The condition is produced by functional shortening of the affected muscle, which limits abduction of the coxofemoral joint, and extension of the stifle and hock.

ii. The distal myotendinous portion of the affected muscle, on the medial aspect of the stifle, is palpably thickened and fibrotic. The affected muscle is determined by tracing the taut band proximally to its origin. The gracilis muscle has its origin on the pubic symphysis, while the semitendinosus muscle has its origin on the caudoventral portion of the lateral angle of the ischiatic tuberosity. If an affected dog is positioned in dorsal recumbency, limited abduction of the coxofemoral joint and extension of the stifle and hock are apparent.

iii. An effective treatment resulting in permanent resolution of lameness has not been established. Medical treatments such as systemic or intralesional steroids, NSAIDs, and acupuncture have been ineffective. Any surgical procedure that disrupts the continuity of the affected muscle is associated with immediate improvement in coxofemoral abduction, increased stifle and hock extension, and resolution of lameness; however, recurrence of lameness and the restrictive fibrous band invariably develops 2–6 months following surgery. Adjunctive post-surgical therapies, such as administration of corticosteroids, NSAIDs, and lathyrogenic agents (d-penicillamine, colchicine), have been ineffective in suppressing fibroplasia and preventing recurrence of lameness.

179 A 5-month-old crossbred dog had a transverse femoral fracture stabilized with multiple intramedullary pins (stack pins). The pins sequentially loosened and were all removed within 6 weeks of the initial fracture repair. The dog was re-examined 2 months postoperatively (179). On palpation, the stifle was rigidly immobilized in extension.

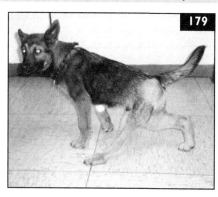

i. What is the name of the condition affecting this dog's hindlimb?

ii. What factors increase the risk of an animal developing this condition?

iii. What measures can be taken to prevent this postoperative complication from occurring?

180 A 7-month-old, 5 kg female Yorkshire terrier sustained simple transverse fractures of the distal third of the radius and ulna. Immediate postoperative radiographs are shown (180a, b).

i. List three technical errors that were committed in applying the fixation in this dog.

ii. According to established guidelines, what is the minimum number of screws that should be used to stabilize each major fracture segment?

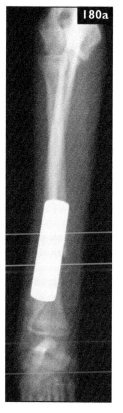
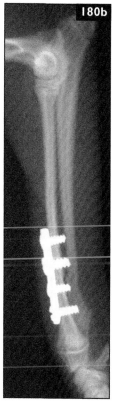

179 i. This dog has quadriceps contracture (also referred to as quadriceps tie-down), a severe form of fracture disease.

ii. The risk of developing quadriceps contracture is highest following femoral fracture in skeletally immature dogs and cats, especially animals <6 months of age. Quadriceps contracture may be unavoidable if resultant from vascular injury sustained at the time of fracture. Unfortunately, most animals develop quadriceps contracture as an adverse sequela to inappropriate coaptation of a fracture, iatrogenic trauma, or inappropriate postoperative care. Multiple intramedullary pins were used to stabilize this dog's transverse femoral fracture, but did not eliminate motion at the fracture site. Premature implant loosening and delayed fracture union ensued, contributing to the development of quadriceps contracture. Factors that further increase the risk of quadriceps contracture include a prolonged delay prior to surgery, and immobilizing the stifle joint in extension following surgery or as a method of fracture management.

iii. Quadriceps contracture may be prevented if the surgery is performed without delay and with atraumatic surgical technique to reduce iatrogenic muscle trauma. Anatomic reduction and stable fracture fixation will encourage limb use. The administration of postoperative analgesia, as well as the application of a 90/90 flexion bandage (see case **229**) followed by early passive stifle range of motion exercises, will also help to decrease the occurrence of this condition.

180 i. The plate is grossly oversized. A 2.7 mm plate was used, when a 1.5/2.0 mm veterinary cuttable plate or a 2.0 mm dynamic compression plate would have been more appropriate in a dog weighing 5 kg. The plate is also too short, resulting in an insufficient number of screws securing each of the major fracture segments. It is also evident from the lateral radiograph that the screws have been shortened. Cutting the end of the screws off to shorten the implants will deform the thread, which will induce damage to the tapped holes in the bone during screw insertion. The consequence will be a poor bone–implant interface, increasing the likelihood of early screw loosening.

ii. Traditional plating technique specifies implant selection based on placing at least 2–3 screws (or engaging 4–6 cortices) on either side of the fracture. However, guidance is not given regarding the ideal working length of the plate. Recent biomechanical data suggest that longer plates with fewer screws provide equivalent strength of fixation compared with standard compression plating techniques, and technical emphasis should be on selecting a plate of adequate length rather than selecting a plate based on the number of screws placed in each fracture segment. Application of a plate that is too short represents one of the most common technical errors made during diaphyseal fracture stabilization.

181 A 3-month-old male English bulldog presented with a mild left forelimb lameness. The dog held the left elbow in partial flexion and there was mild valgus deformity of the left carpus. Mediolateral and craniocaudal radiographs of the elbow were obtained (**181a, b**).

i. What is the diagnosis, and what is the suspected etiopathogenesis of this condition?

ii. Name the breeds of dogs that have been reported to be affected with this condition.

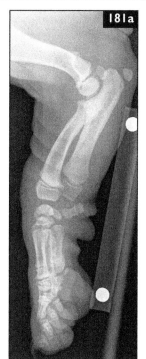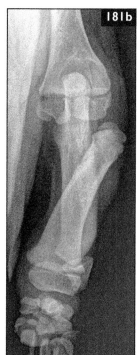

182 An 8-year-old female spayed West Highland white terrier presented with a non-weight-bearing, acute-onset right forelimb lameness. The dog's previous history included 11 months of hind-

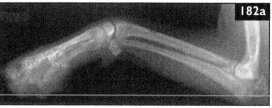

limb pain and a more recent bout of lethargy and depression that improved after steroid administration. On examination the dog was reluctant to bear weight on the hindlimbs and was non-weight bearing on the right forelimb. There was crepitation on palpation of the right elbow. The dog was sedated and a radiograph of the right forelimb was obtained (**182a**).

i. Describe the radiographic abnormalities.

ii. State a diagnosis.

iii. What is the recommended treatment for the most likely diagnosis?

181 i. This puppy has a type I congenital elbow luxation, a condition characterized by caudolateral luxation of the radial head. Type I congenital elbow luxations are presumed to result from hypoplasia of either the medial collateral ligament or the annular ligament. Premature closure of the distal ulnar physis or radial–ulnar synostosis can result in acquired lateral subluxation or luxation of the radial head.
ii. This condition has predominately been reported in larger breed dogs, most notably bulldogs, bull mastiffs, boxers, bull terriers, Staffordshire terriers, Doberman pinschers, collies, golden retrievers and Old English sheepdogs, but has also been reported in a dachshund and a Jack Russell terrier.

182 i. There are multiple lytic radiolucent lesions affecting the humerus, the radius and ulna, and the metacarpal bones. These lesions are well defined, but not circumscribed by a sclerotic margin. There is a pathologic fracture of the olecranon.
ii. The presence of multiple small radiolucencies affecting multiple bones is characteristic of multiple myeloma, which can be confirmed by observation of >5% plasma cells on bone marrow aspirate examination (182b, arrow) and detection of monoclonal gammopathy (IgA or IgG). Flame cells (182c, arrow), a rare abnormal variant of plasma cells, have red staining at the periphery and contain more immunoglobulin than normal plasma cells.
iii. Multiple myeloma can be treated with a chemotherapy regimen of melphalan, cyclophosphamide, and prednisolone. Stabilization of the olecranon fracture should be discussed with the owner, although fracture healing may be complicated because of the dog's underlying disease. Euthanasia or amputation of the limb should also be discussed.

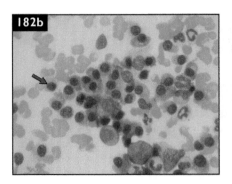

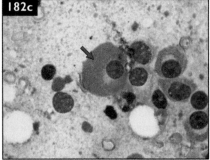

183 An 18-week-old male Staffordshire bull terrier presented with a marked weight-bearing left forelimb lameness. The dog had mild valgus deviation and external rotation of the left distal forelimb and pain was elicited on manipulation of the left elbow. Mediolateral radiographic views of the left (**183a**) and right (**183b**) antebrachii are shown.

i. What is the most likely etiology of this dog's deformity?

ii. What are the clinical implications associated with the radiographic abnormalities affecting this dog's right elbow?

iii. Describe surgical options for re-establishing congruency of this dog's right elbow.

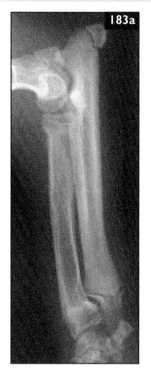
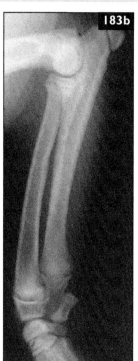

184 A total hip replacement implant system is shown (**184a**).

i. Name the implant prosthesis?

ii. Describe the design features and characteristics of this prosthesis.

iii. What complications are reported in association with the use of this implant system for total hip replacement in dogs?

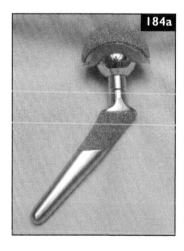

183 i. Asymmetric premature closure of the distal radial physis. The articular surface of the distal radius is angulated in a distomedial-to-proximolateral direction, which typically occurs following eccentric premature closure of the lateral aspect of the distal radial growth plate.

ii. Premature closure of this dog's distal radial growth plate has resulted in a shortened radius. The ulna is unaffected and continued growth of this bone, concurrent with the shortened radius, has resulted in humeroradial subluxation. Fragmentation of the medial coronoid process often occurs in association with distal humeroradial subluxation.

iii. The incongruency could be corrected either indirectly by shortening the ulna or directly by lengthening the radius. Radial lengthening is achieved by performing a radial osteotomy, and then acutely or sequentially distracting the osteotomy until the radius has been lengthened sufficiently to resolve the humeroradial subluxation. Performing a segmental diaphyseal ulnar ostectomy is a relatively simple method that can be used to resolve humeroradial subluxation. A sufficient segment of bone must be removed to restore congruency. The disadvantage of this technique is that the antebrachium is shortened, which can be concerning if the limb segment is already relatively short. Radial lengthening will not cause further limb shortening, but the radius will need stabilization during the healing period.

184 i. The BioMedtrix BFX (cementless) total hip prosthesis. Pictured are the femoral stem, femoral head, and acetabular components.

ii. This is a modular system enabling numerous combinations of the various sizes of each component to be implanted in an individual dog. The femoral stem, composed of cast cobalt chrome (ASTM-F75), is a porous coated implant with cobalt chrome beads (250 nm diameter in three stucco-type layers) to enable bone in-growth. There is a Morse taper on the neck to interface with the femoral head, which ensures a secure connection between these components (**184b**). The femoral head is composed of dense wrought cobalt chrome (ASTM-F799), with a highly

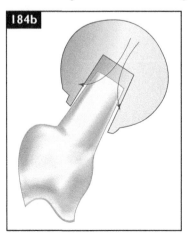

polished surface. The acetabular component consists of a titanium shell (ASTM-F136) with a pre-assembled ultra-high molecular weight polyethylene liner. The shell has a cobalt chrome bead coating similar to that on the stem.

iii. Reported complications include infection, luxation, femoral fracture, sciatic neurapraxia, implant displacement, and implant subsidence.

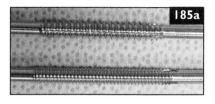

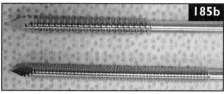

185 Two types of partially threaded pins commonly utilized as fixation pins in external fixator constructs are shown (185a, b). A radiograph of the tibia of a 10-month-old intact male Australian shepherd dog that was attacked by another dog and sustained an open fracture of the tibia is shown (185c).

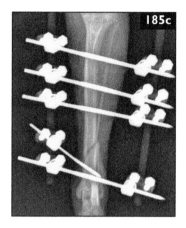

i. What is the correct terminology used to describe each of the pins shown in 185a and 185b?
ii. How would you describe the external fixator construct used to stabilize the fracture in 185c?
iii. Describe how to correctly choose and apply a fixation pin during placement of an external fixator.

186 A 16-month-old female West Highland white terrier presents for a slowly progressive weight-bearing lameness of the left hindlimb that worsens with activity. Palpable crepitus and discomfort can be elicited on extension and abduction of the left coxofemoral joint and the joint has a reduced range of motion. Atrophy of the caudal thigh musculature is also apparent in the left hindlimb. A radiograph of the pelvis is shown (186).

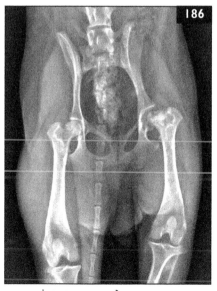

i. What is the diagnosis?
ii. What is the typical signalment of dogs affected with this condition?
iii. What is the etiopathogenesis of this condition?
iv. Describe treatment options for this dog.
v. What is this dog's prognosis following appropriate treatment?

185 i. **185a** depicts two centrally-threaded, positive-profile pins. The upper pin is designed for use in cancellous bone; the lower pin is designed for use in cortical bone. **185b** depicts two end-threaded, positive-profile pins. The upper pin is designed for use in cancellous bone; the lower pin is designed for use in cortical bone.

ii. A five-pin, bilateral, uniplanar modified type II IMEX SK construct. Four centrally-threaded cortical fixation pins and one end-threaded positive-profile fixation pins were used. A single half-pin splintage pin (thus a modified type II construct) was used in the short distal segment: a half-pin can be placed more easily at an angle than a full-pin, avoiding placement of the pin in or too close to the fracture. The half-pin was placed from the medial aspect of the crus because this surface of the tibia has limited overlying musculature.

iii. A minimum of two fixation pins should be used to stabilize each of the major fracture segments, with three or four pins in each segment being considered optimal. The diameter of the pins should not exceed 25–30% of the diameter of the bone at the level at which the pin is placed. Pins should be placed after pre-drilling a pilot hole using a drill bit approximating, but not exceeding, the core diameter of the fixation pin. Pins should be inserted using a high-torque, low-speed drill while protecting the soft tissues.

186 i. Avascular or ischemic necrosis of the femoral head, commonly known as Legg–Calvé–Perthes' disease.

ii. This disease is generally diagnosed in young (4–11 months), small-breed dogs (<10 kg) such as Manchester terriers, miniature pinschers, toy poodles, Lakeland terriers, West Highland white and Cairn terriers. Bilateral involvement occurs in 10–17% of affected dogs.

iii. The disease results from infarction of the proximolateral femoral epiphysis, physis, and metaphysis. The cause of infarction is unknown; proposed theories include hereditary and hormonal factors, trauma, conformational abnormalities, and synovitis, which impair blood flow along the femoral neck. Necrosis of subchondral epiphyseal and metaphyseal bone is followed by revascularization and osseous resorption. Normal weight bearing results in collapse of the mechanically weakened bone, with subsequent deformation of the articular surface, joint incongruency, and development of degenerative joint disease.

iv. Conservative treatment consisting of limited activity and anti-inflammatory drugs can be successful in dogs with limited pain and degenerative changes. Most dogs exhibiting overt clinical lameness will require either a femoral head and neck ostectomy or possibly total hip replacement.

v. Improved limb use after surgical intervention is expected. Dogs with profound, chronic lameness and severe muscle atrophy prior to surgery may be slow to recover following surgery. Improvement can be gradual and may continue to progress for 6–12 months following surgery.

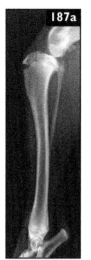
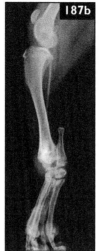
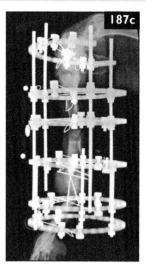

187 A 7-month-old Pyrenean Mountain dog (Great Pyrenees) developed resorption of the right distal tibial epiphysis and talus as a young puppy. The etiology was unknown, but these ano-malies resulted in substantial shortening of the limb and marked abnormalities of the right hock and pes. On examination, the dog did not bear weight on the right hindlimb and there was visible shortening of the crus with swelling, pain, and instability of the hock and a marked external rotation of the right hind paw. Radiographs of the left (187a) and right (187b) distal hindlimbs are shown and the length of the right tibia was 65% that of the left. A pantarsal arthrodesis of the right hock was done and subsequent bifocal lengthening of the right crus was performed using a circular fixator construct. A 4-week postoperative radiograph is shown (187c).
i. What process is being utilized to lengthen this dog's crus?
ii. Define the terms latency period, rate, and rhythm as related to the process being used to lengthen this dog's limb segment.

188 A 2-year-old Irish wolfhound dis-located its prosthetic right hip 14 days after surgery when the dog slipped on the kitchen floor. Revision surgery was performed and external coaptation applied postoperatively for 7 days (188).
i. Identify the type of coaptation applied to this dog's right hindlimb.
ii. What is the primary indication for using this type of external coaptation?
iii. What complications can be asso-ciated with this coaptation device?

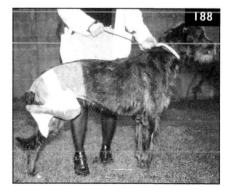

187 i. Distraction osteogenesis. This is the induction of new bone formation, termed regenerate bone, in a gradually widening osteotomy gap created by the controlled, sequential separation of two secured bone segments.

ii. The latency (or delay) period is the time between surgery and the initiation of distraction. This period allows for organization of the hematoma and early vascularization of the fibrous matrix, which can result in better regenerate bone formation. A delay period of several days is usual in human patients; the necessity for a similar latency in young dogs is questionable.

Rate is the total amount of distraction performed each day. Biologic factors such as age, osteotomy location, as well as periosteal and surrounding soft tissue integrity are considered in deciding the rate. Typical distraction rates in dogs range from 0.75–2.0 mm each day, with higher distraction rates typically being used in young dogs. Compliance of the regional soft tissues can become an issue when using higher rates of distraction. Lower distraction rates are advisable in older dogs in order to optimize regenerate bone formation.

Rhythm is the term used to describe the number of incremental lengthenings performed each day during the distraction process. Fractionating the distraction into a higher number of increments (increasing the rhythm) does not affect the biomechanical or histomorphological properties of the regenerate bone, but increasing the rhythm of distraction is beneficial to the regional soft tissues. Rhythms of 6- or 8-hour intervals between distractions have been advocated in dogs and have been associated with less morbidity, particularly flexor contracture, than a once or twice daily rhythm.

188 i. An Ehmer sling has been applied.

ii. Ehmer slings are primarily used to maintain reduction of craniodorsal coxofemoral luxations. The sling can be placed after either open or closed reduction. The Ehmer sling purportedly positions the coxofemoral joint in flexion, internal rotation, and abduction, which helps to maintain reduction by providing maximal acetabular coverage of the femoral head. The sling also prevents weight bearing on the limb, and is typically left in place for 1–3 weeks, allowing for healing and fibrosis of periarticular soft tissues to develop and provide long-term stability to the joint.

iii. The limb in an Ehmer sling is in a forced flexed position and attempts to extend the limb places considerable tension on the tape edges, which can cause pressure necrosis of soft tissues and compromise vascular flow to the distal extremity. The metatarsal region absorbs the majority of the resistance to limb flexion, and adequate padding is essential to prevent ulceration and pressure necrosis from developing. Owners should be instructed on proper maintenance of the bandage and daily monitoring for soft tissue irritation and digital swelling, hypothermia, or discoloration. Severe pressure sores and necrosis from badly maintained or poorly placed Ehmer slings have resulted in limbs having to be amputated.

189 Two bone plates, each made from a different metal, are shown (**189**).
i. What is the composition of each plate?
ii. Define modulus of elasticity.
iii. How do the bending stiffness and fatigue resistance of these two materials compare, in considering similar sized implants?
iv. What process is commonly used during the manufacture of the plate on the femur (A) to improve the implant's stiffness and fatigue resistance?

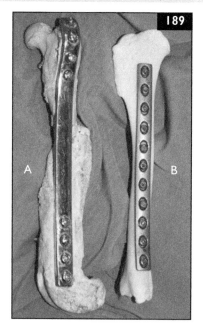

190 A 10-month-old male Labrador retriever is presented with a 6-week history of intermittent, mild, bilateral forelimb lameness, worse on the left than the right. On examination, there is moderate discomfort on full flexion of both elbows, exacerbated by pronation of the antebrachium while the elbow is fully flexed. Radiographs of both elbows demonstrate 1–2 mm smooth osteophytosis on the caudodorsal aspect of the anconeal process, but are considered otherwise unremarkable.

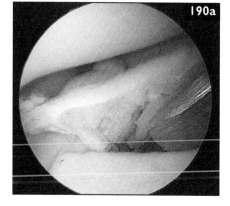

i. Elbow arthroscopy was performed via standard medial arthroscopy portal placement (**190a**). State the diagnosis.
ii. Describe appropriate treatment options for this dog.

189 i. The plate on the femur (A) is manufactured from 316L stainless steel. The plate on the tibia (B) is manufactured from titanium.

ii. Modulus of elasticity (or elastic modulus) is the mathematical description of an object's or substance's tendency to be deformed elastically (i.e. non-permanently) when subjected to an applied load. The elastic modulus of an object is defined by the slope of its stress–strain curve in the elastic deformation region.

iii. The modulus of elasticity for titanium is around half that of 316L stainless steel. This means that titanium deforms more and has a lower stiffness than 316L stainless at a given load. Despite these parameters being lower, titanium has superior fatigue resistance and allows greater elastic deformation compared with 316L stainless steel, which may lead to less stress shielding of bone after implant placement.

iv. The fatigue resistance and stiffness of plates manufactured from 316L stainless steel can be improved by cold working and annealing compared with casting the plate. Excessive contouring of the plate during application causes work-hardening of the alloy and reduces fatigue resistance.

190 i. Fragmentation of the medial coronoid process (MCP). The fragment is located at the radial incisure of the MCP. The humeral condyle is at the top of **190a**, with the radial head to the left and an area of synovitis-associated soft tissue proliferation within the craniomedial joint compartment to the right. The medial aspect of the MCP is visible in the foreground, with the fragment minimally displaced above the adjacent articular surface.

ii. Treatment options include non-surgical, open surgical, and arthroscopic treatments. A recent meta-analysis suggested that arthroscopic management was superior, although limitations regarding the clinical evidence in support of this decision were identified. For both open and arthroscopic surgical options, treatment is focused initially on removal of loose osteochondral fragments, although a rationale has been established for removal of a larger portion of the medial aspect of the MCP due to extension of subchondral pathology beyond the area of arthroscopically visible pathology. Subtotal coronoid ostectomy can be performed open or under arthroscopic guidance, and can be performed using an oscillating saw (**190b, A**), osteotome (**190b, B**), arthroscopic shaver or hand burr. Following osteotomy, the ostectomized fragment is removed from the joint (**190b, C, D**).

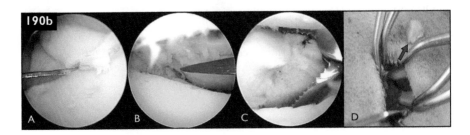

191 A 7-year-old female German shepherd dog had surgery to address severe lameness ascribed to chronic degenerative joint disease of the right elbow that was non-responsive to medical management. Medio-lateral and craniocaudal radiographs of the elbow were obtained 8 weeks after surgery (**191a, b**). The dog was still lame on the right

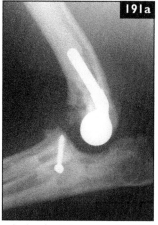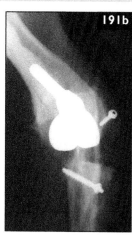

forelimb at this time, although the dog's lameness had improved compared with prior to surgery.

i. What procedure was performed in this dog?

ii. How do the terms constrained and unconstrained apply to the procedure performed in this dog?

iii. What complication is apparent in these radiographs?

iv. What is the success rate for this procedure?

192 This 5-year-old female neutered pointer (**192a**) was evaluated for a right forelimb lameness of several weeks' duration, which had an insidious onset. Mild pain was elicited on manipulation of the left carpus. Cytologic evaluation of synovial fluid obtained from the right carpus was consistent with a clinical diagnosis of mild degenerative joint disease.

i. What is the most likely diagnosis?

ii. Name the breed of dog most commonly affected with this condition.

iii. How should this dog be treated?

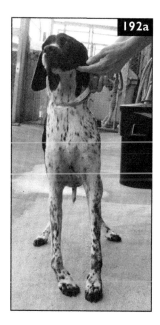

191 i. A total elbow replacement (or arthroplasty) using the BioMedtrix cemented system.
ii. Joint replacement systems are classified based on the mechanical relationship between components. Systems are described as constrained, semi-constrained, or unconstrained. In a constrained system the components lock together, thus providing inherent stability to the system. Constraining the components, however, increases stress on the bone–implant or cement–implant interface, which can lead to loosening. Components of unconstrained systems do not interlock and are dependent on the periarticular soft tissues to maintain stability. Unconstrained systems are less likely to loosen, but have a greater risk of luxation. Components of semi-constrained systems lock together with a 'loose' fit with the aim of providing some inherent stability with limited stress on the bone–implant or cement–implant interface. The BioMedtrix system used in this dog is an unconstrained system.
iii. Widening of the lateral joint space indicates that the lateral collateral ligament prosthesis, placed between the two suture anchors, has failed, resulting in subluxation of the elbow.
iv. Major complications have been reported in 20% of cases (4/20 dogs) and include infection, fracture of the humeral condyle, and lateral luxation. Of the 80% of dogs that did not suffer a major complication there was a significant improvement in limb use, as determined by force plate evaluation 12 weeks following surgery. Limb function continued to improve during the first year following surgery.

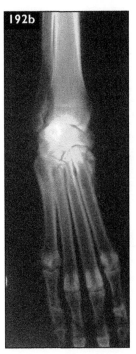
192b

192 i. This dog has a chronic sprain of the lateral collateral ligament of the carpus associated with a carpal varus conformation. This condition has been recognized in middle- to older-aged dogs that present with a history of intermittent to constant forelimb lameness. There is a visible carpal varus deformity with periarticular swelling and fibrosis. Radiographs show periarticular soft tissue swelling and mineralization of this swelling in chronic cases. Osteophytosis and mineralization of intercarpal ligaments also occur. Stress radiographs show laxity in the lateral collateral ligament. A craniocaudal radiograph of this pointer's carpus is shown (**192b**).
ii. Lameness associated with carpal varus has been reported in Border collies and Doberman pinschers.
iii. Mildly affected dogs can be treated by administration of NSAIDs and weight loss when applicable, but the lameness may not completely resolve and is often exacerbated by exercise. Pancarpal arthrodesis can be considered as a surgical option to fully resolve the lameness.

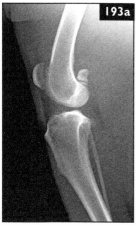 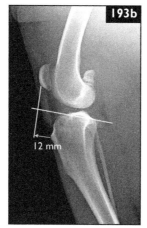 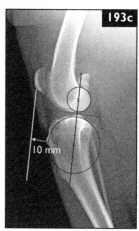

193 A preoperative lateral view radiograph of the stifle joint of a 6-year-old female Labrador retriever with a complete CrCL rupture is shown (**193a**). Two methods of planning a tibial tuberosity advancement (TTA) procedure in this dog are shown (**193b, c**).

i. What angle needs to be measured to properly plan for a TTA procedure?
ii. Describe the different methodologies illustrated in **193b** and **193c**.
iii. Is this preoperative radiograph adequate for preoperative planning for tibial tuberosity advancement?

194 This image (**194a**) shows a contact pressure map from the femorotibial joint of a normal dog's stifle. The use of joint pressure sensing equipment *in vivo* is not yet feasible, so this image was acquired from a cadaver specimen that was axially loaded to simulate the stance phase of walking. The contact map has been superimposed over a representation of the tibial plateau to help orient the reader.

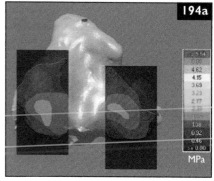

i. Describe the pattern of load transmission in this joint, as depicted by the contact map.
ii. What changes would be expected in the femorotibial contact map of a CrCL-deficient stifle during weight bearing?

193 i. The patellar tendon angle, which is the angle formed by the intersection between a line representing the tibial plateau and a line representing the cranial edge of the patellar tendon, needs to be determined. The objective of the TTA procedure is to achieve a postoperative patellar tendon angle of 90°. A template is used to determine the amount of advancement necessary to achieve this angle.

ii. The two methods of determining the line representing the tibial plateau are illustrated: (1) the traditional method using the tibial plateau slope (**193b**); and (2) alternative method using the common tangent between circles overlying the femoral and tibial condyles (**193c**). The common tangent method is reported to be more accurate.

iii. The positioning is acceptable. The stifle is in an extended position (approximately 135°), there is no cranial translation of the tibia in relation to the femur, and the lateral radiographic positioning is good with superimposition of the femoral condyles and the fabellae.

194 i. There is near-uniform contact pressure distribution in the medial and lateral stifle compartments. The magnitude of the highest contact pressure is low (approximately 2.3 MPa). The contact area between the articular surfaces is also wide, occupying the majority of the medial and lateral tibial condyles.

ii. The primary role of the CrCL is to prevent cranial subluxation of the tibia during weight bearing. During subluxation, the femoral condyles slip caudally on the tibial plateau, distorting surface geometry between the menisci and articular surfaces. An example of contact pressure distributions in a CrCL-deficient stifle under load is shown (**194b**). The contact points have shifted caudally on the tibial plateau, and contact area is markedly reduced in both compartments. In the lateral compartment, the decrease in contact area is not as pronounced as in the medial compartment, because the lateral meniscus has a caudal femoral attachment and is able to conform during subluxation better than the medial meniscus, which is firmly attached to the medial tibial condyle. Peak contact pressures are also much higher than normal (indicated by the red sensels) because the load is transmitted across a smaller region of contact. The alterations contribute to mechanical cartilage degeneration and progressive osteoarthritis.

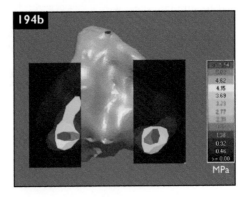

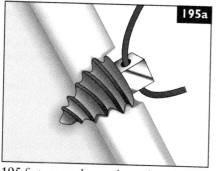
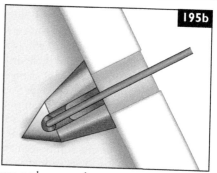

195 Suture anchors, also referred to as tissue or bone anchors, are used to secure soft tissue structures to bone and provide a means for synthetic reconstruction of damaged, excised or traumatically removed tissues. Two types of suture anchor are illustrated (195a, b).

i. Categorize the two anchors based on their insertional location.
ii. What is the primary advantage of the type of suture anchor in 195a?
iii. What is the primary advantage of the type of suture anchor in 195b?

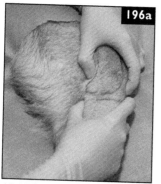
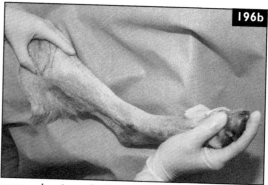

196 These photographs demonstrate palpation of a dog's stifle suspected of having CrCL insufficiency (196a, b).

i. Name the two tests being performed to substantiate the diagnosis of CrCL insufficiency.
ii. Explain why the test illustrated in 196a is generally performed with the stifle positioned in both flexion and extension.
iii. Explain the principles behind the test illustrated in 196b.

195 i. The anchor in **195a** is a transcortical anchor, as the anchor engages the cortex of the bone and resistance to extraction is dependent on the anchor's thread–bone interface. The anchor in **195b** is a subcortical anchor, which is inserted to a subcortical position through a hole drilled in the cortex. Resistance to extraction is dependent on post-insertional changes in the size or shape of the anchor.

ii. Transcortical anchors have superior pull-out strength to subcortical anchors. Variations in the thread design can improve the thread–bone interface and are a major factor in determining pull-out strength.

iii. Subcortical anchors do not protrude beyond the cortical surface of the bone and thus are unlikely to incite soft tissue irritation, which can be a problem when using transcortical anchors. This property is particularly advantageous because suture anchors are most commonly used in periarticular locations, which are subjected to large tissue excursions associated with joint range of motion.

196 i. The photographs illustrate assessing the stifle for cranial drawer (**196a**) and cranial tibial thrust (**196b**), which are often referred to as the tibial compression test.

ii. Cranial drawer should be assessed with the stifle positioned in both flexion and extension because of the CrCL's functional anatomy. The ligament is comprised of two bands. The craniomedial band is taut in flexion and extension whereas the caudolateral band is taut only in extension. The craniomedial band is typically affected in dogs with partial CrCL tears and therefore cranial drawer will only be elicited under these circumstances when the stifle is tested in flexion.

iii. The stifle is subjected to external forces generated during weight bearing as well as internal forces generated by muscle contraction. These external and internal forces result in a cranially directed shear force in the tibia (cranial tibial thrust) due to the fact that the tibial plateau is not oriented perpendicular to the center of motion of the stifle and hock. Cranial tibial thrust is opposed passively by the CrCL and actively by the hamstring muscle group and biceps femoris muscle. CrCL rupture results in cranial translation of the tibia when the joint is loaded. The tibial thrust test mimics this loading by hyperflexion of the hock while the stifle is maintained in extension.

197 Lateral and cranio-caudal radiographs were taken of the right femur of a 10-month-old neutered male hound dog that presented with a 2-day history of non-weight-bearing right hindlimb lameness (**197a, b**). The lameness had an acute onset and developed after the dog ran into a fence post while playing with a littermate.

i. Describe the fracture.

ii. What is the prognosis for continued longitudinal bone growth from this dog's distal femoral physis?

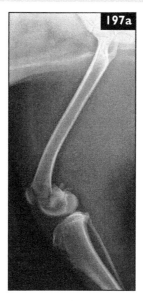
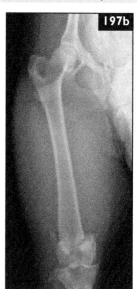

198 A radiograph of the right humerus of a 10-month-old German shepherd dog that had an obvious weight-bearing right forelimb lameness of 5 weeks' duration is shown (**198**). The dog would intermittently hold the right forelimb off the ground when sitting or standing. Pain was elicited on manipulation of the right elbow during the orthopedic examination.

i. Based on the signalment and history, give a list of potential differential diagnoses for this dog's lameness.

ii. Describe the radiographic abnormalities and give a radiographic diagnosis.

iii. What is the prognosis for a dog with this condition?

iv. What would be the most appropriate treatment for this dog?

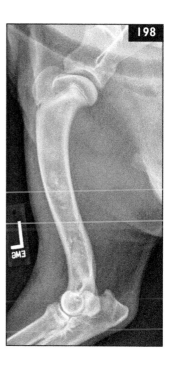

197 i. This dog has a Salter–Harris type II fracture involving the distal femoral physis. The fracture traverses the physis, but propagates into the metaphysis caudally. The condylar segment is displaced slightly caudally, proximally and medially.

ii. The Salter–Harris classification scheme was developed to use as a prognostic indicator for the continued longitudinal bone growth from the affected physis in human patients. In children, the higher the classification number, the worse the prognosis for continued growth. Unfortunately, the prognostic value of the Salter–Harris classification scheme does not apply to dogs. Veterinarians utilize the Salter–Harris classification scheme for descriptive purposes, but most physeal fractures in dogs will result in closure of at least a portion of the growth plate, irrespective of the fracture's Salter–Harris classification or method of fracture stabilization. Histologic evaluation of the growth plates of dogs that had sustained physeal fractures showed there was consistent damage to cells in the proliferative zone of the involved physis, even in dogs with Salter–Harris type I or II fractures. Damage to cells in the proliferative zone will result in closure of the physis, terminating longitudinal bone growth. Nevertheless, the impact of this 10-month-old dog's distal femoral physis closing would be nominal at this point as the dog is approaching skeletal maturity.

198 i. Ununited anconeal process, osteochondrosis of the humeral condyle, fragmented medial coronoid process, incomplete ossification of the humeral condyle, panosteitis, traumatic fracture, and infectious arthritis.

ii. There are ill-defined, patchy areas of increased mineral opacity centered in the medullary cavity of the mid- and distal humeral diaphysis as well as the distal humeral metaphysis. These lesions are somewhat evenly distributed around the nutrient foramen, which is located in the caudal cortex of the distal humeral diaphysis. A focal, well-defined, obliquely oriented radiolucent line is seen extending distally from the level of the nutrient foramen within the metaphyseal medullary opacity; this likely represents the nutrient artery. Although definition of the medial coronoid process is indistinct, the elbow appears congruent without appreciable degenerative joint disease. These abnormalities are consistent with a diagnosis of panosteitis, sometimes also referred to as eosinophilic panosteitis.

iii. Panosteitis is usually self-limiting and typically resolves without treatment. Affected dogs can develop subsequent lesions in other appendicular long bones and owners should be warned that their dog could develop what is described as a 'migrating' or 'shifting limb' lameness.

iv. Pain and lameness can be severe and persist for a prolonged period of time, therefore administration of NSAIDs is often advocated.

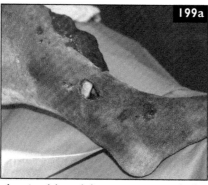

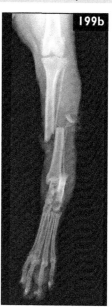

199 A 3-year-old male mixed-breed dog was presented after being hit by a car. On physical examination the dog could not bear weight on the left hindlimb. The crus was swollen and palpably unstable; the fractured tibia was visible through the open wounds (199a). Radiographs of the left crus were obtained; the craniocaudal view image is shown (199b). How would this fracture be classified based on the classification scheme proposed by Gustilo and Anderson?

200 An 18-month-old male neutered chihuahua presented for re-evaluation 3 weeks after having left antebrachial fractures stabilized with a plate on the radius. The dog initially started to bear weight on the left forelimb following surgery and had been using the limb consistently with only a mild lameness before becoming acutely non-weight bearing on the limb the day prior to presentation. A radiograph of the affected limb obtained at the time of re-evaluation is shown (200).
i. Describe the radiographic findings.
ii. What factors may have contributed to these complications?
iii. What anatomic reasons have been suggested for the higher incidence of delayed and non-union radius and ulna fractures in toy breed dogs?

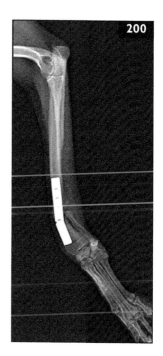

199 This dog has an open fracture as the wound has established direct communication between the fracture and the external environment. Osseous and soft tissue trauma can be severe in open fractures because open fractures are frequently the result of high-energy trauma. Numerous classification schemes have been proposed to categorize open fractures in an attempt to direct treatment protocols or to prognosticate outcomes. The most widely utilized scheme, proposed by Gustilo and Anderson in 1976, categorizes open fractures into three types based on increasing severity of the associated soft tissue damage. Type 1: the skin wound is <1 cm in diameter and has often been caused by penetration from a sharp bone segment. Type 2: the skin wound is typically >1 cm in diameter and often the result of external trauma. Contusion of the soft tissue surrounding the fracture is more severe than in a type 1 fracture. Type 3: the soft tissues surrounding the fracture are severely traumatized with extensive skin, subcutaneous tissue, and muscle injury. There is often severe crushing injury, neurovascular injury, or severe contamination. This dog's tibial fracture would be categorized as a type 3 open fracture based on this classification scheme.

200 i. There has been a loss of reduction and fixation. The 2.0 mm dynamic compression plate, which had been applied to the cranial aspect of the radius, has broken through the screw hole located just distal to the original fracture.
ii. Implant failure can be ascribed to technical, mechanical, or biological factors. Technical error, such as improper selection of an appropriate sized implant, is the most common cause of implant failure. Mechanical failure is typically not the result of the initial loads, but the consequence of cyclic loading that the implants must endure until fracture healing. 'Fatigue failure' typically occurs weeks after surgery and has likely contributed to this dog's complications. Biological factors that prolong fracture healing can result in failure of any implant. The bone must heal in an appropriate time frame to reduce load transmission through the implants. Reasons for biological failure include ischemia and tissue trauma from the injury, improper tissue handling at surgery, anatomic factors, and poor postoperative management.
iii. Small-breed dogs have a decreased vascular density at the distal diaphyseal–metaphyseal junction compared with large-breed dogs. These vascular anomalies may account for the high incidence of complications seen in small-breed dogs following stabilization of radial fractures.

201 A 6-year-old male cat returned home with a non-weight-bearing lameness of the right forelimb. The elbow was swollen and painful. A radiograph of the antebrachium is shown (201).

i. Describe the injury apparent on the radiograph.

ii. These injuries have been classified into types; list the types and classify the fracture in this cat.

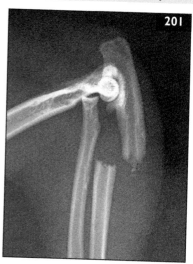

202 Immediate and 2-week postoperative radiographs of a 6-year-old male boxer that has had surgical stabilization of a tibial fracture are shown (202a, b). The dog had a tibial plateau leveling osteotomy performed 2 years ago. The tibial plateau leveling osteotomy plate was removed at the time of fracture repair.

i. What type of plate was used to stabilize this fracture?

ii. How would this plate be described with respect to the implant's function in stabilizing this fracture?

iii. Why did this fracture repair fail?

iv. How does the bending stiffness of a 3.5 mm broad version of the plate utilized in this dog compare with a standard 3.5 mm broad dynamic compression plate?

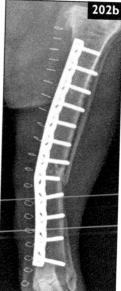

201 i. There is a transverse, mildly comminuted, proximal diaphyseal ulnar fracture with a concurrent cranial luxation of the radial head. This combination of injuries is referred to as a Monteggia fracture. The luxation results from disruption of the annular and interosseous ligaments.

ii. There are four types of Monteggia fracture: type 1, cranial radial head dislocation and ulnar diaphyseal fracture; type 2, caudal radial head dislocation and ulnar diaphyseal fracture; type 3, lateral or craniolateral radial head dislocation and ulnar diaphyseal fracture; and type 4, cranial radial head dislocation associated with ulnar and radial diaphyseal fractures. This cat has sustained a type I fracture, the most common type of Monteggia fracture in cats.

202 i. A limited contact dynamic compression plate (LC-DCP), identified by the scalloped appearance of the surface of the plate in contact with the bone, was used to stabilize this fracture.

ii. The fracture is comminuted and there is a gap between the two major fracture segments on the immediate postoperative radiographs. Therefore, the plate is functioning in a buttress mode.

iii. The fracture was not anatomically reconstructed during surgery, resulting in a functional gap between the two major bone segments. Since the major segments were not in direct contact, there was no load-sharing on the *trans*-cortex (the lateral cortex, opposite the plate). This situation resulted in a bending moment that exceeded the elastic limit of the plate once the dog began to bear weight on the limb.

iv. In one study the mechanical properties of a 3.5 mm broad DCP was found to be equal to that of a 3.5 mm broad LC-DCP when used in a buttress or gap model. Both plates are able to withstand a loading force of approximately three times that of a 30 kg trotting dog. The plate used in this dog was a narrow LC-DCP. If a broad LC-DCP had been used, the construct may have been strong enough to resist the bending moment imposed by weight bearing even with the lack of load-sharing resulting from the presence of a fracture gap at the *trans*-cortex.

203 The type I Monteggia fracture in the cat in case **201** was addressed by stabilizing the ulna with an intramedullary pin and tension band wire in the ulna (**203**).
i. List the important principles to consider when managing a Monteggia fracture.
ii. What functional differences between cats and dogs should be considered when treating this type of injury?

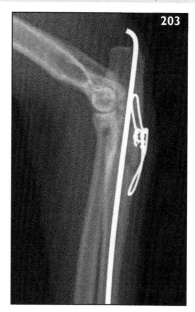

204 A 4-year-old, 3 kg male Pomeranian presented acutely non-weight bearing on the right forelimb after jumping off the sofa. On physical examination the dog held the right forelimb off the ground with the elbow flexed and adducted. The dog's right shoulder region was swollen and manipulation of the joint elicited a marked pain response. The dog was sedated and a radiograph of the right shoulder obtained (**204**).
i. What is the diagnosis?
ii. What are typical signalment and historical features of dogs affected with this condition?
iii. What structures are considered to be the primary stabilizers of the dog's scapulohumeral joint?
iv. Describe appropriate treatment options for this condition.

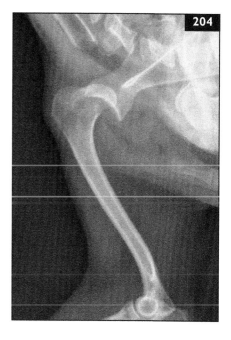

203 i. Surgical intervention is warranted, most commonly open reduction and internal fixation of the ulna using either a pin and tension band wire (**203**) or stabilization with a bone plate. The radial head must be reduced and the integrity of the annular ligament restored. In most instances ligament damage precludes repair with sutures. Therefore, the annular ligament is replaced with a synthetic prosthesis: a suture is placed through a transverse hole drilled in the ulna and circumferentially around the radial head. Alternatively, a positional screw can be placed through both the ulna and the radius to maintain the two bones in close apposition.

ii. Cats have more independent motion between the radius and ulna compared with dogs. Antebrachial pronation and supination are vital in cats for catching prey, climbing, grooming, and self-defence. If a positional screw is placed between the two bones, the screw will limit the normal range of motion and impair function. There is a high risk that the rotational movement will cause the screw to fail or the bone may fracture through the screw hole. If a screw is placed, removal should be planned once healing has occurred (e.g. typically around 6 weeks after surgery).

204 i. This dog has a medial scapulohumeral luxation.

ii. Medial scapulohumeral luxations occur most often in toy and small-breed dogs. While some luxations are congenital or developmental, most occur in middle-aged and older dogs without a history of major trauma. Many dogs have a history of chronic, progressive lameness, which may be due to joint capsule, ligament, or muscular laxity. Associated dysplastic and degenerative abnormalities of the medial glenoid fossa are often present on radiographs.

iii. No single structure is responsible for stability during all phases of joint position. Luxation is, however, only possible with complete disruption of the joint capsule and associated medial (or lateral) glenohumeral ligaments, and these structures are therefore considered the primary static shoulder joint stabilizers. Dynamic stabilizers, which are especially important during movement of the joint, consist of the five 'cuff' muscles: infraspinatus, supraspinatus, subscapularis, teres minor, and biceps brachii muscles.

iv. Appropriate management is dictated by both the etiology and the presence or absence of anatomic abnormalities of the glenoid. True traumatic luxation may be amenable to closed reduction and coaptation in a Spica splint; however, most luxations have chronic underlying soft tissue laxity and require open surgical reduction and augmentation of the medial support structures. Bicipital tendon transposition, prosthetic collateral ligament reconstruction, and capsular imbrication techniques have been described to re-establish medial scapulohumeral joint stability. If there is substantial deformation of the medial glenoid rim, scapulohumeral arthrodesis should be considered.

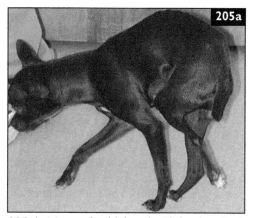
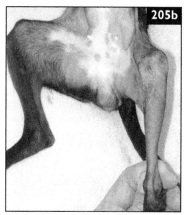

205 A 14-month-old female Chihuahua is shown walking (205a) and positioned in dorsal recumbency (205b). The dog would not bear weight on the left hindlimb, but generally used the right hindlimb when ambulating. Episodically, the dog would only bear weight on the forelimbs (assuming a 'hand-stand' posture), then would sit down suddenly and extend the right hindlimb. The dog could then stand and would again bear weight on the right hindlimb. The left stifle could not be fully extended and the left patella was displaced medially and could not be reduced (205b). The right patella was normally reduced, but was luxated whenever the dog shifted weight to the forelimbs.

i. Describe Putnam's scheme for grading patellar luxations in dogs.
ii. How would each of this dog's patellar luxations be graded according to Putnam's scheme?

206 A 4-year-old female neutered retired racing greyhound presented with a chronic left hindlimb lameness of unknown duration (206a). At presentation the dog was markedly lame and reluctant to bear full weight on the left hindlimb. A firm flexible swelling was palpated proximal to the calcaneus during the orthopedic examination.

i. What terms have been used to describe the posture that the dog is exhibiting?
ii. Describe the mechanism that causes this abnormal stance.
iii. What conditions commonly produce this posture?

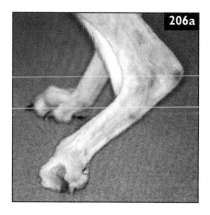

205 i. The scheme is based on a four-tier system, is useful clinically for descriptive purposes and prognosis, and can also be adapted to grade lateral patellar luxations. Grade I: the patella can be manually luxated, but relocates to the trochlear sulcus when released. Grade II: the patella is primarily situated in the trochlear groove, but can be manually luxated or intermittently spontaneously luxates during stifle flexion and extension. The patella remains luxated until it is manually reduced or the stifle is actively flexed and extended. Grade III: the patella is luxated most of the time, but can be manually reduced. The patella, however, readily reluxates when the manual pressure of reduction is released. Grade IV: the patella is luxated all the time and cannot be manually reduced even with the stifle fully extended. Various other classification systems have since been described, but most are adapted from Putnam's system.
ii. This dog would be classified as having a right grade II/IV and a left grade IV/IV medial patellar luxation.

206 i. This posture has been described as clawfoot' or 'eagle's claw'. The clawfoot stance is characterized by hyperflexion of the phalanges and is usually concurrent with increased flexion of the hock ('dropped hock').
ii. This posture is due to relative functional shortening of the intact superficial digital flexor tendon, which results from hock instability. The instability causes the hock to flex during weight bearing, which places pressure on the superficial digital flexor tendon. The resultant tension in the superficial digital flexor tendon causes the characteristic flexion of the digits.
iii. This posture is most often due to partial disruption of the gastrocnemius tendon while the superficial digital flexor tendon remains intact. Fractures of the calcaneus and proximal intertarsal subluxation or tarsometatarsal subluxation also result in a similar posture. This dog had an unusual chronic avulsion fracture of the proximal part of the calcaneus, which resulted in functional compromise of the gastrocnemius tendon (**206b**).

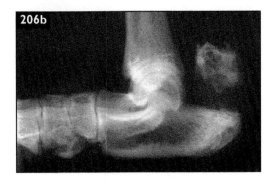

206b

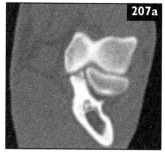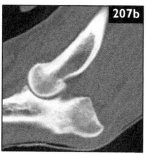

207 A 9-month-old castrated male German shepherd dog presented with a 6-week history of progressive forelimb lameness. On orthopedic examination, pain was elicited on flexion and extension of both elbows. A CT examination of both forelimbs was carried out. Medial parasagittal and axial scans of the left elbow are provided for review (207a, b).

i. Describe the pertinent tomographic abnormalities.
ii. State the diagnosis.
iii. What are the advantages of using CT, rather than plain radiographs, to evaluate dogs in this age group with suspected elbow pathology?

208 Craniocaudal radiographs of the hindlimbs of the 14-month-old female Chihuahua in case 205 are shown (208a, b). The x-ray beam has been centered on the stifles and collimated to include the hips, the stifles, and the tarsi.

i. Describe and explain the radiographic abnormalities.
ii. What surgical procedures would likely be necessary to address this dog's left hindlimb abnormalities?

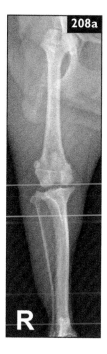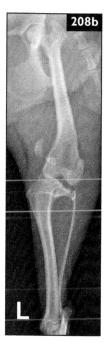

207 i. There is a discrete, triangular, irregularly marginated mineralized fragment associated with the apex of the medial coronoid process (MCP). There is moderate, irregular, periarticular new bone formation consistent with osteophyte formation involving the remainder of the MCP. The subchondral bone of the MCP is hyperattenuating, consistent with sclerosis. Although this scan is displayed in a bone window and level, the soft tissues surrounding the elbow may still be assessed and appear thickened, especially the joint capsule, which can be distinguished from the adjacent periarticular fat.

ii. Fragmented MCP with secondary degenerative joint disease.

iii. Fragmented MCP is one of a triad of developmental orthopedic diseases that affect the elbows of skeletally immature, primarily large- and giant-breed dogs, the other two diseases being ununited anconeal process and osteochondrosis or osteochondritis dissecans. CT has superior accuracy and sensitivity over radiography in identifying fragmentation of the coronoid process, especially when coupled with the results of diagnostic arthroscopy. CT scanning allows visualization of osseous and soft tissue structures without superimposition and the advent of multidetector row CT affords rapid acquisition of high-resolution data sets with sub-millimeter slice thicknesses. In addition, these data can be reformatted into sagittal and dorsal planes, increasing the utility of multidetector row CT in localizing lesions and identifying parenchymal abnormalities within the MCP. Elbow incongruity is purported to be involved in the etiopathogenesis of elbow dysplasia and CT is an accurate means of assessing joint congruency.

208 i. The right hindlimb (**208a**) is relatively normal and can be used for comparison with the left (**208b**). There is ipsilateral distal femoral varus and abnormal femoral condyle development. The left patella is luxated medially. The left tibia is rotated internally relative to the femur as this dog has a grade IV/IV luxation. Internal tibial rotation, evidenced by loss of the normal concave contours of the tibial condyles and exposure of the distal tibiofibular articulation, makes it difficult to distinguish anatomic medial displacement of the tibial tubercle from 'false' displacement due to the radiographic position. Internal tibial rotation also artifactually projects some of the normal tibial procurvatum as apparent proximal tibial valgus. An appropriately positioned craniocaudal (or caudocranial) image is required to identify medial displacement of the tibial tubercle and to accurately measure frontal plane tibial conformation.

ii. Likely procedures would include: (1) medial release of the joint capsule and quadriceps muscle group in order to reduce the patella; (2) trochleoplasty to deepen the trochlear sulcus to improve femoropatellar joint stability; (3) lateral tibial crest transposition to address presumed anatomic medial displacement of the tibial tubercle; (4) lateral capsular and retinacular imbrication to balance soft tissue tension around the patella. Corrective osteotomies of the femur or tibia may be considered, but are less commonly needed in small breeds compared with larger breeds of dog.

209 A stainless steel bone screw is shown (**209**).

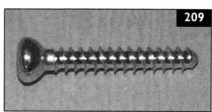

i. What stainless steel alloy is most commonly used to make this implant?
ii. What effect does reducing the carbon content have on stainless steel implants?
iii. How does cold-working of stainless steel affect an implant's material properties?
iv. What are the primary elements in this stainless steel alloy?

210 A dog is shown prepared for gait analysis (**210**).

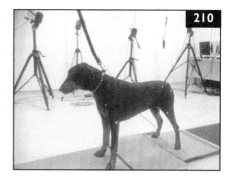

i. What two objective methods of gait assessment are to be performed on this dog?
ii. What variables are measured by these two objective methods of gait assessment?

211 A 14-month-old female chondrodystrophic dog was presented for evaluation of a weight-bearing lameness of the right hindlimb. The owner complained that the dog had an abnormal right hindlimb gait and stood with the right stifle held in an abducted position, which the owner described as a 'cowboy-like' posture. A ventrodorsal radiograph of the dog's hindlimbs is shown (**211**).

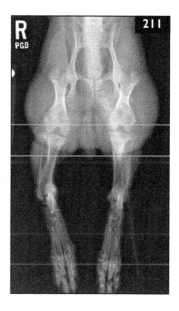

i. What is the diagnosis?
ii. Name the breed of dog most commonly affected with this condition.

209 i. Orthopedic implants are commonly made with medical grade 316L stainless steel: the 300 series alloys are austenitic stainless steel. The L indicates low carbon content.
ii. Reducing the carbon content increases corrosion resistance.
iii. Cold-working stainless steel alters the metallic crystalline lattice, resulting in increased stiffness and yield strength.
iv. The primary elements are iron, chromium, nickel, and molybdenum.

210 i. The two methods are force plate analysis and angular kinematics.
ii. Force plate analysis is a form of linear kinetic assessment that objectively measures the relative and absolute weight applied to a limb. Specifically, force plate analysis measures the subject's ground reaction forces, momentum, breaking and accelerating impulses, and velocity of a limb as the subject stands, walks, trots or runs over the plate. Angular kinematics quantifies the two- and three-dimensional displacement of limb and limb segments about the joints. It is a method of objectively assessing a subject's joint range of motion. The analysis is performed using computer software to analyze captured 'moving' images. The relative two- and three-dimensional motions of a subject's limbs can be used to objectively measure a limb's joint range of motion, amplitude, period, and frequency during various types of motion.

211 i. This dog has a varus deformity of the distal right tibia and fibula, a condition often described as pes varus.
ii. Dachshunds, as was the case in this dog. Affected dogs have eccentric premature closure of the medial portion of the distal tibial physis, which can occur bilaterally. Theoretically, the deformity could develop in any breed as a consequence of trauma that disrupts normal longitudinal growth of the medial portion of the distal tibial physis. Asynchronous medial physeal closure results in development of a subsequent varus deformity of the distal tibia and fibula. While the etiology of this physeal anomaly in dachshunds is unknown, the condition has been shown to have an autosomal mode of inheritance in this breed.

212 Identify the following pieces of equipment (212a–c) used in physical rehabilitation and the primary purpose of each therapeutic modality.

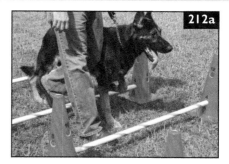

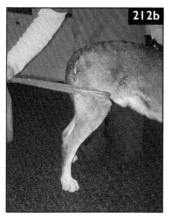

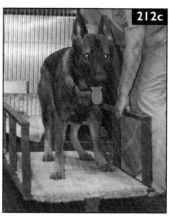

213 i. Briefly describe a plan for correcting the deformity in the dog in case 211 using the center of rotation of angulation (CORA) methodology.
ii. What osteotomy options should be considered to correct this deformity?
iii. A postoperative radiograph of this dog is shown (213a). What method of fixation was used to stabilize this dog's tibia?

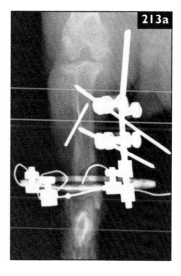

212 (a) Cavaletti rails: used to improve proprioception, increase active limb flexion, encourage limb use, and alter stride length. (b) Therabands: used for isometric muscle strengthening. (c) Wobble boards: used to encourage limb use and improve both proprioception and core strength.

213 i. Using craniocaudal view radiographs of both tibiae, lines tangential to the proximal and distal joint surfaces are created and the location of joint centers identified. On the normal tibia, a line connecting the proximal and distal joint centers is created to identify the mechanical axis. The angles created where the mechanical axis crosses the proximal and distal joint surface lines are measured (**213b**). The angles are transferred to the corresponding joint lines on the deformed tibia, positioned over the joint center, creating two new lines: the proximal and distal mechanical axes. The intersection point of the two lines on the deformed tibia represents the CORA. Deformity correction based on the CORA will result in co-linearity of the proximal and distal mechanical axes, re-establishing a normal spatial relationship between the proximal and distal joint surfaces (**213c**).
ii. A medial opening wedge osteotomy, lateral closing wedge osteotomy, or a dome osteotomy (all centered on the CORA).
iii. A hybrid circular-linear external fixator was used; these constructs are particularly useful for stabilizing the typically short, distal juxta-articular bone segment created when correcting this deformity.

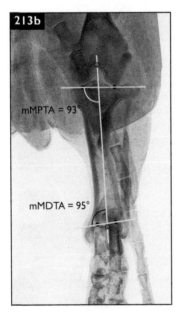
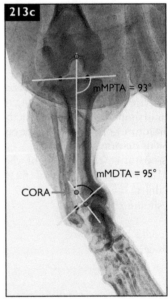

214 A 10-year-old, 38 kg male golden retriever was playing with another dog on the beach when the dog became acutely non-weight-bearing lame on the left hindlimb. On physical exam-ination the dog's left thigh was markedly swollen and pain and crepitus were elicited on manipulation of the left femur. Radiographs of the left femur were obtained (**214a, b**).

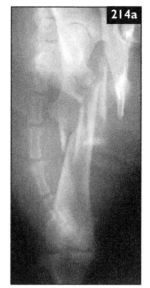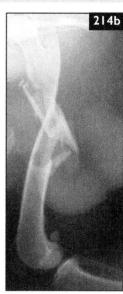

i. Describe the radiographic abnormalities, and provide a tentative diagnosis.

ii. A CBC, serum chemistry panel, and urinalysis were performed. The dog's serum alkaline phosphatase (SAP) was 213 U/l, which is 1.5 times greater than normal. What is the significance of a high SAP in this dog?

iii. What is the prognosis after repair of this fracture?

215 A 20-month-old, 32 kg male greyhound was presented with intermittent right forelimb lameness. The dog had been racing three times a week, but the dog's performance had declined over the past 4 weeks. On orthopedic examination pain was elicited on palpation of the right fourth metacarpal bone. A radiograph of the dog's right fore paw is shown (**215**).

i. Describe the abnormalities present on this radio-graph.

ii. State a diagnosis.

iii. What should the recommended treatment be for this dog?

iv. What could be the consequences if this dog con-tinues to race?

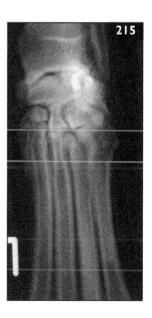

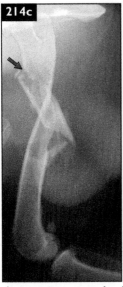

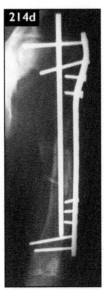

214 i. There is a highly comminuted fracture involving the proximal third of the diaphysis of the femur, with periosteal reaction and adjacent lysis at the proximal extent of the fracture (**214c**, arrow), suggesting possible pre-existing pathology predisposing to fracture. In addition, the reported traumatic incident would be unlikely to result in such a highly comminuted fracture. These historical and radiographic observations, in a 10-year-old dog, should raise suspicions that this fracture is pathologic.

ii. Elevated SAP has been shown to have prognostic significance in dogs with osteosarcoma treated with amputation followed by chemotherapy. In one study, dogs with normal SAP levels before treatment had a median survival time of 12.5 months compared with dogs with elevated SAP concentrations, which have a median survival time of 5.5 months.

iii. In a retrospective study of dogs with pathologic fractures ascribed to osteosarcoma, the fractures were stabilized in 3 dogs (survival times – 113, 109, 534 days). The fracture was stabilized using a plate-rod construct in this golden retriever and the dog was administered postoperative analgesia, but no chemotherapy. The dog used the limb immediately following surgery, but lameness worsened less than 3 weeks following surgery. The limb was re-radiographed at 4 weeks. The tumor had caused massive lysis and destruction of the proximal femur (**214d**) and the dog was euthanized.

215 i. There is increased radiodensity of the mid-diaphysis of the fourth metacarpal bone and a similar smaller area of increased radiodensity is present in the fifth metacarpal bone.

ii. This dog has metacarpal periostitis. Increased bone density occurs as a result of the response to repetitive stress, which causes microfractures in the bone. This condition occurs most commonly in young dogs subjected to extensive training and racing who are not given sufficient time to recover between events.

iii. The dog should be rested to allow the periostitis/stress fracture to heal. Training should then be gradually reinstituted and the dog should race less frequently to allow for more time to recover between races.

iv. If the dog continues to race, a hairline or complete fracture might develop, which would likely require surgical intervention.

216 A 4-year-old Persian cat was presented for recalcitrant elbow pain. The cat had periarticular mineralization around the right elbow and involving the triceps muscle. Initial surgical debridement was performed, but mineralization recurred, range of motion in the joint became markedly reduced, and the cat's pain persisted. The elbow was arthrodesed; post-operative radiographs are shown (216a, b).

i. What angle of fusion is recommended when performing an elbow arthrodesis in a cat?

ii. What postoperative complication has been associated with the use of a plate to stabilize elbow arthrodesis in cats?

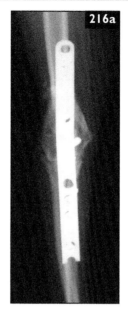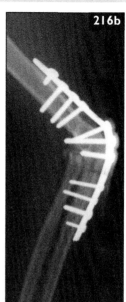

217 A 5-month-old female flat-coated retriever was presented because of persistent left hind-limb lameness. On physical examination the left stifle was painful and effused with pronounced cranial drawer. Mediolateral and caudocranial radiographs of the left stifle are shown (217a).

i. Describe the radiographic abnormalities.

ii. What is the diagnosis?

iii. How could the diagnosis be confirmed?

iv. Describe appropriate treatment for this dog.

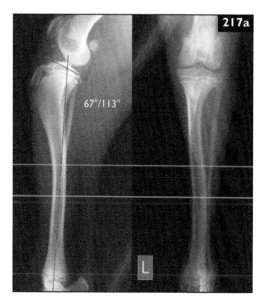

216 i. A cat's elbow should be arthrodesed at approximately 100°. The recommended angle for elbow arthrodesis in dogs is greater (between 130° and 140°). In one case series, less acute angles of fusion (120° and 135°) in two cats resulted in marked circumduction during advancement of the forelimb in the swing phase of the stride. In this cat the angle of elbow fusion was 115°.

ii. Antebrachial fracture at the distal end of the plate through the distal screw hole. In this cat, the most proximal and distal screws are monocortical screws in an attempt to reduce the stress riser effect and therefore minimize the chance of the bone fracturing adjacent to the ends of the plate. The most proximal screw hole was left empty as this end of the plate was not positioned over the humerus. The empty screw hole in the proximal ulna is the result of a stripped bone screw.

217 i. The tibia is cranially subluxated; there is joint effusion causing compression of the infrapatellar fat pad; and there is a well-marginated radiopaque body distal to the patella and in the intercondylar fossa adjacent to the lateral condyle.

ii. With pronounced drawer, effusion, and cranial tibial subluxation evident radiographically, the radiopaque body likely represents avulsion of the origin of the CrCL.

iii. With arthroscopy or via an arthrotomy.

iv. If the avulsion is recent and the ligament has not contracted, the osteochondral fragment can be reattached using a screw and washer or with orthopedic wire

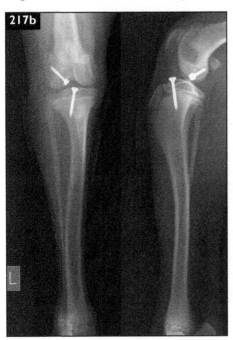

passed through two bone tunnels. Partial tibial epiphysiodesis was also performed in this dog. A screw was inserted via a lateral parapatellar approach into the center of the cranial aspect of the tibial plateau under fluoroscopic guidance. If performed between 5 and 6.5 months of age (7 months in giant breeds), this technique will gradually reduce the slope of the tibial plateau (**217b**) and effectively eliminate tibial thrust; there is cessation of growth of the cranial plateau and continued growth of the caudal plateau.

218 A 7-month-old female Jack Russell terrier presented with a marked left forelimb lameness of gradual onset and 6-weeks chronicity. The dog lived on a farm with a normal sibling and the dogs had a very active lifestyle. On orthopedic examination the anatomy of the left shoulder was palpably abnormal. Manipulation of the scapulohumeral joint elicited crepitus and a pain response. Radiographs of the left scapulohumeral joint were obtained (**218a, b**).

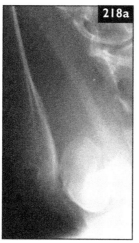
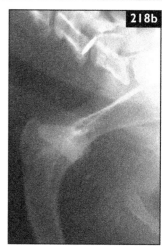

i. What is the diagnosis?
ii. What is the best treatment option in this dog taking into account its active lifestyle?
iii. How successful is the recommended procedure?

219 A 5-year-old male Weimaraner is shown undergoing a tibial plateau leveling osteotomy procedure to address CrCL insufficiency (**219**). What advice regarding environmental modifications should be given to this dog's owner so that the dog's activity can be appropriately managed during the early postoperative convalescent period?

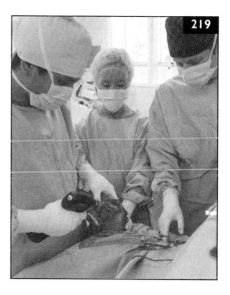

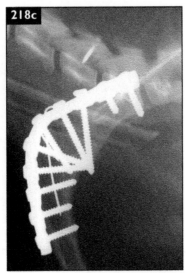

218 i. This dog has a congenital (developmental) shoulder luxation (also termed glenoid dysplasia). The glenoid does not have a normal concave conformation, suggesting that the humeral head has been dislocated for some time, which would hinder normal glenoid development.

ii. The most reasonable treatment option for this dog would be a scapulohumeral arthrodesis (218c). The shoulder was fused at a normal standing angle measured from the contralateral shoulder joint (typically 105–110°).

iii. Shoulder arthrodesis has a good success rate as increased motion of the scapula along the thorax compensates for the loss of motion in the arthrodesed shoulder. In one study the results were good-to-excellent in 87% of the 14 cases in which arthrodesis was performed. This Jack Russell was able to lead a normal active lifestyle after shoulder arthrodesis.

219 Environmental modifications advisable during the early postoperative convalescent period might include: using ramps so the dog will not have to navigate stairs; installing baby gates to restrict the dog to specific areas in the house; and not allowing the dog to walk on slippery surfaces such as wooden or tile floors. The dog should be confined in a kennel when unsupervised and the dog's activity outdoors should be restricted to short walks on a leash. A sling, positioned under the dog's abdomen, may be used to support the dog when walking.

220 Dogs involved in agility often sustain injuries. Veterinarians should have a solid grasp on these sports-related injuries, including how they are sustained, as well as how to treat or potentially prevent such injuries. Therefore, veterinarians treating dogs engaged in agility should have a basic understanding of the sport. Each agility course is different, but contains the same basic types of obstacle: jumps, tunnels, contact obstacles, weave poles, and a pause table or box.

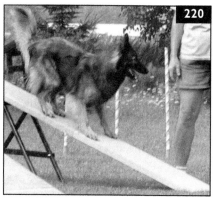

i. What is the significance of the yellow areas on this agility obstacle, and which pieces of agility equipment have these yellow areas (220)?
ii. What is an agility pause table?
iii. What are weave poles?

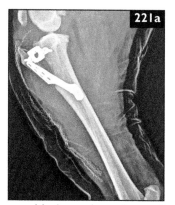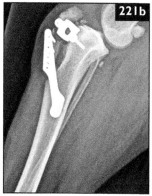

221 A 5-year-old chow chow dog underwent a tibial tuberosity advancement procedure to address a left CrCL injury. An immediate postoperative lateral radiograph is shown (221a). The dog had steadily improved on the limb during the first 3 weeks following surgery, but became acutely lame on the left hindlimb after climbing a flight of stairs. A 4-week postoperative lateral view radiograph is shown (221b).

i. What complications are evident on the 4-week postoperative radiograph?
ii. How common is this complication following tibial tuberosity advancement in dogs?
iii. What surgical technical errors may have predisposed this dog to develop this postoperative complication?

220 i. Some dog agility obstacles are called contact obstacles, because they include yellow contact zones on both ends. To successfully negotiate these obstacles, the dog must place at least one digit in the contact zone. Contact zone rules were created in an effort to protect dogs from injuries. Without the contact zones, dogs might be tempted to jump off an obstacle from too great a height or attempt to mount an obstacle in an unsafe manner. Agility equipment that includes contact zones are the A-frame, the dog walk, and the see-saw.

ii. An agility pause table is a variable height, elevated, 1 m² platform onto which the dog must jump and pause and, depending on the agility organization, may have to sit or lie down for 5 seconds.

iii. Weave poles consist of a series of 5–12 upright poles, which are set up and negotiated in a similar manner to a slalom race. The poles are just under a meter in height and are spaced 45–60 cm apart depending on the event's sponsoring organization. Dogs must weave through the poles and cannot skip a pole. For many dogs, weave poles are one of the most difficult obstacles to master.

221 i. There is a fracture of the tibial tuberosity with dorsal displacement of the proximal portion of the tuberosity. The cage is displaced and there is failure of the most proximal prong of the plate.

ii. In a retrospective study tibial tuberosity fractures accounted for only 1.8% of all reported complications. In that study, 59% of dogs developed one or more postoperative complications, but most complications were minor, such as incisional swelling or bruising.

iii. While some tibial tuberosity fractures can be attributed to excessive physical activity of the dog during the early postoperative convalescent period, most can be ascribed to technical errors made during surgery. On review of this dog's immediate postoperative radiograph, the four-pronged plate that was selected was too short and the cage was placed too distal in the osteotomy. Positioning the cage distally leaves the proximal aspect of the tibial tuberosity unsupported and results in a stress riser effect that can predispose the tibial tuberosity to fracture. While this dog had an acute onset of an obvious lameness, some dogs that fracture the tibial tuberosity exhibit only a mild, transient lameness and minimally displaced fractures will often achieve union without surgical intervention.

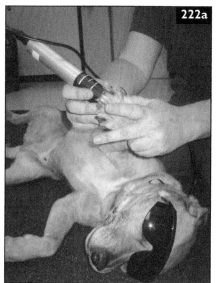

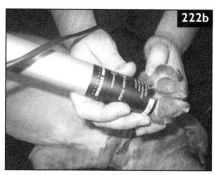

222 This 9-year-old, 27 kg male mixed-breed dog is being treated for a lameness ascribed to chronic meta-carpophalangeal sesamoid disease (**222a, b**).

i. What modality is being used to treat this dog?

ii. Describe how this therapeutic modality mediates pain relief and stimulates wound healing.

iii. How does wavelength affect depth of tissue penetration?

223 A 12-year-old male toy poodle is presented because over the past 4 months the dog has become reluctant to ambulate. On physical exam-ination the dog is noted to have a palmigrade stance in both forelimbs. There is pal-pable soft tissue swelling with crepitus elicited on manipu-lation of both carpi and tarsi. Radiographs of the left carpus are shown (**223a, b**).

i. Describe the radiographic abnormalities.

ii. What differential diagnoses should be considered for this dog?

iii. What additional diagnostic procedures should be performed?

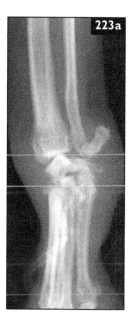

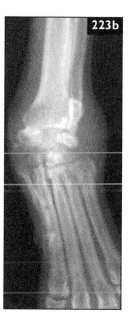

222 i. This dog is being treated with a therapeutic laser.

ii. Photons are emitted from the laser and absorbed by cytochrome C in the mitochondria, resulting in increased cellular metabolism and adenosine triphosphate production. Adenosine triphosphate-dependent membrane pumps are stabilized and cellular proliferation is increased. Pain relief is ascribed to decreased production of inflammatory mediators, such as prostaglandin E_2, tumor necrosis factor, and cyclo-oxygenase-2, as well as reduced edema formation. Other potential mechanisms of pain relief may include increased endogenous opioid production and reduced nerve conduction velocity. Wound healing is enhanced through increased fibroblast proliferation, differentiation, and collagen deposition as well as enhanced neovascularization.

iii. The depth of penetration is directly related to laser wavelength. Wavelengths in the red light spectrum (630–650 nm) will target superficial tissue (wounds), while longer wavelengths (800–905 nm; infrared spectrum) are indicated for treating deeper tissue structures.

223 i. There are focal areas of periarticular osteolysis in the cuboidal carpal bones and proximal metacarpal bones. The middle carpal and carpometacarpal joints are narrowed and indistinct. Moderate soft tissue swelling of the carpus is present. These radiographic abnormalities are consistent with the dog having a chronic severe erosive arthropathy.

ii. With swelling and crepitus reported in both carpi and tarsi, a polyarthropathy is considered most likely. Polyarthropathies can be secondary to tick-borne diseases such as rickettsiosis, Lyme disease, or ehrlichiosis or can be caused be infectious arthritis caused by organisms such as *Leishmania* spp. These diseases have regional geographic distributions and therefore should be considered if the dog is from, or has been to, an area where these diseases are endemic. Erosive polyarthropathies are immune mediated in many dogs, particularly small-breed dogs. Unfortunately, an underlying etiology is infrequently identified and most erosive polyarthropathies are considered idiopathic.

iii. Radiographs of additional affected joints should be obtained. Arthrocentesis of several affected joints should be performed with synovial fluid submitted for cytology as well as culture and sensitivity. A CBC, chemistry, and urinalysis are useful for determining systemic involvement, and consideration should be given to obtaining thoracic and abdominal radiographs. In addition, performing serology for rheumatoid factor and tick-borne diseases should be considered.

224 Immediate postoperative radiographs are shown of the stifle of an 11-month-old wheaten terrier that had undergone a tibial tuberosity transposition as a component of surgery to correct a medial patellar luxation (224a, b).
i. Name the fixation technique used to stabilize the transposed tibial tuberosity.
ii. What is the biomechanical rationale for using this fixation technique?
iii. Ideally, how should the pins be oriented relative to the osteotomy?
iv. What component of this stabilization technique has the greatest effect on the strength of fixation?

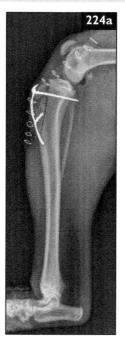
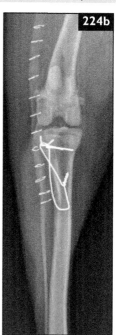

225 A 7-year-old Borzoi presented with a 3-week history of left forelimb lameness. Radiographs of the right antebrachium revealed a lytic lesion affecting the distal metaphysis of the radius. There was also periosteal new bone formation adjacent to this lesion. A bone scan of both antebrachii is shown with the proximal portion of the limbs positioned at the top of the image and the distal portion of the limbs positioned at the bottom of the image (225).
i. Describe the abnormalities and state the most likely diagnosis.
ii. Given the most likely diagnosis, how has this bone scan been helpful in the diagnostic work-up?

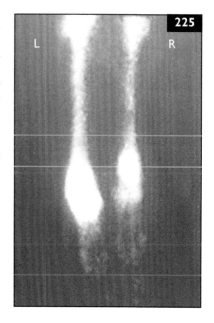

224 i. Pin and tension band wire fixation.

ii. Pin and tension band wire fixation is used to convert distractive forces into compressive forces. In this situation, the quadriceps muscles exert a tensile force on the tibial tuberosity via the patellar tendon. This force, which has both magnitude and direction and thus is a vector, acts to distract the tibial tuberosity proximally. Tension develops in the figure-of-eight tension band wire, which opposes the pull of the quadriceps mechanism, creating a vector force in the opposite direction. The resultant vector of these two opposing forces is directed along the Kirschner wires, thus compressing the osteotomy.

iii. The Kirschner wires should be placed parallel to each other and oriented perpendicular to the osteotomy. This will minimize resistance to the resulting compressive force.

iv. Although both the Kirschner wire diameter and the diameter of the tension band wire affect the strength of the stabilization, the diameter of the latter has the greater effect. Applying the wire in a figure-of-eight pattern results in a stronger fixation than placing the wire in an uncrossed, circular pattern. The location of the distal hole has little effect on fixation strength.

225 i. There is an accumulation of technetium-99m-methylene diphosphonate seen in both distal radial metaphyses, more so in the left radius. The most likely diagnosis is bilateral radial osteosarcoma.

ii. As there was no clinical evidence of pain or lameness in the right forelimb, this bone scan has revealed an additional osteosarcoma lesion. When a second osteosarcoma lesion is found in the metaphysis of a different long bone, this lesion is typically referred to as a 'synchronous primary tumor'. This scenario is in contrast to finding a second lesion in a rib, for example, which would be deemed a metastatic focus (stage III for canine osteosarcoma). The prognosis for dogs with stage III osteosarcoma has been shown to be significantly worse than for dogs that do not have detectable metastasis at the time of diagnosis. While it is not known whether this 'synchronous' tumor represents metastasis or an independent primary neoplastic process or whether the prognosis is worse than it would be for a dog with a solitary lesion, finding a second lesion in the contralateral radius has obvious implications with respect to therapeutic planning. This dog was initially presented as a potential candidate for limb-sparing surgery, but the owner opted for palliative treatment after learning of the second lesion.

226 This image (**226**) shows the medial aspect of the right stifle of a 4-year-old, 41 kg female mastiff that had a tibial plateau leveling osteotomy performed 6 days ago. The dog has placed only a limited amount of weight on the right hindlimb since surgery. On physical examination, the limb had diffuse edematous swelling involving and distal

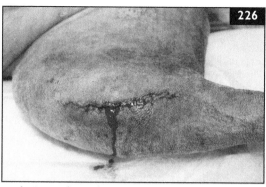

to the stifle and there was purulent drainage from the incision.
i. Describe how surgical site infections (infections that develop anywhere in the operative field following surgical intervention) are classified according to United States Centers for Disease Control guidelines.
ii. What is the reported incidence of surgical site infection in clean general surgery and in clean orthopedic surgery?
iii. List potential risk factors for the development of surgical site infection.

227 A humeral fracture in a 6-month-old female intact Saluki was stabilized with a 6 mm interlocking nail.
i. What complication is evident on these postoperative radiographs (**227a, b**)?
ii. How can complications be minimized when placing an interlocking nail to stabilize diaphyseal humeral fractures in dogs?

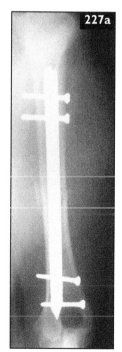
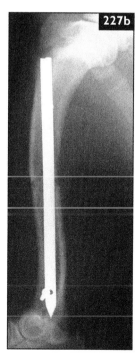

226 i. Surgical site infections are broadly classified into incisional (superficial or deep) and organ or cavity infections. Superficial incisional infections are limited to the skin or subcutaneous tissue and develop within 30 days of surgical intervention. Deep incisional infections extend into underlying tissues such as muscle or fascia and develop within 30 days of surgical intervention if implants were not placed at the time of surgery, or within 1 year if an implant was placed at surgery. Organ or cavity infections can develop in any location of the body manipulated during surgery other than skin, muscle, or fascia, and develop within 30 days of surgical intervention if implants were not placed at the time of surgery, or within 1 year if an implant was placed at surgery.
ii. The incidence ranges from 2% to 4.8% for clean surgical wounds in dogs and cats; 7.1% in clean orthopedic procedures in dogs.
iii. Risk factors include clipping of the skin anytime other than immediately prior to surgery, the use of propofol as an anesthetic induction agent, increasing duration of anesthesia and surgery, increasing number of persons in the operating room, and a dirty surgical site. Corporeal factors such as the animal undergoing surgery being an intact male or the animal having an endocrinopathy have also been associated with an increased risk of surgical site infection.

227 i. The distal screw was not placed through the hole in the nail.
ii. To decrease the occurrence of complications during nail placement, the largest diameter nail that can be accommodated by the medullary canal should be selected. The set screw, which secures the extension to the nail, and the knurled handle, which secures the jig to the extension, need to be tight. If these attachments are not tight, or too much pressure is applied to the jig while drilling the holes for the locking implants, the jig can drift and the holes in the bone may not align with the holes in the nail, as occurred in this dog. The holes in the nail should not be positioned at or adjacent to the fracture site in order to reduce the chance of nail breakage. Bolts should be used instead of screws. Bolts have a larger core diameter than corresponding diameter screws and are less susceptible to cyclic failure. If only one locking implant (screw or bolt) is placed in the proximal humerus, that implant should be placed distal to the greater tubercle so the locking implant engages dense cortical bone; this reduces the risk of implant loosening and subsequent fracture collapse. In problematic fractures, consideration can be given to adjunctive stabilization such as articulating the nail with an external fixator or using hybrid interlocking nail bolt/external skeletal fixator pins, or using an alternative implant system altogether.

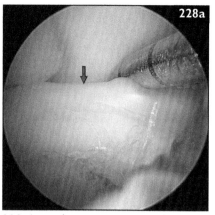
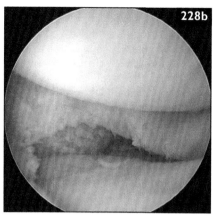

228 An arthroscopic image of the caudal horn of a dog's medial meniscus that has sustained a vertical longitudinal tear is shown (**228a**, arrow). A partial meniscectomy was performed to remove the damaged parenchyma (**228b**, post partial meniscectomy).
i. What is the effect of performing a partial medial meniscectomy on femorotibial contact pressures and meniscal strain?
ii. Why is meniscal function dependent on this structure's viscoelastic properties?

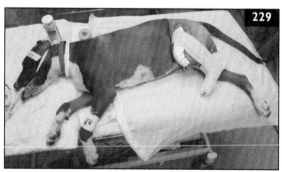

229 A 10-month-old dog had a bandage placed on its hindlimb following open reduction and stabilization of a distal femoral fracture (**229**).
i. Name this coaptation bandage.
ii. Describe the purpose of applying this bandage following open reduction and internal fixation of a femoral fracture.

228 i. Partial meniscectomy involves removing the axial portion of the meniscus. When pathology is confined to the axial portion of the meniscus, the peripheral rim of meniscal parenchyma as well as the cranial and caudal meniscotibial ligaments can be preserved. Excising 30% of the width from the axial circumference of the meniscus has no significant effect on contact mechanics. Hemimeniscectomy, in which the entire caudal horn of the medial meniscus is excised, results in an 87% increase in peak contact pressures in the medial compartment. Excising 30% of the meniscus results in a 38% decrease in medial meniscal strain, and excising 75% of the meniscus results in a 69% decrease in medial meniscal strain.
ii. The menisci are composed of fibrocartilage with a composition of 75% water and 25% collagen. When loaded, water is forced to flow through the matrix and redistribute within or effuse from the parenchyma. The high frictional drag forces associated with the water flow through the porous-permeable solid matrix give rise to time-dependent viscoelastic behaviors such as creep and stress relaxation. The significance of the viscoelastic behavior of the meniscus is that when the joint is loaded for long periods, the contact area increases, thereby reducing the stress per unit area of the articular cartilage. Proteoglycan content influences the viscoelastic behavior of the meniscus because the highly polar glycosaminoglycan chains bind water and counteract fluid flow.

229 i. A 90/90 flexion bandage has been placed on this dog's hindlimb.
ii. The function of a 90/90 flexion bandage is to maintain the stifle in flexion and the quadriceps muscle group in an elongated position. The name 90/90 is derived from the positioning of the stifle and hock joints, which are maintained in approximately 90° flexion. The bandage is applied to prevent the development of quadriceps contracture (also referred to as quadriceps tie-down), a debilitating form of fracture disease most commonly associated with distal diaphyseal or physeal femoral fractures in skeletally immature dogs and cats. This bandage is generally applied following open reduction and internal fixation of femoral fractures in skeletally immature animals to maintain the quadriceps muscles in an extended position. The bandage is typically maintained for 5–7 days postoperatively.

230 An 8-year-old male Labrador retriever presented initially with a history of mild intermittent lameness of the left forelimb of 12 weeks' duration. During the orthopedic examination, pain was elicited on manipulation of the left carpus, but there was no appreciable swelling of the joint. The dog was treated with exercise restriction and administration of an NSAID. The dog initially improved, but 12 weeks later re-presented with an acute-onset marked lameness of the left forelimb. Pain and swelling were isolated to the left carpus. Carpal radiographs were obtained (**230a, b**).

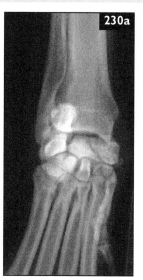 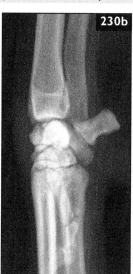

i. What is the diagnosis?
ii. What is the proposed etiology of this condition?
iii. How should this dog be treated?
iv. In what breeds has this condition most commonly been reported?

231 A 7-year-old female German shepherd dog that worked as a guide dog for a blind person presented with a 6-month history of an intermittent weight-bearing lameness of the right forelimb. The dog wore a harness when working and the owner could appreciate an asymmetry in the dog's gait with uneven pull. Orthopedic examination revealed mild resentment to right shoulder manipulation and palpation over the greater tubercle, but no other abnormalities. A mediolateral radiograph of the right scapulohumeral joint is shown (**231a**).

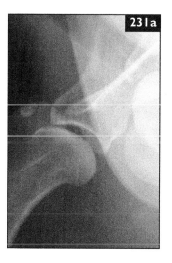

i. What abnormality is present on the radiograph?
ii. What additional radiographic view would be most useful to localize the lesion?
iii. What is the proposed pathogenesis for this lesion?
iv. How often is this lesion seen in shoulder radiographs of dogs that are not lame?
v. What is the recommended treatment for this condition?

230 i. This dog has a fracture of the radial carpal bone.

ii. The radial carpal bone develops from three separate centers of ossification and one proposal suggests that these centers do not fuse. The cartilage remnants predispose the radiocarpal bone to fracture through these areas of incomplete ossification. An alternative possibility is that the fracture is a stress fracture, as fractures have been seen in bones that had a normal appearance on prior radiographs. The primary fracture line most commonly extends in a proximolateral-to-distomedial direction (**230a**). A small dorsal fragment was also recognized in this dog (**230b**). The bone usually fractures into three pieces with the fragments or fracture surfaces appearing yellow and sclerotic at surgery, consistent with a chronic fracture.

iii. Although reduction and stabilization of these fractures using interfragmentary compression have been attempted, results have uniformly been poor, with most fractures failing to obtain union. Pancarpal arthrodesis has been advocated as a primary treatment for radiocarpal bone fractures, particularly chronic fractures, because of the guarded prognosis associated with repair.

iv. The breeds most commonly reported include boxers, Labrador retrievers and springer spaniels.

231 i. There is a small area of mineralization in the region of the tendon of insertion of the supraspinatus muscle.

ii. A cranioproximal-to-craniodistal view of the bicipital groove can help determine whether the area of mineralization may impinge on the biceps brachii tendon (**231b**).

iii. The cause of supraspinatus mineralization is not proven, but various theories exist including aging, overuse, trauma, and hypoxia secondary to hypovascularity of the supraspinatus tendon. At the point that the supraspinatus tendon crosses over the greater tubercle, vascular compromise may cause hypoxia and promote chondroid metaplasia and soft tissue mineralization.

iv. In one study, there were six dogs with bilateral radiographic signs of calcifying

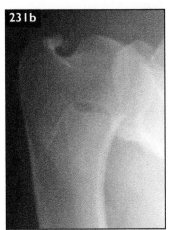

tendinopathy, although the dogs only had unilateral lameness. In another study, 11/12 dogs with bilateral abnormalities only had unilateral lameness.

v. Surgical excision of the affected portion of the tendon resulted in good limb function in 16/19 dogs with follow-up in one study. This German shepherd dog was treated by surgical excision of the mineralized parenchyma. The lameness resolved and the dog was able to return to being a fully functional guide dog.

232 A 5-year-old male springer spaniel presented with a right forelimb lameness that the owner ascribed to the dog perpetually digging in the garden. On physical examination, there was swelling localized to the medial aspect of the right carpus. Mild pain could be elicited on flexion of the right carpus and firm direct palpation over the swelling. Radiographs of both carpi were obtained (232a, right; 232b, left).

i. State the most likely diagnosis.

ii. Describe appropriate treatment options for this dog.

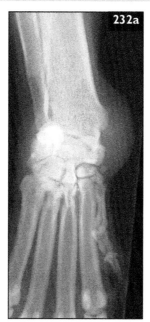
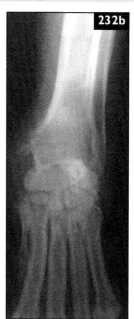

233 A procedure developed for extracapsular stabilization of CrCL-deficient stifles in dogs is illustrated (233).

i. Name the procedure.

ii. What are the reported advantages of this stabilization method compared with the traditional lateral fabellotibial suture stabilization methods?

iii. What are the potential disadvantages associated with this procedure?

iv. Describe the anatomic landmarks recommended for initiating the femoral and tibial tunnels on the lateral aspect of the stifle.

v. What adjacent anatomic structures must be protected when drilling the tibial tunnel in preparation for placement of the prosthesis?

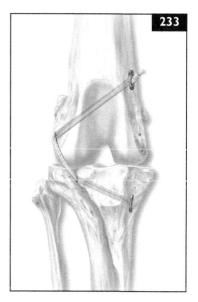

232 i. This dog has stenosing tenosynovitis of the abductor pollicus longus tendon. The condition causes chronic forelimb lameness in dogs. The lesion is similar to de Quervain's tenosynovitis in people and is thought to be caused by repetitive movements of the carpus. Dogs usually have a firm soft tissue swelling medial and proximal to the carpus. Radiographs of the carpus are characterized by a deep radiolucent medial radial sulcus and osseous proliferations medial and slightly cranial to the distal radius. Ultrasonographic examination of the swelling medial to the carpus is characterized by an irregular hypoechoic abductor pollicis longus tendon. The abductor pollicis longus tendon sheaths may be fluid filled and all tendon sheaths are thickened. Enthesopathy of the abductor pollicis longus tendon is present in some dogs.

ii. Conservative management consisting of exercise restriction and avoiding digging should be initially instituted. If these measures are not successful, steroids (methylprednisolone acetate) can be injected around the tendon. Finally, if the lameness does not resolve, surgical release of the tendon from its groove can be done by incising the retaining retinaculum.

233 i. The TightRope CCL, which utilizes multifilament polyethylene fibertape passed through femoral and tibial bone tunnels as a lateral extracapsular prosthesis. The prosthesis is secured medially on both the femur and tibia using a toggle and button, respectively.

ii. A correctly placed TightRope CCL prosthesis is more isometric than a traditional fabellotibial suture. It provides bone-to-bone fixation of the prosthesis, which provides stronger fixation and allows for less plastic deformation in the system. The TightRope CCL was developed to be inserted in a minimally invasive manner.

iii. Use of a braided non-absorbable material increases the potential of post-operative infection. The positions of the bone tunnels do not yield a truly isometric prosthesis with respect to stifle kinematics, so some cyclic elongation of the material may occur.

iv. The femoral bone tunnel should be initiated immediately distal to the lateral fabellofemoral condylar junction, 2 mm cranial to the caudal surface of the lateral femoral condyle. The tibial bone tunnel should be initiated in the caudal aspect of the muscular groove of the tibia, 2 mm distal to the articular surface of the tibia.

v. The long digital extensor tendon, the caudal band of the sartorius muscle, and the medial collateral ligament.

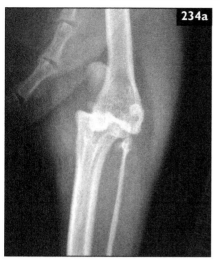
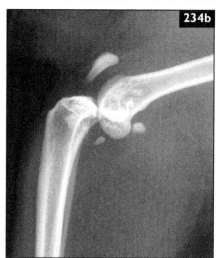

234 Lateral and craniocaudal radiographs (234a, b) of the left stifle of a 6-year-old male cat that was found by the owner stuck hanging in a chain link fence by this limb are shown.
i. Describe this cat's injury.
ii. What would be the recommended treatment for this cat?

235 An 8-year-old mixed-breed dog was presented for evaluation of a right forelimb lameness. The lameness was first noted 4 weeks earlier and the severity of the lameness had progressed to the point that the dog now only intermittently placed weight on the affected limb. During the orthopedic examination a pigmented interdigital mass was found between the third and fourth digits (235a). Cytological evaluation of an aspirate of the mass was characterized by a loosely arranged population of pleomorphic cells that contained variable numbers of dark green-to-black, intracytoplasmic granules.
i. What is the most likely diagnosis?
ii. Discuss the biological behavior of this tumor and the diagnostic staging that should be performed.
iii. Describe appropriate treatment.

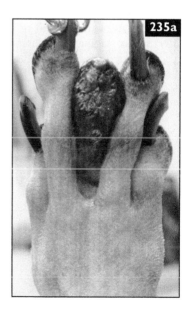

234 i. The stifle is luxated. Stifle luxations are typically the result of multiple ligamentous injuries leading to gross instability, and the injury is often referred to as a deranged stifle. The medial collateral ligament and both cruciate ligaments are often ruptured, although in some animals the lateral collateral ligament is also damaged. Concurrent injury to the joint capsule, menisci, and periarticular muscles and tendons may also be present.

ii. Treatment should begin with surgical exploration of the joint to assess the ligamentous structures, articular cartilage, and menisci. Severely damaged structures are excised. The joint is lavaged and then stabilized using either a transarticular pinning method, extracapsular suture stabilization, and/or a transarticular external fixator. Arthrodesis can be considered if damage to the articular cartilage is severe, reconstruction of the supporting ligamentous structures is impossible, or if the luxation is chronic and untreated. Amputation may even be considered if severe vascular compromise or neurologic injury is present.

235 i. Based on the gross appearance and the cytologic description, this mass is most likely a malignant melanoma.

ii. While melanomas of the haired skin are generally benign, tumors involving the digits or nail bed usually have a more aggressive behavior. In addition to performing cytology of an aspirate from the primary tumor, the local lymph node should be aspirated, even if the node is not enlarged, to evaluate for metastatic disease. Additionally, thoracic radiographs should be performed to evaluate for evidence of pulmonary metastatic disease. Ideally, CT of the lungs would also be performed, as it is more sensitive for detection of pulmonary metastases.

iii. This dog should be treated with partial amputation of the paw. Consideration should be given to removal of the ipsilateral popliteal lymph node, which will allow proper staging of the tumor. Removal of the lymph node may also reduce the

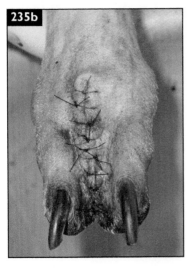

residual tumor burden, which may improve the efficacy of adjuvant therapy, such as administration of a melanoma vaccine. While there is still controversy regarding the efficacy of immunotherapy in dogs with malignant melanoma, this option is often offered to clients. This dog was treated by amputation of digits III and IV together with the interdigital mass (**235b**).

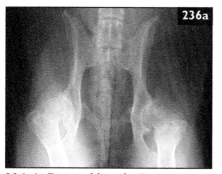
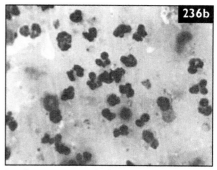

236 A 7-year-old male Bernese mountain dog presented for evaluation of a non-weight-bearing left hindlimb lameness of 3 days' duration. On physical examination, marked pain was elicited on manipulation of the left coxofemoral joint. The dog had a history of diarrhea 2 weeks prior to the occurrence of lameness. A ventrodorsal radiograph of the extended hips were taken with the dog anesthetized (**236a**). This shows marked degenerative joint disease, with periarticular osteophytosis, joint mice, and hip subluxation, likely secondary to hip dysplasia. Joint fluid was aspirated from the left hip and submitted for cytologic examination (**236b**), culture, and sensitivity.

i. Develop a list of differential diagnoses that should be considered with a dog presenting with this history and physical examination abnormalities.
ii. Describe the cytologic abnormalities and state the most likely cause of this dog's acute-onset lameness.
iii. What is the prognosis for this dog achieving a full recovery?

237 A 7-year-old female spayed rottweiler is presented for difficulty rising and climbing steps and is increasingly reluctant to exercise. The dog has advanced osteoarthritis of both elbows secondary to elbow dysplasia, which was addressed arthroscopically at 11 months of age. The dog also had bilateral tibial plateau leveling osteotomies several years ago to address CrCL insufficiency. On physical examination there were palpable abnormalities in both elbows and both stifles and pain could be elicited in these joints consistent with chronic arthritis. The dog was also markedly obese (**237**). Biochemistry and urinary profiles are within normal limits.

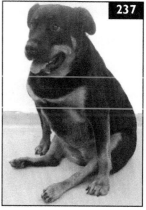

i. What advice should be given to the client regarding their dog's weight?
ii. What obstacles are inherent to implementing a weight loss program?
iii. How should this dog's weight loss program be structured?

236 i. Differential diagnoses should include luxation, fracture, neoplasia, sepsis, and acute inflammation associated with trauma such as a sprain. Degenerative joint disease and osteoarthritis of the hip are unlikely to cause acute pain and non-weight-bearing lameness unless there has been an acute exacerbating inflammatory event such as infection or a sprain of a chronically arthritic joint.

ii. The joint fluid contains a high percentage of neutrophils with foamy cytoplasm. Although organisms are not present, the high predominance of neutrophils in association with this dog's history and clinical abnormalities make septic arthritis the most likely diagnosis.

iii. The prognosis is guarded. Dogs often develop septic arthritis in joints with pre-existing osteoarthritic changes, as was the case in this dog. In this dog, synovial fluid was injected into blood culture medium in an aseptic manner immediately after arthrocentesis. *Escherichia coli* was cultured. A 6-week course of cephalexin was administered based on the results of the antibiotic sensitivity. The lameness improved within 48 hours and after 6 weeks the owner felt that the dog's function was satisfactory. Surgical options such as femoral head and neck excision had been discussed with the owner if pain and lameness persisted or function deteriorated.

237 i. The client needs to be convinced of the serious consequences associated with obesity and a program implemented to reduce their dog's weight. The advantages of weight reduction and the adverse effects of obesity and associated diseases must be explained. Discussion can center around longevity, quality of life, and the owner's responsibility to keep their dog in a healthy condition.

ii. Owners are often not aware, or are in denial, that their pet is overweight. It is the veterinarian's responsibility to identify the problem, convince owners of its seriousness, and motivate them to implement a dietary and lifestyle change. Complicating the situation is the fact that owners of obese dogs are often obese and inactive. Weight loss will not occur unless owners recognize the problem and are willing to take corrective steps.

iii. Formulation of a program for achieving weight reduction consists of: (1) setting a goal for the amount of weight to lose; (2) calculating a precise daily calorie intake; (3) selecting a specific food and feeding method; (4) defining exercise requirements; (5) monitoring the progress of weight loss; (6) adjusting calories, food, and exercise as necessary; and (7) stabilizing the dog's calorie intake as the dog loses weight to ensure that weight is not regained.

238 A 1-year-old spayed female Great Pyrenees mountain dog (238a) was evaluated because the dog had difficulty rising and had an abnormal hindlimb gait. The owners first noted these problems when the dog was 6 months of age. During physical examination the dog shifted the majority of its weight forward to the forelimbs both while standing and when walking. The dog's hindlimbs had a 'knock-kneed' appearance (genu valgum) when viewed from behind. Grade III/IV lateral patellar luxations were present in both stifles. The dog also had external torsion of the distal hindlimbs arising in the tarsometatarsal region. A craniocaudal radiograph of the right femur is shown (238b).

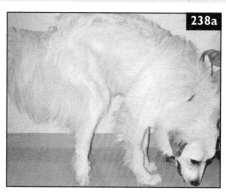

i. Describe the radiographic abnormalities.
ii. The dog underwent surgery and during exploration of the right stifle, a Steinmann pin (238c) was placed in alignment with the anatomic longitudinal axis of the dog's femoral sulcus.

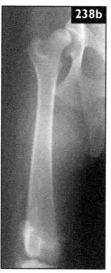

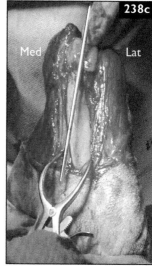

What femoral conformational abnormality is most evident in this image?

239 A screw and plate are shown (239).
i. Name the plate pictured in this image.
ii. Describe the plate's advantageous properties with respect to the implant's intended use.

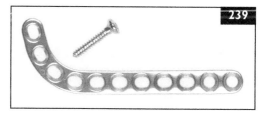

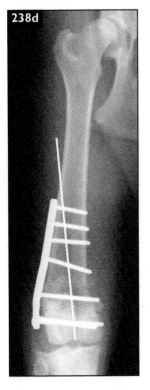

238d

238 i. The femur is slightly externally rotated as evidenced by the prominent lesser trochanter, complete superimposition of the lateral fabella on the distal femur, and the absence of medial fabella bisection by the medial femoral cortex. Generally, this radiographic position artifactually increases apparent femoral varus (or in this dog, decreased valgus) and lateralizes the patella. Even though this radiograph is poorly positioned, distal femoral valgus is evident and the patella is luxated laterally, consistent with the physical examination. There is also subluxation of the femoral head and mild osteophyte formation along the femoral neck.

ii. Distal femoral valgus was confirmed at surgery by placing the Steinmann pin in alignment with the longitudinal axis of the femoral trochlear sulcus (238c). The pin clearly extends medial to the femoral diaphysis. Normal dogs have a degree of distal femoral varus, and a line representing the distal femoral anatomic axis would extend proximally towards the lateral margin of the greater trochanter, as seen in this dog's postoperative radiograph, in which the distal femoral conformation was normalized by performing a closing wedge ostectomy, stabilized with a distal femoral osteotomy plate (238d).

239 i. A femoral supracondylar plate.
ii. The plate is designed for the stabilization of distal femoral fractures in cats: the curved or 'hockey stick' shape facilitates application of the plate to the femoral condyle, allowing placement of an increased number of screws in the condylar segment compared with the number of screws that could be placed if a conventional straight plate were applied. The plate shown is the short version; a longer plate is available that can extend to the proximal metaphyseal region of a cat's femur and can be used to stabilize supracondylar fractures with diaphyseal involvement.

240 An 18-month-old, 48 kg male entire Anatolian shepherd dog was presented with bilateral hindlimb conformational abnormalities, which were worse in the right hindlimb. The owner presented the dog for treatment when the dog was 10 months of age. Mediolateral and craniocaudal radiographs of the dog's right hindlimb were obtained (240a, b). The dog's limb prepared for corrective surgery is shown (240c).

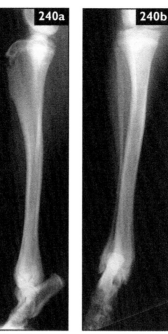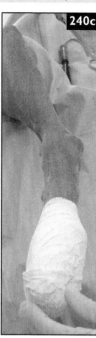

i. What is the diagnosis?
ii. In which breeds has this condition been most commonly reported?
iii. Discuss the purported underlying pathogenesis of this condition.
iv. What surgical techniques have been described for treating dogs affected with this condition?

241 This arthroscopic image (241) shows the lateral compartment of the shoulder of a 4-year-old male working Labrador retriever presented for a chronic weight-bearing lameness of the right forelimb that is exacerbated by activity. Arthroscopy was performed with the limb in a hanging position.
i. What is your diagnosis?
ii. What arthroscopic portal would have been used to obtain this image?
iii. What surgical options have been reported to treat this condition in dogs?

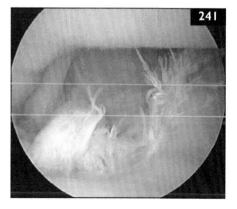

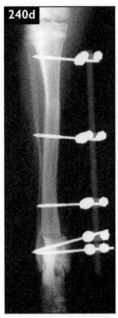 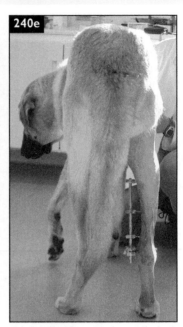

240 i. This dog has valgus deformity of the distal crus, also called tibial valgus.
ii. Shetland sheepdogs and rottweilers are overrepresented.
iii. Asymmetric closure or growth of the distal tibial metaphysis late in affected dogs' skeletal development may be responsible for the development of tibial valgus.
iv. Surgical treatment involves either a closing wedge ostectomy, in which a small triangle of bone is excised to definitively correct the deformity, or an opening osteotomy, in which the ends of the bone segments are asymmetrically separated after a simple osteotomy, to correct the angulation. Effective stabilization of the osteotomy or ostectomy can be challenging because of the short length of the distal juxta-articular segment. Various types of bone plate and external fixator have been used in addressing these deformities. In this dog a closing wedge ostectomy of the tibia was done, leaving the fibula intact, and a unilateral linear fixator was applied (**240d**). The dog is shown weight bearing on the limb the day following surgery (**240e**). A bilateral frame may have been more appropriate given the size of this dog.

241 i. This dog has a rupture of the lateral glenohumeral ligament.
ii. The craniomedial portal was used to evaluate the lateral compartment of the scapulohumeral joint.
iii. Arthroscopic-assisted or open capsulorrhaphy using screws or anchors and prosthetic sutures would be the most likely surgical options. Scapulohumeral arthrodesis could be an option, but only if there was extensive concurrent shoulder pathology.

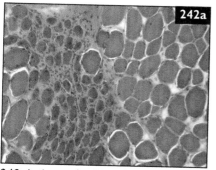

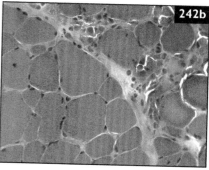

242 A 6-month-old male Labrador retriever puppy was presented for evaluation because the owner had noted that the dog had difficulty going down stairs, showed episodic hindlimb lameness and was not as active as its littermates. The litter was intended to produce working dogs and both the sire and dam had field trial pedigrees. No abnormalities were found on physical or orthopedic examination. Blood work was performed and revealed elevated serum alanine aminotransferase (ALT, 545 U/L; reference 0–40), aspartate aminotransferase (AST, 350 U/L; reference 0–40) and creatine kinase (CK, 33,368 U/L; reference 0–200) activities. Biopsies were obtained from the vastus lateralis and triceps brachii muscles and evaluated in frozen sections (242a [magnification x20], 242b [magnification x40]).

i. What is the relevance of the elevated enzyme activities?

ii. What are the predominant pathologic abnormalities present in the muscle biopsy specimens?

iii. The elevated enzyme activities and pathologic changes are characteristic of which group of diseases?

iv. What other organ systems should be evaluated in this puppy?

243 A ventrodorsal postoperative radiograph of a 2-year-old female neutered rottweiler that underwent an open surgical reduction and stabilization of a traumatic craniodorsal right coxofemoral joint luxation is shown (243).

i. What surgical procedure has been performed?

ii. In a cadaveric biomechanical study by Baltzer *et al.* (2001), what was the conclusion regarding implant types and suture materials used for this procedure?

iii. What percentage of dogs can be expected to reluxate following this procedure?

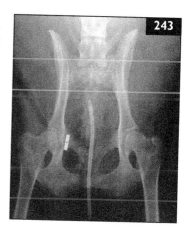

242 i. CK levels are a marker of myofiber damage and used to diagnose muscle diseases. Activity is moderately to markedly increased in necrotizing, inflammatory, and dystrophic myopathies, and usually normal or only mildly increased in non-inflammatory muscle diseases. Persistently elevated CK activity warrants muscle biopsy. Other enzymes, such as ALT and AST, may be increased with myofiber damage, but lack the tissue specificity of CK.

ii. A large cluster of basophilic regenerating fibers with prominent internal nuclei (**242a**) and degenerating fibers (**242b**) are present. Cellular infiltrates are limited to macrophages phagocytizing necrotic debris. A degenerative rather than an inflammatory myopathy should be considered.

iii. Muscle biopsy is critical in establishing a diagnosis. The pattern of muscle fiber degeneration and regeneration in association with a very high CK activity is typical of muscular dystrophies. Muscular dystrophies are a heterogeneous group of inherited, degenerative, mostly non-inflammatory disorders characterized by progressive muscle weakness and wasting. Several forms of muscular dystrophy have been identified in dogs. Dystrophin deficiency has been described in Labrador retrievers. In this puppy the diagnosis was confirmed by immunohistochemistry and immunoblotting. Clinical severity is variable and this dog had a mild form of disease.

iv. Cardiomyopathy, sometimes fatal, can be associated with muscular dystrophies. A full cardiac evaluation should be performed if muscular dystrophy is diagnosed.

243 i. A toggle rod has been used to stabilize the coxofemoral luxation.

ii. A mechanical comparison of toggle pins fashioned from 1.0 mm Kirschner wires and 4.5 mm diameter cannulated toggle rods implanted into acetabula found no significant differences between the two implants for any of the parameters tested. The mechanical properties of braided polyester, woven polyester, and monofilament polybutester suture materials were compared and braided polyester had the best *in-vitro* mechanical properties of the suture materials tested.

iii. In one study, 7 of 62 (11%) of dogs reluxated following open reduction and toggle rod placement. Reluxation was more likely if the duration of surgery exceeded 2 hours; however, many of these dogs had multiple orthopedic injuries, which were addressed during the same anesthetic episode. Another study, which evaluated the use of toggle rods to manage coxofemoral luxations in dogs with multiple orthopedic injuries, reported that 3 of 14 (21%) dogs reluxated. Two of these dogs had hip dysplasia, which likely contributed to reluxation.

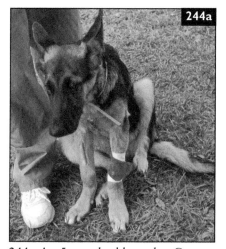
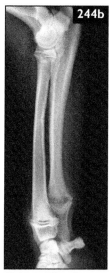
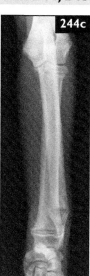

244 A 5-month-old male German shepherd dog presented with lameness and distal limb swelling of all four limbs (**244a**). The dog was mildly depressed, with a reduced appetite, and was reluctant to ambulate. On physical examination there was firm symmetrical swelling of both distal radii and ulnae. There was concurrent mild swelling of the distal tibiae and fibulae. Digital pressure applied to the swollen regions evoked a marked pain response. Mediolateral and craniocaudal radiographs of the right antebrachium are shown (**244b, c**).

i. What is the diagnosis?
ii. What eponym is used to describe the linear metaphyseal radiolucency adjacent to the physes?
iii. What eponym is used to describe the radiodense area surrounding the linear metaphyseal radiolucency?
iv. What is this dog's prognosis?

245 This 5-year-old, 32 kg male Louisiana Catahoula leopard dog is receiving therapy for an iliopsoas muscle strain (**245**).
i. What therapy is this dog receiving?
ii. What therapeutic effects does this rehabilitative modality provide in the treatment of muscle strains?
iii. What effect does altering the applied frequency (Hz) have on depth of penetration?

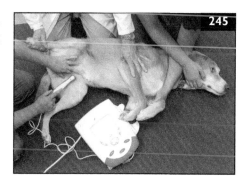

244 i. This dog has metaphyseal osteopathy, commonly referred to as hypertrophic osteodystrophy.

ii. The linear metaphyseal radiolucency is referred to as the Trummerfeld zone. Extensive necrosis of the normal mesenchymal elements with an infiltration of inflammatory cells (principally neutrophils) can be seen if this lesion is examined histologically. The radiolucent metaphyseal zone is a consequence of trabecular resorption in the infiltrated area.

iii. The radiodense area surrounding the Trummerfeld zone is referred to as the white line of Frankel. This is a consequence of trabecular collapse and mineralization of trabecular hemorrhage.

iv. The prognosis is guarded. Periods of malaise and pain can recur with subsequent bouts, which can continue until the dog reaches skeletal maturity. Fractures have been reported through the metaphyses in affected dogs. The inflammation can result in premature complete or asymmetric growth plate closure, which can cause conformational limb deformity such as distal antebrachial valgus, procurvatum, and external rotation. Radius curvus, which develops due to retarded longitudinal bone growth of the distal ulnar physes, may improve as the metaphyseal osteopathy resolves and does not necessarily require surgical management.

245 i. This dog is receiving therapeutic ultrasound.

ii. This modality is used for deep tissue heating and non-thermal effects such as cavitation and acoustic microstreaming. Therapeutic ultrasound has been shown to stimulate fibroblast activity, increase protein synthesis, improve blood flow, and aid in soft tissue and bone healing.

iii. The depth of tissue penetration is determined by the ultrasound frequency. At a frequency of 1 MHz, sound waves will reach depths of 2–5 cm and at a frequency of 3 MHz, energy will be absorbed at a shallower depth (1–2 cm). The frequency also determines the rate of absorption and therefore rate of heating: at a frequency of 3 MHz, tissues will heat three times faster than at a frequency of 1 MHz.

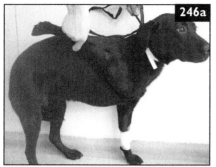
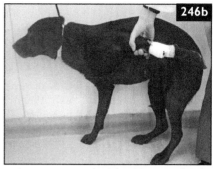

246 A 6-year-old male working Labrador retriever presented with a history of right forelimb lameness. The dog initially became acutely lame on the limb 6 months previously, but the lameness improved within 3 weeks without specific treatment. The dog then developed a chronic lameness in the same limb of 6 weeks' duration. A complete orthopedic examination was performed. The dog had pain associated with manipulation of the metacarpophalangeal joint of digit II of the right fore paw. No pain was elicited on right shoulder manipulation. Photographs were taken of the dog during right (**246a**) and left shoulder manipulation (**246b**).
i. What is abnormal regarding the maneuver being performed in these two images?
ii. State a diagnosis.
iii. What treatment should be advised for this dog?

247 A 4-year-old, 22 kg male English springer spaniel became acutely lame in the left forelimb after jumping across a ditch. On physical examination the dog's left elbow was swollen and painful to manipulation. Preoperative and postoperative craniocaudal radiographs of the humerus are shown (**247a, b**).
i. Describe the fracture.
ii. List three approaches that could have been used to perform open reduction and stabilization of this fracture.

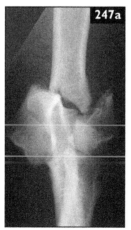
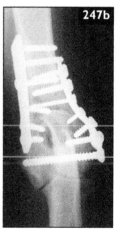

iii. What are the advantages and disadvantages of each of these approaches?

246 i. The dog's right elbow can be completely extended while the right shoulder is fully flexed, allowing the paw to be elevated dorsal to the level of the dog's vertebral column without eliciting an adverse response from the dog. This motion is restricted in the left forelimb.

ii. The ability to fully flex the shoulder while the ipsilateral elbow is fully extended can only occur if there is loss or disruption of concurrent extensor function in the scapulohumeral joint and flexor function in the elbow associated with a complete rupture of the biceps brachii tendon. These abnormalities are pathognomonic for complete rupture of the biceps brachii tendon.

iii. The rupture of the biceps brachii tendon was an incidental finding; pain was not elicited on manipulation of the shoulder. Treatment is usually not necessary if the injury is chronic, as in this dog. Tenodesis may aid recovery for dogs with acute injuries. The ruptured tendon is secured to the proximal humerus using a spiked staple or screw and spiked washer. Investigation of the right metacarpophalangeal joint of digit II of the right fore paw revealed a fragmented sesamoid (II), which was removed at surgery. Lameness resolved within 4 weeks of surgery and the dog was able to return to work.

247 i. This dog has sustained an intracondylar fracture of the distal humerus. The supracondylar components of this dog's fracture are oblique and fractures with this configuration are often referred to as 'Y' fractures. If the epicondylar components of the fracture were transverse rather than oblique, the fracture would be referred to as a 'T' fracture.

ii. Intracondylar fractures of the distal humerus can be approached caudally via olecranon osteotomy or via triceps tenotomy. Alternatively, combined medial and lateral approaches to the distal humerus can be used without disrupting the triceps mechanism.

iii. While an olecranon osteotomy affords excellent exposure of the distal humerus, this approach is associated with a very high incidence of postoperative complications. A triceps tenotomy also affords excellent exposure, but there are concerns regarding healing of the sutured tenotomy in a dog of this size. Combined medial and lateral approaches afford sufficient exposure for fracture reduction and stabilization with less periarticular soft tissue dissection and fewer postoperative complications. In this dog, combined medial and lateral approaches were used to reduce the fracture and place the implants.

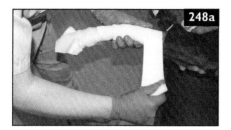

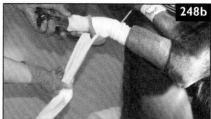

248 A dog is receiving regional analgesia in preparation for resection of a mass from a digital pad. A catheter has been inserted into the cephalic vein. The catheter is placed as far distally and as close to the surgical site as possible and then secured firmly. After exsanguination of the limb with an Esmarch's bandage

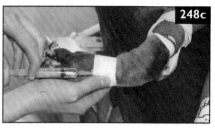

(248a), a tourniquet is applied proximal to the catheter and the Esmarch's bandage removed (248b). Lidocaine is then injected through the catheter over a period of 90 seconds (248c).

i. What method of analgesia is being used in this dog?
ii. When using this technique, how long should it take for the limb to become analgesed?
iii. How does the technique work?
iv. How long can a tourniquet be safely left in place?

249 An 8-year-old, 50 kg male castrated mixed-breed dog presented with chronic weight-bearing right forelimb lameness. Pain could be elicited on manipulation of the right elbow, especially when digital pressure was applied distal to the medial epicondyle of the humerus.
i. Describe the radiographic abnormalities (249a, b).
ii. What is the purported

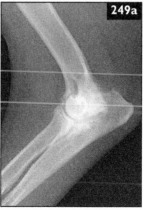

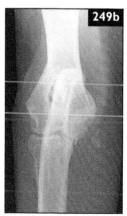

etiology of the radiodense structure located adjacent to the humeral condyle?
iii. What further diagnostic imaging might be useful in establishing the cause of this dog's lameness?

248 i. Intravenous regional analgesia is being performed on this dog.

ii. Analgesia of the distal limb should develop within 15 minutes. Analgesia initially develops distally and then extends proximally – opposite to what occurs with a nerve block.

iii. The site of action is controversial, with some studies claiming that the main effect is on smaller nerves and sensory nerve endings, while others show that main nerve trunks are primarily affected. Ischemia of tissues may also contribute to the analgesic effect.

iv. Most recommendations are for a maximum period of 1.5–2 hours in dogs. The main concern is ischemic muscle damage, although nerve injury is also a concern. In humans, there is a three-fold increase in the incidence of nerve injury for every 30 minutes that the tourniquet is in place. Other reported physiological effects include hypertension and, upon release, small increases in serum potassium concentrations, acidosis, and hyperlactatemia. Once the tourniquet has been released, sensory and motor function return within a few minutes.

249 i. There is ulnar notch sclerosis and osteophytosis, particularly on the cranial aspect of the radial head and in the caudal aspect of the joint. There is a rounded mineralized structure located distomedial to the medial epicondyle on the craniocaudal view radiograph.

ii. The etiology of the soft tissue mineralization, located within the tendons of the antebrachial flexor muscles, which originate on the medial epicondyle of the humerus, is poorly understood. The condition has been referred to as ununited medial epicondyle, a type of elbow dysplasia involving mineralized flexor tendons, metaplasia of the flexor tendons, and medial epicondylitis of the elbow. Several etiologies have been proposed: (1) failure of the ossification center of the medial epicondyle to fuse with the distal humerus; (2) osteochondrosis; (3) traumatic avulsion of the flexor tendons from the medial epicondyle; and (4) dystrophic mineralization of the flexor tendons due to chronic inflammation or overuse. The condition can be associated with other causes of elbow dysplasia and osteoarthritis.

iii. Further evaluation could include CT to evaluate the elbow for primary causes of osteoarthritis, such as a fragmented medial coronoid process.

250 Mediolateral and cranio-caudal radiographs of the stifle joint of a small-breed dog are shown (250a, b).

i. Describe the radiographic abnormality present.

ii. What breed of dog is this abnormality observed in most commonly?

iii. What other conditions may have a similar radiographic appearance?

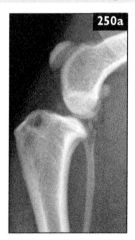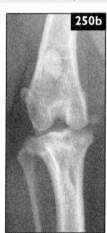

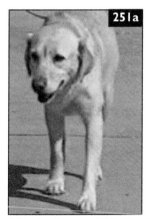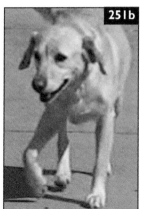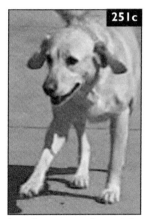

251 An 8-year-old Labrador retriever presented 6 weeks after a transient right forelimb lameness episode was noted after a weekend of bird hunting. Over the subsequent 6 weeks the dog developed an abnormal stance and gait: the dog stood and sat with the right forelimb externally rotated. When walking and trotting the right forelimb had a shortened stride length and was circumducted during the swing phase of advancement (251a–c). Palpation of the right forelimb revealed that the humerus was mechanically fixed in an externally rotated position at the shoulder, with mild atrophy of the supraspinatus and infraspinatus muscles. The infraspinatus muscle felt firm on direct palpation.

i. What is the most likely diagnosis based on the dog's signalment, history, and characteristic stance and gait abnormalities?

ii. What is the recommended treatment for this dog?

iii. What is the prognosis for this dog's return to its intended function (hunting)?

250 i. There is distal displacement of the medial fabella of the head of the gastro-cnemius muscle.

ii. In one study, displacement of the medial fabella was observed in 70% of West Highland white terriers evaluated. Displacement of the fabella is considered a normal anatomic variation in small-breed dogs and was found in 9% of other small-breed dogs evaluated. The condition is uncommon in large-breed dogs.

iii. Pathologic fabellar displacement has also been described in dogs and may have a similar radiographic appearance. Traumatic avulsion of the medial or lateral head of the gastrocnemius muscle can result in distal displacement of the fabella. Avulsion of the lateral fabella has also been observed after placement of fabellar-tibial sutures for extracapsular stabilization of CrCL-deficient stifles.

251 i. This dog has infraspinatus contracture. This condition is thought to be caused by trauma to the musculotendinous unit incurred during strenuous activity. Injury to the muscle is thought to cause vascular damage, resulting in ischemia, which leads to the subsequent fibrotic contracture.

ii. Surgery involving infraspinatus tenotomy or partial tenectomy with release of associated adhesions should be recommended. This is accomplished via a craniolateral approach to the shoulder, with retraction of the cranial head of the acromial deltoid muscle to expose the tendon of insertion of the infraspinatus muscle. Transection of the tendon and any associated adhesions should restore a normal range of motion to the affected shoulder.

iii. The dog should regain normal function with appropriate surgical treatment and postoperative rehabilitation.

252 A 6-month-old male rottweiler presents with a 1-month history of intermittent weight-bearing lameness of the left hindlimb. The dog had an erect hindlimb stance. Both tarsi had palpable effusion and pain was elicited on palpation of the tarsi.

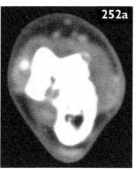

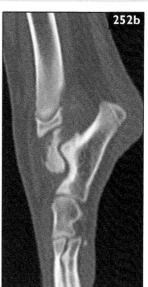

CT of the tarsi was performed. Transverse 2 mm thick slices in soft tissue (**252a**) and bone windows at the level of the proximal aspect of the left talocrural joint and a sagittal 1 mm thick reformatted image in a bone window (**252b**) at the level of the lateral trochlear ridge of the left tarsus are shown.

i. Describe the CT abnormalities.
ii. What is the tentative diagnosis?
iii. What relationship does the size of the lesion have to the clinical signs?

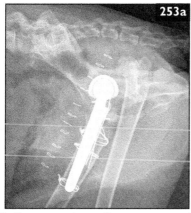

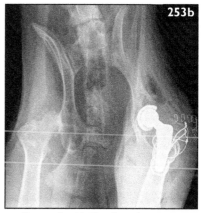

253 Shown are immediate postoperative radiographs (**253a, b**) of an 11-month-old, 21 kg cross-breed dog that presented with a history of hindlimb lameness and hip pain. Total hip replacement was performed using a BioMedtrix BFX (cementless) total hip prosthesis.

i. What intraoperative complications have occurred?
ii. What risk factors predispose to these complications when using this total hip system?

252 i. There is a large, irregularly marginated subchondral bone defect in the central portion of the lateral trochlear ridge. The subchondral bone is sclerotic. A thin, curvilinear, well-marginated, mineralized attenuating body is located dorsal to this defect and is separated from the subjacent bone by a hypoattenuating line. Marked intracapsular soft tissue swelling is present within the tarsocrural joint.
ii. This dog has a large osteochondritis dissecans lesion of the lateral trochlear ridge of the left talus. A similar, but smaller lesion was found in the right tarsus.
iii. In one study the size of the subchondral bone lesion was found to have a direct positive correlation with the severity of lameness.

253 i. The placement of multiple cerclage wires around the proximal femur suggests that a fissure fracture developed in the proximal femur during surgery. This fissure may have occurred during preparation of the femoral canal, during seating of the femoral prosthesis or during attempted reduction of the prosthesis. The pins and tension band wire fixation associated with the greater trochanter suggest that the greater trochanter required stabilization to the proximal femur. The absence of a visible trochanteric osteotomy suggests that the greater trochanter may have avulsed during attempted reduction.
ii. Age is a risk factor, with older dogs being predisposed to femoral fracture. A low femoral canal flare index, in which the medullary canal is cylindrical rather than champagne flute shaped, predisposes to proximal femoral fissure fracture. The dorsal luxation of the contralateral hip provides supportive evidence that reduction of the prosthetic hip was likely challenging, increasing the probability that the greater trochanter avulsed through the physis. Postoperative hip luxation has been shown to be more likely following total hip replacement surgery in dogs with pre-existing luxated dysplastic hips.

254 These are 6-week postoperative radiographs (**254a, b**) of a dog that had a cranial tibial wedge ostectomy to address CrCL insufficiency.

i. What small breed of dog has been reported as commonly having steep tibial plateau angles and thus be prone to developing CrCL insufficiency?

ii. List three disadvantages associated with performing a cranial tibial wedge ostectomy compared with other tibial osteotomy procedures.

iii. Critique this dog's radiographs.

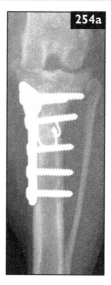
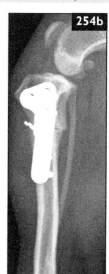

255 A 6-year-old female Shetland sheepdog presented with a 4-week history of hindlimb lameness. The dog had a plantigrade stance and palpable instability at the calcaneoquartal joint. Pre- and postoperative radiographs are shown (**255a, b**). A tarsometatarsal arthrodesis was performed and stabilized with a locking compression plate.

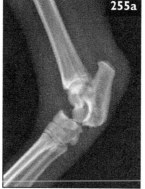
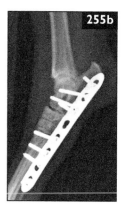

i. What are the four surgical tenets that should be adhered to when performing an arthrodesis?

ii. What vascular structure can be injured and result in postoperative plantar necrosis when performing a tarsometatarsal arthrodesis?

iii. This photograph was taken during application of the plate (**255c**). Name the instrument identified by the arrow.

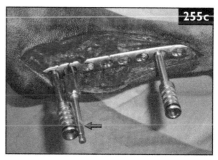

254 i. West Highland white terrier, a breed that has been reported as often having tibial plateau angles in excess of 30°. This is purported to be secondary to alteration in growth of the proximal tibial physis. This dog was a West Highland white terrier and the tibial plateau angle was measured as 31° prior to surgery.

ii. Three disadvantages associated with performing a cranial tibial wedge osteotomy are: variability in postoperative tibial plateau angles; the potential for creating patella baja; and shortening of the tibia.

iii. The alignment of the tibia is good and the slope of the tibial plateau has been reduced to 11°. The ostectomy has yet to achieve union, but there does not appear to be any loss of reduction or fixation. There are still fragments of cortico-cancellous bone graft, macerated pieces of the excised wedge that were implanted at surgery, visible on the lateral radiograph. There is some new bone formation on the distal pole of the patella, the cranial tibial plateau, and the fabellae consistent with mild degenerative joint disease.

255 i. The four surgical tenets for performing an arthrodesis are: (1) The articular cartilage should be debrided to expose the underlying subchondral bone; (2) cancellous bone graft should be implanted in the debrided joint space to accelerate osseous union; (3) the arthrodesis should be immobilized with stable, if not rigid, fixation; and (4) the involved limb segment should be fused at a functional angle.

ii. Damage to the perforating metatarsal artery has been implicated as the cause of postoperative plantar necrosis following hock arthrodesis. This vessel emerges dorsally between the base of the second and third metatarsal bones. The artery's dorsomedial location adjacent to the tarsometatarsal joint explains why there is a risk of inducing plantar necrosis in cases in which a plate is applied medially or if aggressive debridement of the tarsometatarsal joint is performed.

iii. The intraoperative photograph demonstrates the use of a push-pull device to temporarily stabilize the plate along the lateral surface of the pes in order to maintain the implant's position before and during screw placement.

References

1

Chanoit C, Singhani NN, Marcellin-Little DJ *et al.* (2010) Comparison of five radiographic views for assessment of the medial aspect of the humeral condyle in dogs with osteochondritis dissecans. *Am J Vet Res* **71**:780–783.

Wosar MA, Lewis DD, Neuwirth L *et al.* (1999) Radiographic evaluation of elbow joints before and after surgery in dogs with possible fragmented medial coronoid process. *J Am Vet Med Assoc* **214**:52–58.

2

Campbell BG, Wootton JA, Krook L *et al.* (1997) Clinical signs and diagnosis of osteogenesis imperfecta in three dogs. *J Am Vet Med Assoc* **211**:183–187.

Evason MD, Taylor SM, Bebchuk TN (2007) Suspect osteogenesis imperfecta in a male kitten. *Can Vet J* **48**:296–298.

3

Johnson KA (2009) Locking plates – the ultimate implant? *Vet Comp OrthopTraumatol* **22**:I–II.

Moed BR, Grimshaw CS, Segina DN (2012) Failure of locked design-specific plate fixation of the pubic symphysis: a report of six cases. *J Orthop Trauma* **26**:e71–75.

Schutz M, Sudkamp NP (2003) Revolution in plate osteosynthesis: new internal fixator systems. *J Orthop Sci* **8**:252–258.

4

Leach D, Sumner-Smith G, Dagg AI (1977) Diagnosis of lameness in dogs: a preliminary study. *Can Vet J* **18**:58–63.

Scott H, Witte P (2011) Investigation of lameness in dogs. 1. Forelimb. *In Practice* **233**:20–27.

5

Runge J, Kelly S, Gregor T *et al.* (2010) Distraction index as a risk factor for osteoarthritis associated with hip dysplasia in four large dog breeds. *J Small Anim Pract* **51**:264–269.

Smith G, Biery D, Gregor T (1990) New concepts of coxofemoral joint stability and the development of a clinical stress-radiographic method for quantitating hip joint laxity in the dog. *J Am Vet Med Assoc* **196**:59–70.

6

Liu SK, Dorfman HD, Patnaik AK (1974) Primary and secondary bone tumours in the cat. *J Small Anim Pract* **15**:141–156.

Bitetto WV, Patnaik AK, Schrader SC *et al.* (1987) Osteosarcoma in cats: 22 cases (1974–1984). *J Am Vet Med Assoc* **190**:91–93.

Heldmann E, Anderson M, Wagner-Mann C (2000) Feline osteosarcoma: 145 cases (1990–1995). *J Am Anim Hosp Assoc* **36**:518–521.

7

Miller J, Beale BS (2008) Tibiotarsal arthroscopy: applications and long-term outcome in dogs. *Vet Comp Orthop Traumatol* **21**:159–165.

References

Gielen I, van Bree H, Van Ryssen B *et al*. (2002) Radiographic, computed tomographic and arthroscopic findings in 23 dogs with osteochondrosis of the tarsocrural joint. *Vet Rec* **150**:442–447.

8

Watson ADJ, Adams WM, Thomas CB (1995) Craniomandibular osteopathy in dogs. *Compend Contin Educ Pract Vet* **17**:911–922.

Padgett GA, Mostosky UVC (1986) The mode of inheritance of craniomandibular osteopathy in West Highland White Terrier dogs. *Am J Med Genet* **25**:9–13.

9

Riser WH, Shirer JF (1965) Normal and abnormal growth of the distal foreleg in large and giant breeds. *J Am Vet Radiol Soc* **6**:50–64.

Johnson KA (1981) Retardation of endochondral ossification at the distal ulnar growth plate in dogs. *Aust Vet J* **57**:474–478.

Hazewinkel HAS, Goedegebuure SA, Poulos PW *et al*. (1985) Influences of chronic calcium excess on the skeletal development of growing Great Danes. *J Am Anim Hosp Assoc* **21**:377–391.

10

Radasch RM (1999) Biomechanics of bone and fractures. *Vet Clin North Am Small Anim Pract* **29**:1045–1082.

Burstein AH, Currey J, Frankel VH *et al*. (1972) Bone strength. The effect of screw holes. *J Bone Joint Surg Am* **54**:1143–1156.

11

Clements DN, Gear RN, Tattersall J *et al*. (2004) Type I immune-mediated polyarthritis in dogs: 39 cases (1997–2002). *J Am Vet Med Assoc* **224**:1323–1327.

Werner L, Bright J (1983) Drug-induced immune hypersensitivity disorders in two dogs treated with trimethoprim sulfadiazine: case reports and drug challenge studies. *J Am Anim Hosp Assoc* **19**:731–734.

12

McLaughlin R (2002) Feline stifle disease. *Vet Clin North Am Small Anim Pract* **32**:963–982.

McLaughlin RM (1998) Arthrodesis. In: *Manual of Internal Fixation in Small Animals*, 2nd edn. (eds. WO Brinker, ML Olmstead, G Sumner-Smith *et al*.) Springer-Verlag, Berlin, pp. 247–254.

Kowaleski MP, Boudrieau RJ, Pozzi A (2012) Stifle joint. In: *Veterinary Surgery: Small Animal*. (eds. KM Tobias, SA Johnston) Saunders/Elsevier, St Louis, pp. 906–998.

13

Kraft S, Ehrhart EJ, Gall D *et al*. (2007) Magnetic resonance imaging characteristics of peripheral nerve sheath tumors of the canine brachial plexus in 18 dogs. *Vet Radiol Ultrasound* **48**:1–7.

Kippenes H, Gavin PR, Bagley RS *et al*. (1999) Magnetic resonance imaging features of tumors of the spine and spinal cord in dogs. *Vet Radiol Ultrasound* **40**:627–633.

Brehm DM, Vite CH, Steinberg HS *et al*. (1995) A retrospective evaluation of 51 cases of peripheral nerve sheath tumors in the dog. *J Am Anim Hosp Assoc* **31**:349–359.

14

De Haan JJ, Goring RL, Beale BS (1994) Evaluation of polysulfated glycosaminoglycan for the treatment of hip dysplasia in dogs. *Vet Surg* **23**:177–181.

15

Liptak JM, Ehrhart N, Santoni BG (2006) Cortical bone graft and endoprosthesis in the distal radius of dogs: a biomechanical comparison of two different limb-sparing techniques. *Vet Surg* **35**:150–160.

16

Rose SA, Peck JN, Tano CA *et al.* (2011) Effect of a locking triple pelvic osteotomy plate on screw loosening in 26 dogs. *Vet Surg* **41**:156–162.

Rose SA, Bruecker KA, Petersen SW *et al.* (2011) Use of locking plate and screws for triple pelvic osteotomy. *Vet Surg* **41**:114–120.

Hosgood G, Lewis DD (1993) Retrospective evaluation of fixation complications of 49 pelvic osteotomies in 36 dogs. *J Small Anim Pract* **34**:123–130.

17

Kramer M, Gerwing M, Sheppard C *et al.* (2001) Ultrasonography for the diagnosis of diseases of the tendon and tendon sheath of the biceps brachii muscle. *Vet Surg* **30**:64–71.

18

Chalman JA, Butler HC (1985) Coxofemoral joint laxity and the Ortolani sign. *J Am Anim Hosp Assoc* **21**:671–676.

Ginja MMD, Gonzalo-Orden JM, Melo-Pinto P *et al.* (2008) Early hip laxity examination in predicting moderate and severe hip dysplasia in Estrela mountain dogs. *J Small Anim Pract* **49**:641–646.

Puerto DA, Smith GK, Gregor TP *et al.* (1999) Relationship between results of the Ortolani method of hip joint palpation and distraction index, Norberg angle, and hip score in dogs. *J Am Vet Med Assoc* **214**:497–501.

19

Kapatkin A, Howe-Smith R, Shofer F (2000) Conservative versus surgical treatment of metacarpal and metatarsal fractures in dogs. *Vet Comp Orthop Traumatol* **13**:123–127.

Johnson AL (2003). Current concepts in fracture reduction. *Vet Comp Orthop Traumatol* **16**:59–66.

Meeson RL, Davidson C, Arthurs GI (2011) Soft-tissue injuries associated with cast application for distal limb orthopaedic conditions. *Vet Comp Orthop Traumatol* **24**:126–131.

20

Marcellin-Little DJ, DeYoung DJ, Ferris KK *et al.* (1994) Incomplete ossification of the humeral condyle in spaniels. *Vet Surg* **23**:475–487.

21

Braden TD (1976) Fascia lata transplant for repair of chronic achilles tendon defects. *J Am Anim Hosp Assoc* **12**:800–805.

King M, Jerram R (2003) Achilles tendon rupture in dogs. *Compend Contin Educ Pract Vet* **25**:613–619.

Corr SA, Draffan D, Kulendra E *et al.* (2010) Retrospective study of Achilles mechanism disruption in 45 dogs. *Vet Rec* **167**:407–411.

References

22

Welches CD, Scavelli TD (1990) Transarticular pinning to repair luxation of the stifle joint in dogs and cats: a retrospective study of 10 cases. *J Am Anim Hosp Assoc* **26**:207–214.

Keeley B, Glyde M, Guerin S *et al.* (2007) Stifle joint luxation in the dog and cat: the use of temporary intraoperative transarticular pinning to facilitate joint reconstruction. *Vet Comp Orthop Traumatol* **20**:198–203.

Bruce WJ (1999) Stifle joint luxation in the cat: treatment using transarticular external skeletal fixation. *J Small Anim Pract* **40**:482–488.

23

Alleman AR, Bain PJ (2000) Diagnosing neoplasia: the cytologic criteria for malignancy. *Vet Med* **95**:204–223.

Neihaus SA, Locke JE, Barger AM *et al.* (2011) A novel method of core aspirate cytology compared to fine-needle aspiration for diagnosing canine osteosarcoma. *J Am Anim Hosp Assoc* **47**:317–323.

24

Fries CL, Remedios AM (1995) The pathogenesis and diagnosis of canine hip dysplasia: a review. *Can Vet J* **36**:494–497.

25

Selcer RR, Bubb WJ, Walker TL (1991) Management of vertebral column fractures in dogs and cats: 211 cases (1977–1985). *J Am Vet Med Assoc* **198**:1965–1968.

Wheeler JL, Lewis DD, Cross AR *et al.* (2007) Closed fluoroscopic-assisted spinal arch external skeletal fixation for the stabilization of vertebral column injuries in five dogs. *Vet Surg* **36**:442–448.

Bruce CW, Brisson BA, Gyselinck K (2008) Spinal fracture and luxation in dogs and cats – a retrospective evaluation of 95 cases. *Vet Comp Orthop Traumatol* **21**:280–284.

26

Andreoni AA, Guerrero TG, Hurter K *et al.* (2010) Revision of an unstable HELICA endoprosthesis with a Zurich cementless total hip replacement. *Vet Comp Orthop Traumatol* **23**:177–181.

Kim JY, Hayashi K, Garcia TC *et al.* (2011) Biomechanical evaluation of screw-in femoral implant in cementless total hip system. *Vet Surg* **41**:94–102.

Hach V, Delfs G (2009) Initial experience with a newly developed cementless hip endoprosthesis. *Vet Comp Orthop Traumatol* **22**:153–158.

27

Heffron LE, Campbell JR (1978) Morphology, histology and functional anatomy of the canine cranial cruciate ligament. *Vet Rec* **102**:280–283.

Arnoczky SP, Marshall JL (1977) The cruciate ligaments of the canine stifle: an anatomical and functional analysis. *Am J Vet Res* **38**:1807–1814.

28

Wilson JW, Belloli DM, Robbins T (1985) Resistance of cerclage to knot failure. *J Am Vet Med Assoc* **187**:389–391.

Blass CE, Piermattei DL, Withrow SJ
et al. (1986) Static and dynamic
cerclage wire analysis. *Vet Surg*
15:181–184.

29

Suter PF, Carb AV (1969) Shoulder
arthrography in dogs – radiographic
anatomy and clinical application. *J
Small Anim Pract* **10**:407–413.

Barthez PY, Morgan JP (1993) Bicipital
tenosynovitis in the dog – evaluation
with positive contrast arthrography.
Vet Radiol Ultrasound **34**:325–330.

30

Clarke SP, Jermyn K, Carmichael
S (2007) Avulsion of the triceps
tendon insertion in a cat. *Vet Comp
Orthop Traumatol* **20**:245–247.

Liehmann L, Lorinson D (2006)
Traumatic triceps tendon avulsion in
a cat. *J Small Anim Pract* **47**:94–97.

Davies JV, Clayton Jones DG (1982)
Triceps tendon rupture in the dog
following corticosteroid injection. *J
Small Anim Pract* **23**:779–787.

32

Venzin C, Ohlerth S, Koch D et al.
(2004) Extracorporeal shockwave
therapy in a dog with chronic
bicipital tenosynovitis. *Schweiz Arch
Tierheilkd* **146**:136–141.

Stobie D, Wallace LJ, Lipowitz AJ
et al. (1995) Chronic bicipital
tenosynovitis in dogs: 29 cases
(1985–1992). *J Am Vet Med Assoc*
207:201–207.

Bruce WJ, Burbidge HM, Bray JP et
al. (2000) Bicipital tendinitis and
tenosynovitis in the dog: a study of
15 cases. *NZ Vet J* **48**:44–52.

33

Nielsen C, Pluhar E (2005) Diagnosis
and treatment of hind limb muscle
strain injuries in 22 dogs. *Vet Comp
Orthop Traumatol* **18**:247–253.

34

Pozzi A, Lewis DD (2009) Surgical
approaches for minimally invasive
plate osteosynthesis in dogs. *Vet
Comp Orthop Traumatol* **22**:316–
320.

Hudson CC, Pozzi A, Lewis DD
(2009) Minimally invasive plate
osteosynthesis: applications and
techniques in dogs and cats. *Vet Comp
Orthop Traumatol* **22**:175–182.

35

Payne J, McLaughlin RM, Silverman E
(2005) Comparison of normograde
and retrograde intramedullary
pinning of feline tibias. *J Am Anim
Hosp Assoc* **41**:56–60.

Pardo AD (1994) Relationship of
tibial intramedullary pins to canine
stifle joint structures: a comparison
of normograde and retrograde
insertion. *J Am Anim Hosp Assoc*
30:369–374.

36

MacAuley DC (2001) Ice therapy: how
good is the evidence? *Int J Sports
Med* **22**:379–384.

Rexing J, Dunning D, Siegel AM et al.
(2010) Effects of cold compression,
bandaging, and microcurrent
electrical therapy after cranial
cruciate ligament repair in dogs. *Vet
Surg* **39**:54–58.

References

37

Shelton GD, Schule A, Kass PH (1997) Risk factors for acquired myasthenia gravis in dogs: 1,154 cases (1991–1995). *J Am Vet Med Assoc* **211**:1428–1431.

Dewey CW, Bailey CS, Shelton GD *et al.* (1997) Clinical forms of acquired myasthenia gravis in dogs: 25 cases (1988–1995). *J Vet Intern Med* **11**:50–57.

38

Cook JL, Cook CR, Tomlinson JL (1997) Scapular fractures in dogs: epidemiology, classification, and concurrent injuries in 105 cases (1988–1994). *J Am Anim Hosp Assoc* **33**:528–532.

39

Cogar SM, Cook CR, Curry SL *et al.* (2008) Prospective evaluation of techniques for differentiating shoulder pathology as a source of forelimb lameness in medium and large breed dogs. *Vet Surg* **37**:132–141.

Cook JL, Renfro DC, Tomlinson JL *et al.* (2005) Measurement of angles of abduction for diagnosis of shoulder instability in dogs using goniometry and digital image analysis. *Vet Surg* **34**:463–468.

40

Deneuche AJ, Viguier E (2002) Reduction and stabilization of a supraglenoid tuberosity avulsion under arthroscopic guidance in a dog. *J Small Anim Pract* **43**:308–311.

41

Farese JP, Kirpensteijn J, Kik M *et al.* (2009) Canine appendicular chondrosarcoma: biologic behavior and survival of 25 cases treated with amputation: a Veterinary Society of Surgical Oncology retrospective study. *Vet Surg* **38**:914–919.

42

Mahoney PN, Lamb CR (1996) Articular, periarticular and juxtaarticular mineralised bodies in the dog and cat: a radiologic review. *Vet Radiol Ultrasound* **37**:3–19.

43

Johnson KA, Muir P, Nicoll RG *et al.* (2000) Asymmetric adaptive modeling of central tarsal bones in racing greyhounds. *Bone* **27**:257–263.

Tomlin JL, Lawes TJ, Blunn GW *et al.* (2000) Fractographic examination of racing greyhound central (navicular) tarsal bone failure surfaces using scanning electron microscopy. *Calcif Tissue Int* **67**: 260–266.

44

Johnson JM, Johnson AL, Pijanowski GJ *et al.* (1997) Rehabilitation of dogs with surgically treated cranial cruciate ligament-deficient stifles by use of electrical stimulation of muscles. *Am J Vet Res* **58**:1473–1478.

45

Johnson AL, Broaddus KD, Hauptman JG *et al.* (2006) Vertical patellar position in large-breed dogs with clinically normal stifles and large-breed dogs with medial patellar luxation. *Vet Surg* **35**:78–81.

Mostafa AA, Griffon DJ, Thomas MW *et al.* (2008) Proximodistal alignment of the canine patella: radiographic evaluation and association of medial and lateral patellar luxation. *Vet Surg* 37:201–211.

Johnson AL, Probst CW, DeCamp CE *et al.* (2001) Comparison of trochlear block recession and trochlear wedge recession for canine patellar luxation using a cadaver model. *Vet Surg* 30:140–150.

46

Canapp SO (2007) The canine stifle. *Clin Tech Small Anim Pract* 22:195–207.

Edge-Hughes L (2007) Hip and sacroiliac disease: selected disorders and their management with physical therapy. *Clin Tech Small Anim Pract* 22:183–194.

47

Talcott KW, Schulz KS, Kass PH *et al.* (2002) In vitro biomechanical study of rotational stabilizers of the canine elbow joint. *Am J Vet Res* 63:1520–1526.

O'Brien MG, Boudrieau RJ, Clark GN (1992) Traumatic luxation of the cubital joint (elbow) in dogs: 44 cases (1978–1988). *J Am Vet Med Assoc* 201:1760–1765.

Farrell M, Draffan D, Gemmill T *et al.* (2007) In vitro validation of a technique for assessment of canine and feline elbow joint collateral ligament integrity and description of a new method for collateral ligament prosthetic replacement. *Vet Surg* 36:548–556.

48

Stern L, McCarthy R, King R *et al.* (2007) Imaging diagnosis: discospondylitis and septic arthritis in a dog. *Vet Radiol Ultrasound* 48:335–337.

49

Robertson SA, Taylor PM, Sear JW (2003) Systemic uptake of buprenorphine by cats after oral mucosal administration. *Vet Rec* 152:675–678.

50

Vaughan LC (1992) Flexural deformity of the carpus in puppies. *J Small Anim Pract* 33:381–384.

Cetinkaya MA, Yardimci C, Sa lam M (2007) Carpal laxity syndrome in forty-three puppies. *Vet Comp Orthop Traumatol* 20:126–130.

51

Reems MR, Beale BS, Hulse DA (2003) Use of a plate-rod construct and principles of biological osteosynthesis for repair of diaphyseal fractures in dogs and cats: 47 cases (1994–2001). *J Am Vet Med Assoc* 223:330–335.

Uhl JM, Segui B, Kapatkin AS *et al.* (2008) Mechanical comparison of 3.5 mm broad dynamic compression plate, broad limited-contact dynamic compression plate, and narrow locking compression plate systems using interfragmentary gap models. *Vet Surg* 37:663–673.

Sumner-Smith G, Cawley AJ (1970) Nonunion of fractures in the dog. *J Small Anim Pract* 11:311–325.

References

52

Ness MG (2009) The effect of bending and twisting on the stiffness and strength of the 3.5 SOP implant. *Vet Comp Orthop Traumatol* **22**:132–136.

53

McLaughlin R, Roush JK (1995) A comparison of two surgical approaches to the scapulohumeral joint in dogs. *Vet Surg* **24**:207–214.

Howard PE (1984) Luxation of the canine shoulder joint to maximize exposure for treatment of osteochondritis dissecans. *Vet Surg* **13**:15–17.

Tomlinson J, Constantinescu G, McClure R *et al.* (1986) Caudal approach to the shoulder joint in the dog. *Vet Surg* **15**:294–299.

55

Roy RG, Wallace LJ, Johnson GR (1994) A retrospective long-term evaluation of ununited anconeal process excision on the canine elbow. *Vet Comp Orthop Traumatol* **7**:94–97.

Fox SM, Burbidge HM, Bray JC *et al.* (1996) Ununited anconeal process: lag-screw fixation. *J Am Anim Hosp Assoc* **32**:52–56.

Pettitt RA, Tattersall J, Gemmill T *et al.* (2009) Effect of surgical technique on radiographic fusion of the anconeus in the treatment of ununited anconeal process. *J Small Anim Pract* **50**:545–548.

56

Muir P, Johnson KA (1996) Fractures of the proximal ulna in dogs. *Vet Comp Orthop Traumatol* **9**:88–94.

57

Reif U, Dejardin LM, Probst CW (2004) Influence of limb positioning and measurement method on the magnitude of the tibial plateau angle. *Vet Surg* **33**:368–375.

Vecchio NE, Hosgood G, Vecchio LE *et al.* (2012) Changes in tibial plateau angles after tibial plateau-levelling osteotomy in dogs with cranial cruciate deficiency. *NZ Vet J* **60**:9–13.

Headrick JF, Cook JL, Helphrey M *et al.* (2007) A novel radiographic method to facilitate measurement of the tibial plateau angle in dogs. A prospective clinical study. *Vet Comp Orthop Traumatol* **20**:24–28.

58

Canapp SO, Cross AR, Brown MP *et al.* (2005) Examination of synovial fluid and serum following intravenous injections of hyaluronan for the treatment of osteoarthritis in dogs. *Vet Comp Orthop Traumatol* **18**:169–174.

Smith G Jr, Myers SL, Brandt KD *et al.* (2005) Effect of intraarticular hyaluronan injection on vertical ground reaction force and progression of osteoarthritis after anterior cruciate ligament transection. *J Rheumatol* **32**:325–334.

Kuroki K, Cook JL, Kreeger JM (2002) Mechanisms of action and potential uses of hyaluronan in dogs with osteoarthritis. *J Am Vet Med Assoc* **221**:944–950.

59

Morello E, Vasconi E, Martano M *et al.* (2005) Pasteurized tumoral autograft and adjuvant chemotherapy for the treatment of canine distal radial osteosarcoma: 13 cases. *Vet Surg* **32**:539–544.

60
Boemo CM, Eaton-Wells RD (1995) Medial displacement of the tendon of origin of the biceps brachii muscle in 10 greyhounds. *J Small Anim Pract* **36**:69–73.

61
Owen MR, Langley-Hobbs SJ, Moores AP *et al.* (2004) Mandibular fracture repair in dogs and cats using epoxy resin and acrylic external skeletal fixation. *Vet Comp Orthop Traumatol* **17**:189–197.

62
Tafti AK, Hanna P, Bourque AC (2005) Calcinosis circumscripta in the dog: a retrospective pathological study. *J Vet Med A Physiol Pathol Clin Med* **52**:13–17.
Joffe DJ (1996) Calcinosis circumscripta in the footpad of a dog. *Can Vet J* **37**:161–162.
Stampley A, Bellah JR (1990) Calcinosis circumscripta of the metacarpal pad in a dog. *J Am Vet Med Assoc* **196**:113–114.

63
Hammel SP, Pluhar GE, Novo RE *et al.* (2006) Fatigue analysis of plates used for fracture stabilization in small dogs and cats. *Vet Surg* **35**:573–578.
Perren SM (1991) The concept of biological plating using the limited contact-dynamic compression plate (LC-DCP). Scientific background,design and application. *Injury* **22**:1–41.
Perren SM, Klaue K, Pohler O *et al.* (1990) The limited contact dynamic compression plate (LC-DCP). *Arch Orthop Trauma Surg* **109**:304–310.

64
Engelke E, Pfarrer C, Waibl H (2011) Anatomy of the collateral ligaments of the feline elbow joint: functional implications. *Anat Histol Embryol* **40**:80–88.

65
Farrell M, Draffan D, Gemmill T *et al.* (2007) *In vitro* validation of a technique for assessment of canine and feline elbow joint collateral ligament integrity and description of a new method for collateral ligament prosthetic replacement. *Vet Surg* **36**:548–556.
Farrell M, Thomson DG, Carmichael S (2009) Surgical management of traumatic elbow luxation in two cats using circumferential suture prostheses. *Vet Comp Orthop Traumatol* **22**:66–69.

66
Campbell JR (1976) The technique of fixation of fractures of the distal femur using Rush pins. *J Small Anim Pract* **17**:323–329.
Whitney WO, Schrader SC (1987) Dynamic intramedullary crosspinning technique for repair of distal femoral fractures in dogs and cats: 71 case (1981–1985). *J Am Vet Med Assoc* **191**:1133–1138.

67
Claes LE, Heigele CA, Neidlinger-Wilker C *et al.* (1998) Effects of mechanical factors on the fracture healing process. *Clin Orthop Rel Res* **255S**:S132–147.
Perren SM (1979) Physical and biological aspects of fracture healing with special reference to internal fixation. *Clin Orthop Rel Res* **138**:175–196.

References

Pauwels F (1960) Eine neue theorie über den einfluß mechanischer reize auf die differenzierung der stutzgewebe. *Z Anat Entwicklungsgesch* **121**:478–515.

68
Pozzi A, Hildreth BE, Rajala-Schultz PJ (2008) Comparison of arthroscopy and arthrotomy for the diagnosis of medial meniscal pathology: an ex-vivo study. *Vet Surg* **37**:749–755.

69
Monk LM, Preston CA, McGowan CM (2006) Effects of early intensive postoperative physiotherapy on limb function after tibial plateau leveling osteotomy in dogs with deficiency of the cranial cruciate ligament. *Am J Vet Res* **67**:529–536.

Shono T, Masumoto K, Fujishima K *et al.* (2007) Gait patterns and muscle activity in the lower extremities of elderly women during underwater treadmill walking against water flow. *J Physiol Anthropol* **26**:579–586.

Burnett JM, Wardlaw JL (2012) Physical rehabilitation for veterinary practices. *Today's Vet Pract* **2**:14–20.

70
Langenbach A, Giger U, Green P *et al.* (1998) Relationship between degenerative joint disease and hip joint laxity by use of distraction index and Norberg angle measurement in a group of cats. *J Am Vet Med Assoc* **213**:1439–1443.

Liska WD (2010) Micro total hip replacement for dogs and cats: surgical techniques and outcomes. *Vet Surg* **39**:797–810.

72
Basher AWP, Walter MC, Newton CD (1986) Coxofemoral luxation in the dog and cat. *Vet Surg* **15**:356–362.

Bone DL, Walker M, Cantwell HD (1984) Traumatic coxofemoral luxation in dogs: results of repair. *Vet Surg* **13**:263–270.

Evers P, Johnston GR, Wallace LJ (1997) Long-term results of treatment of traumatic coxofemoral joint dislocation in dogs: 64 cases (1973–1992). *J Am Vet Med Assoc* **210**:59–64.

73
Graupmann-Kuzma A, Valentine BA, Shubitz LF *et al.* (2008) Coccidioidomycosis in dogs and cats: a review. *J Am Anim Hosp Assoc* **44**:226–235.

Johnson LR, Herrgesell EJ, Davidson AP *et al.* (2003) Clinical, clinicopathologic, and radiographic findings in dogs with coccidioidomycosis: 24 cases (1995–2000). *J Am Vet Med Assoc* **222**:461–466.

Heinritz CK, Gilson SD, Soderstrom MJ *et al.* (2005) Subtotal pericardectomy and epicardial excision for treatment of coccidioidomycosis-induced effusive-constrictive pericarditis in dogs: 17 cases (1999–2003). *J Am Vet Med Assoc* **227**:435–440.

74
Kinzel S, Hein S, von Scheven C *et al.* (2002) 10 years experience with denervation of the hip joint capsule for treatment of canine hip joint dysplasia and arthrosis. *Berl Munch Tierarztl Wochenschr* **115**:53–56.

Schmaedecke A, Saut JP, Ferrigno CR (2008) A quantitative analysis of the nerve fibres of the acetabular periosteum of dogs. *Vet Comp Orthop Traumatol* **21**:413–441.

Ferringo CRA, Schmaedecke A, Oliveira LM *et al.* (2007) Acetabular denervation of the cranial and dorsal aspect of the acetabular joint for treatment of hip dysplasia in dogs. One year evulation of 97 dogs. *Pesquisa Veterinária Brasileira* **28**:333–340.

76

Dunn ME, Blond L, Letard D *et al.* (2007) Hypertrophic osteopathy associated with infective endocarditis in an adult boxer dog. *J Small Anim Pract* **48**:99–103.

Lee JH, Lee JH, Yoon HY *et al.* (2012) Hypertrophic osteopathy associated with pulmonary adenosquamous carcinoma in a dog. *J Vet Med Sci* **74**:667–672.

Liptak JM, Monnet E, Dernell WS *et al.* (2004) Pulmonary metastatectomy in the management of four dogs with hypertrophic osteopathy. *Vet Comp Oncol* **2**:1–12.

77

Zahn K, Frei R, Wunderle D *et al.* (2008) Mechanical properties of 18 different AO bone plates and the clamp-rod internal fixation system tested on a gap model construct. *Vet Comp Orthop Traumatol* **21**:185–194.

Zahn K, Matis U (2004) The clamp rod internal fixator – application and results in 120 small animal fracture patients. *Vet Comp Orthop Traumatol* **17**:110–120.

78

Vernon FF, Olmstead ML (1983) Femoral head fractures resulting in epiphyseal fragmentation. Results of repair in 5 dogs. *Vet Surg* **12**:123–126.

DeAngelis M, Hohn RB (1968) The ventral approach to excision arthroplasty of the femoral head. *J Am Vet Med Assoc* **152**:135–138.

79

McCartney W, Carmichael S (2000) Talar neck fractures in five cats. *J Small Anim Pract* **41**:204–206.

80

Shires PK, Hulse DA, Kearney MT (1985) Carpal hyperextension in two-month-old pups. *J Am Vet Med Assoc* **186**:49–52.

81

Colborne GR, Innes JF, Comerford, EJ *et al.* (2005) Distribution of power across the hind limb joints in Labrador Retrievers and Greyhounds. *Am J Vet Res* **66**:1563–1571.

Comerford EJ, Tarlton JF, Avery NC *et al.* (2006) Distal femoral intercondylar notch dimensions and their relationship to composition and metabolism of the canine anterior cruciate ligament. *Osteoarth Cartil* **14**:273–278.

82

McAnulty JF, Lenehan TM, Maletz LM (1986) Modified segmental spinal instrumentation in repair of spinal fractures and luxations in dogs. *Vet Surg* **15**:143–149.

References

Ullman SL, Boudrieau RJ (1993) Internal skeletal fixation using a Kirschner apparatus for stabilization of fracture/luxations of the lumbosacral joint in six dogs: a modification of the transilial pin technique. *Vet Surg* **22**:11–17.

83

Moores AP, Owen MR, Fews D *et al.* (2004) Slipped capital femoral epiphysis in dogs. *J Small Anim Pract* **45**:602–608.

Dupuis J, Breton L, Drolet R (1997) Bilateral epiphysiolysis of the femoral heads in two dogs. *J Am Vet Med Assoc* **210**:1162–1165.

84

Cook JL, Renfro DC, Tomlinson JL *et al.* (2005) Measurement of angles of abduction for diagnosis of shoulder instability in dogs using goniometry and digital image analysis. *Vet Surg* **34**:463–468.

85

McNicholas WT, Wilkens BE, Blevins WE *et al.* (2002) Spontaneous femoral capital physeal fractures in adult cats: 26 cases (1996–2001). *J Am Vet Med Assoc* **221**:1731–1736.

Queen J, Bennett D, Carmichael S *et al.* (1998) Femoral neck metaphyseal osteopathy in the cat. *Vet Rec* **142**:159–162.

86

Wallace AM, De La Puerta B, Trayhorn D *et al.* (2009) Feline combined diaphyseal radial and ulnar fractures. A retrospective study of 28 cases. *Vet Comp OrthopTraumatol* **22**:38–46.

87

Streppa HK, Singer MJ, Budsberg SC (2001) Applications of local antimicrobial delivery systems in veterinary medicine. *J Am Vet Med Assoc* **219**:40–48.

Sayegh AI, Moore RM (2003) Polymethylmethacrylate beads for treating orthopedic infections. *Comp Cont Educ Pract* **25**:788–795.

Henry SL, Gregory AH, Seligson D (1993) Long-term implantation of gentamycin-polymethylmethacrylate antibiotic beads. *Clin Orthop Relat Res* **295**:47–53.

88

Bader HL, Ruhe AL, Wang LW *et al.* (2010) An ADAMTSL2 founder mutation causes Musladidn–Lueke syndrome, a heritable disorder of Beagle dogs, featuring stiff skin and joint contractures. *PLoS ONE* **5**(9):e12817.doi:10.1371/journal.pone.0012817.

89

Jermyn K, Roe SC (2011) Influence of screw insertion order on compression generated by bone plates in a fracture model. *Vet Comp Orthop Traumatol* **6**:403–407.

Ya'ish FMM, Nanu AM, Cross AT (2011) Can DCP and LCP plates generate more compression? The effect of multiple eccentrically placed screws and their drill positioning guides. *Injury* **42**:1095–1100.

90

Craig LE, Julian ME, Ferracone JD (2002) The diagnosis and prognosis of synovial tumors in dogs: 35 cases. *Vet Pathol* **39**:413–414.

91

Kerwin SC, Lewis DD, Hribernik TN (1992) Diskospondylitis associated with *Brucella canis* infection in dogs: 14 cases (1980–1991). *J Am Vet Med Assoc* **201**:1253–1257.

Schultz RM, Johnson EG, Wisner ER *et al.* (2008) Clinicopathologic and diagnostic imaging characteristics of systemic aspergillosis in 30 dogs. *J Vet Intern Med* **22**:851–859.

Berry WL, Leisewitz AL (1996) Multifocal *Aspergillus terreus* discospondylitis in two German Shepherd dogs. *J S Afr Vet Assoc* **67**:222–228.

92

Farese JP, Milner R, Thompson MS *et al.* (2004) Stereotactic radiosurgery for treatment of osteosarcomas involving the distal limb in dogs. *J Am Vet Med Assoc* **225**:1567–1572.

93

Manley PA, Adams WM, Danielson KC *et al.* (2007) Long-term outcome of juvenile pubic symphysiodesis and triple pelvic osteotomy in dogs with hip dysplasia. *J Am Vet Med Assoc* **230**:206–210.

Patricelli AJ, Dueland RT, Adams WM *et al.* (2002) Juvenile pubic symphysiodesis in dysplastic puppies at 15 and 20 weeks of age. *Vet Surg* **31**:435–444.

Vezzoni A, Dravelli G, Vezzoni L *et al.* (2008) Comparison of conservative management and juvenile pubic symphysiodesis in the early treatment of canine hip dysplasia. *Vet Comp Orthop Traumatol* **21**:267–279.

94

Johnson KA, Lomas GR, Wood AK (1984) Osteomyelitis in dogs and cats caused by anaerobic bacteria. *Aust Vet J* **61**:57–61.

95

Weber BG, Cech O (1976) *Pseudarthrosis: Pathophysiology, Biomechanics, Therapy and Results.* Hans Huber, Bern, pp. 1–323.

Hamilton MH, Langley Hobbs SJ (2005) Use of the AO veterinary mini 'T'-plate for stabilisation of distal radius and ulna fractures in toy breed dogs. *Vet Comp Orthop Traumatol* **18**:18–25.

Muir P (1997) Distal antebrachial fractures in toy-breed dogs. *Compend Contin Educ Pract Vet* **19**:137–145.

96

Lujan Feliu-Pascual A, Shelton GD, Targett MP *et al.* (2006) Inherited myopathy of Great Danes. *J Small Anim Pract* **47**:249–254.

Chang KC, McCulloch ML, Anderson TJ *et al.* (2010) Molecular and cellular insights into a distinct myopathy of Great Dane dogs. *Vet J* **183**:322–327.

97

Ost PC, Dee JF, Dee LG *et al.* (1987) Fractures of the calcaneus in the racing Greyhound. *Vet Surg* **16**:53–59.

98

Guille AE, Lewis DD, Anderson TP *et al.* (2004) Evaluation of surgical repair of humeral condylar fractures using self-compressing Orthofix pins in 23 dogs. *Vet Surg* **33**:314–322.

References

Daubs BM, McLaughlin RM, Silverman E *et al.* (2007) Evaluation of compression generated by self-compressing Orthofix bone pins and lag screws in simulated lateral humeral condylar fractures. *Vet Comp Orthop Traumatol* 20:175–179.

Vida JT, Pooya H, Vasseur PB *et al.* (2005) Biomechanical comparison of orthofix pins and cortical bone screws in a canine humeral condylar fracture model. *Vet Surg* 34:491–498.

100
Jones JC, Banfield CM, Ward DL (2000) Association between postoperative outcome and results of magnetic resonance imaging and computed tomography in working dogs with degenerative lumbosacral stenosis. *J Am Vet Med Assoc* 216:1769–1774.

101
Heikel HVA (1959) Aplasia and hypoplasia of the radius. *Acta Orthop Scand Suppl* 39:1–155.

Lockwood A, Montgomery R, McEwen V (2009) Bilateral radial hemimelia, polydactyly and cardiomegaly in two cats. *Vet Comp Orthop Traumatol* 22:511–513.

Twole HA, Breur GJ (2004) Dysostoses of the canine and feline appendicular skeleton. *J Am Vet Med Assoc* 225:1685–1692.

102
Hampshire VA, Doddy FM, Post LO *et al.* (2004) Adverse drug event reports at the United States Food and Drug Administration Center for Veterinary Medicine. *J Am Vet Med Assoc* 225:533–536.

Wallace JL, Fiorucci S (2003) A magic bullet for mucosal protection... and aspirin is the trigger. *Trends Pharmacol Sci* 24:323–326.

103
Scott H (2005) Repair of long bone fractures in cats. *In Practice* 27:390–397.

Fruchter AM, Holmberg DL (1991) Mechanical analysis of the veterinary cuttable plate. *Vet Comp Orthop Traumatol* 4:116–119.

104
Guerrero TG, Montavon PM (2005) Medial plating for carpal panarthrodesis. *Vet Surg* 34:153–158.

105
Duffy AL, Hackett TB (2010) Canine pedal injury resulting from metal landscape edging. *J Vet Emerg Crit Care* 20:533–536.

Gelberman RH, Siegel DB, Woo SL *et al.* (1991) Healing of digital flexor tendons: importance of the interval from injury to repair. A biomechanical, biochemical, and morphological study in dogs. *J Bone Joint Surg Am* 73:66–75.

106
Wenger S (2004) Brachial plexus block using electrolocation for pancarpal arthrodesis in a dog. *Vet Anaesth Anal* 31:272–275.

Trumpatori BJ, Carter JE, Hash J *et al.* (2010) Evaluation of a midhumeral block of the radial, ulnar, musculocutaneous and median (RUMM block) nerves for analgesia of the distal aspect of the thoracic limb in dogs. *Vet Surg* 39:785–796.

References

107

Denny HR, Barr ARS (1991) Partial carpal and pancarpal arthrodesis in the dog: a review of 50 cases. *J Small Anim Pract* **32**:329–334.

Willer RL, Johnson KA, Turner TM *et al.* (1990) Partial carpal arthrodesis for third degree carpal sprains: a review of 45 carpi. *Vet Surg* **19**:334–340.

108

Montgomery RD, Long IR, Milton JL *et al.* (1989) Comparison of aerobic culturette, synovial membrane biopsy and blood culture medium in detection of canine bacterial arthritis. *Vet Surg* **18**:300–303.

109

Fitzpatrick N, Yeadon R, Smith TJ *et al.* (2009) Techniques of application and initial clinical experience with sliding humeral osteotomy for treatment of medial compartment disease of the canine elbow. *Vet Surg* **38**:261–278.

110

Tomlinson J, Fox D, Cook JL *et al.* (2007) Measurement of femoral angles in four dog breeds. *Vet Surg* **36**:593–598.

Palmer RH, Ikuta CL, Cadmus JM (2011) Comparison of femoral angulation measurement between radiographs and anatomic specimens across a broad range of varus conformations. *Vet Surg* **40**:1023–1028.

Swiderski JK, Palmer RH (2007) Long-term outcome of distal femoral osteotomy for treatment of combined distal femoral varus and medial patellar luxation: 12 cases (1999–2004). *J Am Vet Med Assoc* **231**:1070–1075.

111

Ryan TM, Platt SR, Llabres-Diaz FJ *et al.* (2008) Detection of spinal cord compression in dogs with cervical intervertebral disc disease by magnetic resonance imaging. *Vet Rec* **163**:11–15.

Forterre F, Konar M, Tomek A *et al.* (2008) Accuracy of the withdrawal reflex for localization of the site of cervical disk herniation in dogs: 35 cases (2004–2007). *J Am Vet Med Assoc* **232**:559–563.

Dallman MJ, Palettas P, Bojrab MJ (1992) Characteristics of dogs admitted for treatment of cervical intervertebral disk disease: 105 cases (1972–1982). *J Am Vet Med Assoc* **200**:2009–2011.

112

Lewis DD, Stubbs WP, Neuwirth L *et al.* (1997) Results of screw/wire/polymethylmethacrylate fixation for acetabular fracture repair in 14 dogs. *Vet Surg* **26**:223–234.

Stubbs WP, Lewis DD, Miller GJ *et al.* (1998) A biomechanical evaluation and assessment of reduction for two methods of acetabular osteotomy fixation in dogs. *Vet Surg* **27**:429–437.

Lanz OI, Lewis DD, Madison JB *et al.* (1998) A biomechanical comparison of composite fixation and veterinary acetabular plates for stabilization of acetabular osteotomies in dogs loaded in three-point bending fashion. *Vet Comp Orthop Traumatol* **11**:152–157.

114

Daly WR (1978) Femoral head and neck fractures in the dog and cat: a review of 115 cases. *Vet Surg* **7**:29–38.

References

115

Edgerton BC, An KN, Morrey BF (1990) Torsional strength reduction due to cortical defects in bone. *J Orthop Res* **8**:851–855.

Egger EL (1983) Static strength of six external skeletal fixation configurations. *Vet Surg* **12**:130–136.

Bouvy BM, Markel MD, Chelikani S *et al.* (1993) Ex vivo biomechanics of Kirschner–Ehmer external skeletal fixation applied to canine tibiae. *Vet Surg* **22**:194–207.

116

Paul HA, Bargar WL, Coster I (1987) Approach to the canine coxofemoral joint, body of the ilium, and ischium by osteotomy of the greater trochanter. *J Am Anim Hosp Assoc* **23**:71–74.

Whitelock RG, Dyce J, Houlton JEF (1997) Repair of femoral trochanteric osteotomy in the dog. *J Small Anim Pract* **38**:195–199.

117

Ehrhart N (2005) Longitudinal bone transport for treatment of primary bone tumors in dogs: technique description and outcome in 9 dogs. *Vet Surg* **34**:24–34.

118

Arnbjerg J, Bindseil E (1994) Patella fractures in cats. *Feline Pract* **22**:31–35.

Langley-Hobbs SJ (2009) Survey of 52 fractures of the patella in 34 cats. *Vet Rec* **164**:80–86.

Langley-Hobbs SJ, Ball S, McKee WM (2009) Transverse stress fractures of the proximal tibia in 10 cats with non-union patellar fractures. *Vet Rec* **164**:425–430.

119

Fjeld TO (1992) Osteochondrodysplastic dwarfism in the dog. Clinical and radiographic findings. Case Histories. *Eur J Compan Anim Pract* **3**:31–36.

120

Gorse MJ, Purington PT, Penwick RC *et al.* (1990) Talocalcaneal luxation. An anatomical and clinical study. *Vet Surg* **19**:429–434.

121

Danielson KC, Fitzpatrick N, Muir P *et al.* (2006) Histomorphometry of fragmented medial coronoid process in dogs: a comparison of affected and normal coronoid processes. *Vet Surg* **35**:501–509.

Fitzpatrick N, Yeadon R (2009) Working algorithm for treatment decision making for developmental disease of the medial compartment of the elbow in dogs. *Vet Surg* **38**:285–300.

122

Cohen L, Israeli I, Levi S *et al.* (2012) Normograde and retrograde pinning of the distal fragment in feline humeral fractures. *Vet Surg* **41**:604–610.

Langley-Hobbs SJ, Straw M (2005) The feline humerus: an anatomical study with relevance to external skeletal fixation and intramedullary pin placement. *Vet Comp Orthop Traumatol* **18**:1–6.

123

De La Puerta B, Emmerson T, Moores AP *et al.* (2008) Epoxy putty external skeletal fixation for fractures of the four main metacarpal and metatarsal bones in cats and dogs. *Vet Comp Orthop Traumatol* **21**:451–456.

Fitzpatrick N, Riordan JO, Smith TJ *et al.* (2011) Combined intramedullary and external skeletal fixation of metatarsal and metacarpal fractures in 12 dogs and 19 cats. *Vet Surg* **40**:1015–1022.

124

Spodnick GJ, Berg J, Rand WM *et al.* (1992) Prognosis for dogs with appendicular osteosarcoma treated by amputation alone: 162 cases (1978–1988). *J Am Vet Med Assoc* **200**:995–999.

Lascelles BDX, Dernell WS, Correa MT *et al.* (2005) Improved survival associated with postoperative wound infection in dogs treated with limb-salvage surgery for osteosarcoma. *Ann Surg Oncol* **12**:1073–1083.

125

Geisen V, Weber K, Hartmann K (2009) Vitamin D-dependent hereditary rickets type I in a cat. *J Vet Intern Med* **23**:196–199.

Henik RA, Forrest LJ, Friedman AL (1999) Rickets caused by excessive renal phosphate loss and apparent abnormal vitamin D metabolism in a cat. *J Am Vet Med Assoc* **215**:1644–1649, 1620–1621.

Tanner E, Langley-Hobbs SJ (2005) Vitamin D-dependent rickets type 2 with characteristic radiographic changes in a 4-month-old kitten. *J Feline Med Surgery* **7**:307–311.

126

Voss K, Geyer H, Montavon PM (2003) Antebrachial luxation in a cat: a case report and anatomical study of the medial collateral ligament. *Vet Comp Orthop Traumatol* **16**:266–270

127

Verhoeven GEC, Coopman F, Duchateau L *et al.* (2009) Interobserver agreement on the assessability of standard ventrodorsal hip-extended radiographs and its effect on agreement in the diagnosis of canine hip dysplasia and on routine FCI scoring. *Vet Radiol Ultrasound* **50**:259–263.

Risler A, Klauer JM, Keuler NS *et al.* (2009) Puppy line, metaphyseal sclerosis, and caudolateral curvilinear and circumferential femoral head osteophytes in early detection of canine hip dysplasia. *Vet Radiol Ultrasound* **50**:157–166.

128

Renberg WC, Goring RL, de Haan JJ (1996) Repair of diaphyseal radius and ulna fractures using a modified type I external skeletal fixator and ulnar intramedullary pin. *Vet Comp Orthop Truamatol* **9**:29–35.

Okrasinski EB, Pardo AD, Graehler RA (1991) Biomechanical evaluation of acrylic external skeletal fixation in dogs and cats. *J Am Vet Med Assoc* **199**:1590–1593.

Roe S, Keo T (1997) Epoxy putty for free-form external skeletal fixators. *Vet Surg* **26**:472–477.

129

Vanini R, Olmstead ML, Smeak DD (1988) An epidemiological study of 151 distal humeral fractures in dogs and cats. *J Am Anim Hosp Assoc* **24**:531–536.

Lefebvre JB, Robertson TR, Baines SJ *et al.* (2008) Assessment of humeral length in dogs after repair of Salter–Harris Type IV fracture of the lateral part of the humeral condyle. *Vet Surg* **37**:545–551.

References

130

McChesney AE, Stephens LC, Lebel J *et al*. (1980) Infiltrative lipoma in dogs. *Vet Pathol* **17**:316–322.

Bergman PJ, Withrow SJ, Straw RC *et al*. (1994) Infiltrative lipoma in dogs: 16 cases (1981–1992). *J Am Vet Med Assoc* **205**:322–324.

McEntee MC, Thrall DE (2001) Computed tomographic imaging of infiltrative lipoma in 22 dogs. *Vet Radiol Ultrasound* **42**:221–225.

131

Fischer H, Norton J, Kobluk LN *et al*. (2004) Surgical reduction and stabilization for repair of femoral capital physeal fractures in cats: 13 cases. *J Am Vet Med Assoc* **224**:1478–1482.

Culvenor JA, Black AP, Lorkin KF *et al*. (1996) Repair of femoral capital physeal injuries in cats – 14 cases. *Vet Comp Orthop Traumatol* **9**:182–185.

132

Baker SG, Roush JK, Unis MD *et al*. (2010) Comparison of four commercial devices to measure limb circumference in dogs. *Vet Comp Orthop Traumatol* **23**:406–410.

133

Burton NJ, Owen MR (2007) Treatment of a shoulder luxation in a forelimb amputee dog. *Vet Comp Orthop Traumatol* **20**:146–149.

Liehmann L, Lorinson D (2006) Traumatic triceps tendon avulsion in a cat. *J Small Anim Pract* **47**:94–97.

134

McKee WM, May C, Macias C *et al*. (2004) Pantarsal arthrodesis with a customised medial or lateral bone plate in 13 dogs. *Vet Rec* **154**:165–170.

Theoret MC, Moens NMM (2007) The use of veterinary cuttable plates for carpal and tarsal arthrodesis in small dogs and cats. *Can Vet J* **48**:165–168.

135

Burger M, Forterre F, Brunnberg L (2004) Surgical anatomy of the feline sacroiliac joint for lag screw fixation of sacroiliac fracture-luxation. *Vet Comp Orthop Traumatol* **17**:146–151.

Shales C, Moores A, Kulendra E *et al*. (2010) Stabilization of sacroiliac luxation in 40 cats using screws inserted in lag fashion. *Vet Surg* **39**:696–700.

Shales C, White L, Langley-Hobbs SJ (2009) Feline sacroiliac luxation: anatomic study of dorsoventral articular surface angulation and safe corridor for placement of screws used for lag fixation. *Vet Surg* **38**:343–348.

136

Fettig AA, McCarthy RJ, Kowaleski MP (2002) Intertarsal and tarsometatarsal arthrodesis using 2.0/2.7-mm or 2.7/3.5-mm hybrid dynamic compression plates. *J Am Anim Hosp Assoc* **38**:364–369.

Whitelock R, Dyce J, Houlton JEF (1999) Metacarpal fractures associated with pancarpal arthrodesis in dogs. *Vet Surg* **28**:25–30.

137

Powers BE, LaRue SM, Withrow SJ (1988) Jamshidi needle biopsy for diagnosis of bone lesions in small animals. *J Am Vet Med Assoc* **193**:205–214.

Wykes PM, Powers BE, Withrow SJ (1985) Closed biopsy for diagnosis of long bone tumors: accuracy and results. *J Am Anim Hosp Assoc* **21**:485–494.

138

Johnson KA (1987) Accessory carpal bone fractures in the racing greyhound: classification and pathology. *Vet Surg* **16**:60–64.

Johnson KA, Piermattei DL, Davis PE (1988) Characteristics of accessory carpal bone fractures in 50 racing greyhounds. *Vet Comp Orthop Traumatol* **2**:104–107.

Johnson KA, Dee JF, Piermattei DL (1989) Screw fixation of accessory carpal bone fractures in racing greyhounds: 12 cases (1981–1986). *J Am Vet Med Assoc* **194**:1618–1625.

139

Langley-Hobbs SJ, Meeson RL, Hamilton MH *et al.* (2009) Feline ilial fractures: a prospective study of dorsal plating and comparison with lateral plating. *Vet Surg* **38**:334–342.

Hamilton MH, Evans DA, Langley-Hobbs SJ (2009) Feline ilial fractures: assessment of screw loosening and pelvic canal narrowing after lateral plating. *Vet Surg* **38**:326–333.

Meeson R, Corr S (2011) Management of pelvic trauma: neurological damage, urinary tract disruption and pelvic fractures. *J Feline Med Surg* **13**:347–361.

140

Cook JL, Tomlinson JL, Reed AL (1999) Fluoroscopically guided closed reduction and internal fixation of fractures of the lateral portion of the humeral condyle: prospective clinical study of the technique and results in ten dogs. *Vet Surg* **28**:315–321.

141

Theyse LFH, Voorhout G, Hazewinkel HAW (2005) Prognostic factors in treating antebrachial growth deformities with a lengthening procedure using a circular external skeletal fixation system in dogs. *Vet Surg* **34**:424–435.

142

Murphy TP, Hill CM, Kapatkin AS *et al.* (2001) Pullout properties of 3.5-mm AO/ASIF self-tapping and cortex screws in a uniform synthetic material and in canine bone. *Vet Surg* **30**:253–260.

143

Abelson AL, McCobb EC, Shaw S *et al.* (2009) Use of wound soaker catheters for the administration of local anesthetic for post-operative analgesia: 56 cases. *Vet Anaesth Analg* **63**:597–602.

144

Lewis DD, Radasch RM, Beale BS *et al.* (1999) Initial clinical experience with the IMEX™ Circular External Skeletal Fixation System. Part II: Use in bone lengthening and correction of angular and rotational deformities. *Vet Comp Orthop Traumatol* **12**:118–127.

References

Sereda CW, Lewis DD, Radasch RM et al. (2009) Descriptive report of antebrachial growth deformity correction in 17 dogs from 1999–2007, using hybrid linear-circular external fixator constructs. *Can Vet J* 50:723–732.

145

Dorea HC, McLaughlin RM, Cantwell HD et al. (2005) Evaluation of healing in feline femoral defects filled with cancellous autograft, cancellous allograft or Bioglass. *Vet Comp Orthop Traumatol* 18:157–168.

Kerwin SC, Lewis DD, Elkins AD et al. (1996) Deep-frozen allogenic cancellous bone grafts in 10 dogs: a case series. *Vet Surg* 25:18–28.

146

Petazzoni M, Urizzi A, Verdonck B et al. (2010) Fixin internal fixator: concept and technique. *Vet Comp Orthop Traumatol* 23:250–253.

147

Kramer A, Walsh P, Seguin B (2008) Hemipelvectomy in dogs and cats: technique overview, variations, and description. *Vet Surg* 37:413–419.

148

Lees GE, Sautter JH (1979) Anemia and osteopetrosis in a dog. *J Am Vet Med Assoc* 175:820–824.

Maley JR, Dvorak LD, Bahr A (2010) What is your diagnosis? Osteopetrosis. *J Am Vet Med Assoc* 236:287–288.

149

Rahal SC, De Biasi F, Vulcano LC et al. (2000) Reduction of humeroulnar congenital elbow luxation in 8 dogs by using the transarticular pin. *Can Vet J* 41:849–853.

Campbell CR (1971) Luxation and ligamentous injuries of the elbow of the dog. *Vet Clin North Am* 1:429–440.

Milton JL, Horne RD, Bartels JE (1979) Congenital elbow luxation in the dog. *J Am Vet Med Assoc* 175:572–582.

150

Saunders HM, Jezyk PK (1991) The radiographic appearance of canine congenital hypothyroidism: skeletal changes with delayed treatment. *Vet Radiol* 32:171–177.

Bojanic K, Acke E, Jones BR (2011) Congenital hypothyroidism of dogs and cats: a review. *NZ Vet J* 59:115–122.

Lieb AS, Grooters AM, Tyler JW et al. (1997) Tetraparesis due to vertebral physeal fracture in an adult dog with congenital hypothyroidism. *J Small Anim Pract* 38:364–367.

151

Radasch RM, Lewis DD, McDonald D (2008) Pes varus correction in 13 Dachshunds using a 1-A hybrid linear-circular external fixator. *Vet Surg* 37:71–81.

Sereda CW, Lewis DD, Radasch RM et al. (2009) Descriptive report of antebrachial growth deformity correction in 17 dogs from 1999–2007, using hybrid linear-circular external fixator constructs. *Can Vet J* 50:723–732.

152

Read RA, Black AP, Armstrong SJ *et al.* (1992) Incidence and clinical significance of sesamoid disease in Rottweilers. *Vet Rec* **130**:533–535.

Daniel A, Read RA, Cake MA (2008) Vascular foramina of the metacarpophalangeal sesamoids of Greyhounds and their relationship to sesamoid disease. *Am J Vet Res* **69**:716–721.

Mathews KG, Koblik PD, Whitehair JG *et al.* (2001) Fragmented palmar metacarpophalangeal sesamoids in dogs: a long-term evaluation. *Vet Comp Orthop Traumatol* **14**:7–14.

155

Vezzoni A, Boiocchi L, Vezzoni L *et al.* (2010) Double pelvic osteotomy for the treatment of hip dysplasia in young dogs. *Vet Comp Orthop Traumatol* **23**:444–452.

Punkie JP, Fox DB, Tomlinson JL *et al.* (2011) Acetabular ventroversion with double pelvic osteotomy versus triple pelvic osteotomy: a cadaveric study in dogs. *Vet Surg* **40**:555–562.

156

Bergh MS, Gilley RS, Shofer FS *et al.* (2006) Complications and radiographic findings following cemented total hip replacement: a retrospective evaluation of 97 dogs. *Vet Comp Orthop Traumatol* **19**:172–179.

Ota J, Cook JL, Lewis DD *et al.* (2005) Short-term aseptic loosening of the femoral component in canine total hip replacement: effects of cementing technique on cement mantle grade. *Vet Surg* **34**:345–352.

Hirose S, Otsuka H, Morishima T (2012) Outcomes of Charnley total hip arthroplasty using improved cementing with so-called second- and third-generation techniques. *J Orthop Sci* **17**:118–123.

157

Sissener TR, Whitelock RG, Langley-Hobbs SJ (2009) Long-term results of transarticular pinning for surgical stabilisation of coxofemoral luxation in 20 cats. *J Small Anim Pract* **50**:112–117.

158

Balara JM, McCarthy RJ, Kiupel M *et al.* (2009) Clinical, histologic, and immunohistochemical characterization of wart-like lesions on the paw pads of dogs: 24 cases (2000–2007). *J Am Vet Med Assoc* **274**:1555–1558.

Guilliard MJ, Segboer I, Shearer DH (2010) Corns in dogs; signalment, possible aetiology and response to surgical treatment. *J Small Anim Pract* **52**:162–168.

159

Allen MJ, Leone KA, Lamonte K *et al.* (2009) Cemented total knee replacement in 24 dogs: surgical technique, clinical results, and complications. *Vet Surg* **38**:555–567.

Liska WD, Doyle ND (2009) Canine total knee replacement: surgical technique and one-year outcome. *Vet Surg* **38**:568–582.

160

Adamantos S, Boag A (2007) Thirteen cases of tetanus in the dog. *Vet Rec* **161**:298–302.

References

Langner KFA, Schenk HC, Leithaeuser C et al. (2011) Localised tetanus in a cat. *Vet Rec* **169**:126.

Sanford JP (1995) Tetanus: forgotten but not gone. *New Eng J Med* **332**:812–813.

161

Cook JL, Hudson CC, Kuroki K (2008) Autogenous osteochondral grafting for treatment of stifle osteochondrosis in dogs. *Vet Surg* **37**:311–321.

Gudas R, Kalesinskas RJ, Kimtys V et al. (2005) A prospective randomized clinical study of mosaic osteochondral autologous transplantation versus microfracture for the treatment of osteochondral defects in the knee joint in young athletes. *Arthroscopy* **21**:1066–1075.

162

Muir P, Johnson KA, Markel MD (1995) Area moment of inertia for comparison of implant cross-sectional geometry and bending stiffness. *Vet Comp Orthop Traumatol* **8**:146–152.

163

Moores AP (2011) Maxillomandibular external skeletal fixation in five cats with caudal jaw trauma. *J Small Anim Pract* **52**:38–41.

Nicholson I, Wyatt J, Radke H et al. (2010) Treatment of caudal mandibular fracture and temporomandibular joint fracture-luxation using a bi-gnathic encircling and retaining device. *Vet Comp Orthop Traumatol* **23**:102–108.

164

Muir P, Johnson KA, Markel MD (1995) Area moment of inertia for comparison of implant cross-sectional geometry and bending stiffness. *Vet Comp Orthopaed* **8**:146–152.

165

Nelligan MR, Wheeler JL, Lewis DD et al. (2007) Bilateral correction of metatarsal rotation in a dog using circular external skeletal fixation. *Aust Vet J* **85**:332–336.

Petazzoni M, Piras A, Jaeger GH et al. (2009) Correction of rotational deformity of the pes with external skeletal fixation in four dogs. *Vet Surg* **38**:506–514.

166

Sammarco JI, Conzemius MG, Perkowski SZ et al. (1996) Postoperative analgesia for stifle surgery: a comparison of intra-articular bupivacaine, morphine, or saline. *Vet Surg* **25**:59–69.

167

Samoy Y, Van Ryssen B, Van Caelenberg A et al. (2008) Single-phase bone scintigraphy in dogs with obscure lameness. *J Small Anim Pract* **49**:444–450.

168

Mahn MM, Cook JL, Cook CR et al. (2005) Arthroscopic verification of ultrasonographic diagnosis of meniscal pathology in dogs. *Vet Surg* **34**:318–323.

Theiman KM, Tomlinson JL, Fox DB et al. (2006) Effect of meniscal release on rate of subsequent meniscal tears and owner-assessed outcome in dogs with cranial cruciate disease treated with tibial plateau leveling osteotomy. *Vet Surg* **35**:705–710.

169
Salter RB, Harris WR (1963) Injuries to the epiphyseal plate. *J Bone Joint Surg Am* **45**:587–622.

170
Jermyn K, Roe SC (2011) Influence of screw insertion order on compression generated by bone plates in a fracture model. *Vet Comp Orthop Traumatol* **6**:403–407.

171
Lantz GC, Cantwell HD (1986) Intermittent open-mouth lower jaw locking in five dogs. *J Am Vet Med Assoc* **188**:1403–1405.

Hazewinkel HAW, Koole R, Voorhout G (1993) Mandibular coronoid process displacement: signs, causes, treatment. *Vet Comp Orthop Traumatol* **6**:29–35.

Robins G, Grandage J (1977) Temporomandibular joint dysplasia and open-mouth jaw locking in the dog. *J Am Vet Med Assoc* **171**:1072–1076.

172
Kona-Boun JJ, Cuvelliez S, Troncy E (2006) Evaluation of epidural administration of morphine or morphine and bupivacaine for postoperative analgesia after premedication with an opioid analgesic and orthopedic surgery in dogs. *J Am Vet Med Assoc* **229**:1103–1112.

173
Laverty PH, McClure SR (2002) Initial experience with extracorporeal shock wave therapy in six dogs. Part 1. *Vet Comp Orthop Traumatol* **15**:177–183.

Venzin C, Ohlerth S, Koch D *et al.* (2004) Extracorporeal shockwave therapy in a dog with chronic bicipital tenosynovitis. *Schweiz Arch Tierheilkd* **146**:136–141.

174
Harryssom OLA, Cormier DR, Marcellin-Little DJ *et al.* (2003) Rapid prototyping for treatment of canine limb deformities. *Rapid Prototyping J* **9**:37–42.

Dismukes DI, Fox DB, Tomlinson JL *et al.* (2008) Use of radiographic measures and three-dimensional computed tomographic imaging in surgical correction of an antebrachial deformity in a dog. *J Am Vet Med Assoc* **232**:68–73.

Wendleburg KM, Lewis DD, Sereda CW *et al.* (2011) Use of an interlocking nail-hybrid fixator construct for distal femoral deformity correction in three dogs. *Vet Comp Orthop Traumatol* **24**:236–245.

175
Kirpenstein J, Straw RC, Pardo AD (1994) Partial and total scapulectomy in the dog. *J Am Anim Hosp Assoc* **30**:313–319.

Norton C, Drenen CM, Emms SG (2006) Subtotal scapulectomy as the treatment for scapular tumour in the dog: a report of six cases. *Aust Vet J* **84**:364–366.

References

176

Bennett RA, Egger EL, Histand M *et al*. (1987) Comparison of the strength and holding power of 4 pin designs for use with half pin (type I) external skeletal fixation. *Vet Surg* **16**:207–211.

Aron DN, Toombs JP, Hollingsworth SC (1986) Primary treatment of severe fractures by external skeletal fixation: threaded pins compared with smooth pins. *J Am Anim Hosp Assoc* **22**:659–670.

Beck AL, Pead MJ (2003) The use of Ellis pins (negative profile tip-threaded pins) in external skeletal fixation in dogs and cats. *Vet Comp Orthop Traumatol* **16**:223–231.

177

Gorse MJ, Purinton PT, Penwick RC *et al*. (1990) Talocalcaneal luxation: an anatomic and clinical study. *Vet Surg* **19**:429–434.

Macias C, McKee WM, May C (2000) Talocalcaneal luxation with plantar displacement of the head of the talus in a dog and a cat. *Vet Rec* **147**:743–745.

178

Lewis DD, Shelton GD, Piras A *et al*. (1997) Gracilis or semitendinosus myopathy in eighteen dogs. *J Am Anim Hosp Assoc* **33**:177–188.

179

Bardet JF, Hohn RB (1983) Quadriceps contracture in dogs. *J Am Vet Med Assoc* **183**:680–685.

Fries CL, Binnington AG, Cockshutt JR (1988) Quadriceps contracture in four cats: a complication of internal fixation of femoral fractures. *Vet Comp Orthop Traumatol* **2**:91–96.

180

Tornkvist H, Hearn TC, Schatzker J (1996) The strength of plate fixation in relation to the number and spacing of bone screws. *J Orthop Traumatol* **10**:204–208.

181

Clark KJ, Jerram RM, Walker AM (2010) Surgical management of suspected congenital luxation of the radial head in three dogs. *NZ Vet J* **58**:103–109.

Fafard AR (2006) Unilateral congenital elbow luxation in a Dachshund. *Can Vet J* **47**:909–912.

Spadari A, Romagnoli N, Venturini A (2001) A modified Bell-Tawse procedure for surgical correction of congenital elbow luxation in a Dalmatian puppy. *Vet Comp Orthop Traumatol* **14**:210–213.

182

Matus RE, Leifer CE, MacEwen EG *et al*. (1986) Prognostic factors for multiple myeloma in the dog. *J Am Vet Med Assoc* **188**:1288–1292.

183

Balfour RJ, Boudrieau RJ, Gores BR (2000) T-plate fixation of distal radial closing wedge osteotomies for treatment of angular limb deformities in 18 dogs. *Vet Surg* **29**:207–217.

Preston CA (2000) Distraction osteogenesis to treat premature distal radial growth plate closure in a dog. *Aust Vet J* **78**:387–391.

Guthrie S, Pead M (1992) A complication arising after surgical correction of short radius syndrome. *J Small Anim Pract* **33**:24–26.

184
Ganz SM, Jackson J, VanEnkevort B (2010) Risk factors for femoral fracture after canine press-fit cementless total hip arthroplasty. *Vet Surg* 39:688–695.

185
Toombs JP, Bronson DG, Ross D *et al.* (2003) The SK external fixation system: description of components, instrumentation and application techniques. *Vet Comp Orthop Traumatol* 16:76–81.
Clary EM, Roe SC (1996) In vitro biomechanical and histological assessment of pilot hole diameter for positive-profile external skeletal fixation pins in canine tibiae. *Vet Surg* 25:453–462.

186
Trostel CT, Pool RR, McLaughlin RM (2003) Canine lameness caused by developmental orthopedic disease; panosteitis, Legg–Calvé–Perthes Disease and hypertrophic osteodystrophy. *Comp Contin Educ Pract Vet* 25:282–293.
Lee R, Fry PD (1969) Some observations on the occurrence of Legg–Calvé–Perthes' disease (coxaplana) in the dog, and an evaluation of excision arthroplasty as a method of treatment. *J Small Anim Pract* 10:309–317.
Roperto F, Papparella S, Crovace A (1992) Legg–Calvé–Perthes disease in dogs: histological and ultrstructural investigations. *J Am Anim Hosp Assoc* 28:156–162.

187
Lewis DD, Radasch RM, Beale BS *et al.* (1999) Initial clinical experience with the IMEX™ Circular External Skeletal Fixation System. Part II: use in bone lengthening and correction of angular and rotational deformities. *Vet Comp Orthop Traumatol* 12:118–127.
Ehrhart N (2005) Longitudinal bone transport for treatment of primary bone tumors in dogs: a classification of the technique and summary of nine cases. *Vet Surg* 34:24–34.
McCartney WT (2008) Limb lengthening in three dogs using distraction rates without a latency period. *Vet Comp Orthop Traumatol* 21:446–450.

188
Fox SE (1998) External coaptation bandages: How and when to use them. *Vet Med* 83:153–164.

189
Blake CA, Boudrieau RJ, Torrance BS *et al.* (2011) Single cycle to failure in bending of three standard and five locking plates and plate constructs. *Vet Comp Orthop Traumatol* 24:408–417.

190
Evans RB, Gordon-Evans WJ, Conzemius MG (2008) Comparison of three methods for the management of fragmented medial coronoid process in the dog. A systematic review and meta-analysis. *Vet Comp Orthop Traumatol* 21:106–109.

References

Fitzpatrick N, Smith TJ, Evans RB et al. (2009) Subtotal coronoid ostectomy for treatment of medial coronoid disease in 263 dogs. *Vet Surg* 38:233–245.

Burton NJ, Owen MR, Kirk LS et al. (2011) Conservative versus arthroscopic management for medial coronoid process disease in dogs: a prospective gait evaluation. *Vet Surg* 40:972–980.

191

Conzemius MG, Aper RL, Corti LB (2003) Short-term outcome after total elbow arthroplasty in dogs with severe naturally occurring osteoarthritis. *Vet Surg* 32:545–552.

Conzemius M (2009) Nonconstrained elbow replacement in dogs. *Vet Surg* 38:279–284.

192

Gemmill TJ, Bennett D, Carmichael S (2006) Chronic disruption of the lateral collateral ligament complex of the carpus in two dogs. *Vet Rec* 158:25.

Langley-Hobbs SJ, Hamilton MH, Pratt JN (2007) Radiographic and clinical features of carpal varus associated with chronic sprain of the lateral collateral ligament complex in 10 dogs. *Vet Comp OrthopTraumatol* 20:324–330.

193

Dennler R, Kipfer N, Tepic S et al. (2006) Inclination of the patellar ligament in relation to flexion angle in stifle joints of dogs without degenerative joint disease. *Am J Vet Res* 67:1849–1854.

194

Andriacchi TP, Mündermann A, Smith RL et al. (2004) A framework for the in vivo pathomechanics of osteoarthritis at the knee. *Ann Biomed Eng* 32:447–457.

Isaac DI, Meyer EG, Haut RC (2008) Chondrocyte damage and contact pressures following impact on the rabbit tibiofemoral joint. *J Biomech Eng* 130:041018.

Kim SE, Pozzi A, Banks SA et al. (2009) Effect of tibial plateau leveling osteotomy on femorotibial contact mechanics and stifle kinematics. *Vet Surg* 38:23–32.

195

Robb JL, Cook JL, Carson W (2005) In vitro evaluation of screws and suture anchors in metaphyseal bone of the canine tibia. *Vet Surg* 34:499–508.

196

Carobbi B, Ness MG (2009) Preliminary study evaluating tests used to diagnose canine cranial cruciate ligament failure. *J Small Anim Pract* 50:224–226.

197

Johnson JM, Johnson AL, Eurell AC (1994) Histological appearance of naturally occurring canine physeal fractures. *Vet Surg* 23:81–86.

198

Kasström H, Olsson SE, Suter PF (1972) Panosteitis in the dog. A radiographic, scintimetric and trifluorochrome investigation. *Acta Radiol* (Suppl) 319:15–23.

Muir PM, Dubielzig RR, Johnson KA (1996) Panosteitis. *Compend Contin Educ Pract Vet* 18:29–33.

Schawalder P, Andres HU, Jutzi K *et al*. (2002) Canine panosteitis: an idiopathic bone disease investigated in the light of a new hypothesis concerning pathogenesis. Part 1: Clinical and diagnostic aspects. *Schweiz Arch Tierheilkd* **144**:115–130.

199
Gustilo RB, Anderson JT (1976) Prevention of infection in the treatment of one thousand and twenty-five open fractures of long bones: retrospective and prospective analyses. *J Bone Joint Surg Am* **58**:453–458.

Tillson DM (1995) Open fracture management. *Vet Clin North Am Small Anim Pract* **25**:1093–1110.

200
Welch JA, Boudrieau RJ, DeJardin LM (1997) The intraosseous blood supply of the canine radius: implications for healing of distal fractures in small dogs. *Vet Surg* **26**:57–61.

Brianza SZM, Delise M, Ferraris MM *et al*. (2006) Cross-sectional geometrical properties of distal radius and ulna in large, medium and toy breed dogs. *J Biomech* **39**:302–311.

201
Irubetagoyena I, Lopez T, Autefage A (2011) Type IV Monteggia fracture in a cat. *Vet Comp Orthop Traumatol* **24**:483–486.

Bush M, Owen M (2009) Type-IV variant Monteggia fracture with concurrent proximal radial physeal fracture in a Domestic Shorthaired Cat. *Vet Comp Orthop Traumatol* **22**:225–228.

202
Uhl JM, Seguin B, Kapatkin AS *et al*. (2008) Mechanical comparison of 3.5 mm broad dynamic compression plate, limited-contact dynamic compression plate, and narrow locking compression plate systems using interfragmentary gap models. *Vet Surg* **37**:663–673.

203
Schwarz PD, Schraeder SC (1984) Ulnar fractures and dislocation of the proximal radial epiphysis in the dog and cat. A review of 28 cases. *J Am Vet Med Assoc* **185**:190–194.

204
Vasseur PB (1983) Clinical results of surgical correction of shoulder luxation in dogs. *J Am Vet Med Assoc* **182**:503–505.

Fowler DJ, Presnell KR, Holmberg DL (1987) Scapulohumeral arthrodesis: results in seven dogs. *J Am Anim Hosp Assoc* **24**:667–672.

Sidaway BK, McLaughlin RM, Elder SH *et al*. (2004) Role of the tendons of the biceps brachii and infraspinatus muscles and the medial glenohumeral ligament in the maintenance of passive shoulder joint stability in dogs. *Am J Vet Res* **65**:1216–1222.

205
Roush JK (1993) Canine patellar luxation. *Vet Clin North Am Small Anim Pract* **23**:855–868.

Putnam RW (1968) *Patellar luxation in the dog*. Dissertation. Veterinary College, University of Guelph.

References

206

Reinke JD, Mughannam AJ, Owens JM (1993) Avulsion of the gastrocnemius tendon in 11 dogs. *J Am Anim Hosp Assoc* **29**:410–418.

207

Groth AM, Benigni L, Moores AP *et al.* (2009) Spectrum of computed tomographic findings in 58 canine elbows with fragmentation of the medial coronoid process. *J Small Anim Pract* **50**:15–22.

Holsworth IG, Wisner ER, Scherrer WE *et al.* (2005) Accuracy of computerized tomographic evaluation of canine radio-ulnar incongruence in vitro. *Vet Surg* **34**:108–111.

208

Johnson AL, Probst CW, DeCamp CE *et al.* (2001) Comparison of trochlear block recession and trochlear wedge recession for canine patellar luxation using a cadaver model. *Vet Surg* **30**:140–150.

Arthurs GI, Langley-Hobbs SJ (2006) Complications associated with corrective surgery for patellar luxation in 109 dogs. *Vet Surg* **35**:559–566.

209

Syrett BC, Davis EE (1979) In vivo evaluation of a high-strength, high-ductility stainless steel for use in surgical implants. *J Biomed Mater Res* **13**:543–556.

Chrzanowski W, Armitage DA, Knowles JC *et al.* (2008) Chemical, corrosion and topographical analysis of stainless steel implants after different implantation periods. *J Biomater App* **23**:51–71.

210

Wolf A, Senesh M (2011) Estimating joint kinematics from skin motion observation: modeling and validation. *Comput Methods Biomech Biomed Engin* **1**:1–8.

Oosterlinck M, Bosmans T, Gasthuys F *et al.* (2011) Accuracy of pressure plate kinetic asymmetry indices and their correlation with visual gait assessment scores in lame and non-lame dogs. *Am J Vet Res* **72**:820–825.

212

Burnett JM, Wardlaw JL (2012) Physical rehabilitation for veterinary practices. *Today's Vet Pract* **2**:14–20.

213

Johnson SG, Hulse DA, Van Gundy TE *et al.* (1989) Corrective osteotomy for pes varus in the Dachshund. *Vet Surg* **18**:373–379.

Radasch RM, Lewis DD, McDonald DE *et al.* (2008) Pes varus correction in Dachshunds using a hybrid external fixator. *Vet Surg* **37**:71–81.

Petazzoni M, Nicetto T, Vezzoni A *et al.* (2012) Treatment of pes varus using locking plate fixation in seven Dachshund dogs. *Vet Comp Orthop Traumatol* **25**:231–238.

214

Garzotto CK, Berg J, Hoffmann WE *et al.* (2000) Prognostic significance of serum alkaline phosphatase activity in canine appendicular osteosarcoma. *J Vet Intern Med* **14**:587–592.

Boulay JP, Wallace LJ, Lipowitz LJ (1987) Pathological fracture in the long bones in the dog. *J Am Anim Hosp Assoc* **23**:297–303.

References

Bhandal J, Boston SE (2011)
Pathological fracture in dogs
with suspected or confirmed
osteosarcoma. *Vet Surg* **40**:423–430.

215
Johnson KA, Skinner GA, Muir
P (2001) Site specific adaptive
remodeling of Greyhound
metacarpal cortical bone subjected
to asymmetric cyclic loading. *Am J
Vet Res* **62**:787–793.

Bellenger CR, Johnson KA, Davis PE
et al. (1981) Fixation of metacarpal
and metatarsal fractures in
greyhounds. *Aust Vet J* **57**:205–211.

216
Moak PC, Lewis DD, Roe SC *et
al.* (2000) Arthrodesis of the
elbow in three cats. *Vet Comp
OrthopTraumatol* **13**:149–153.

de Haan JJ, Roe SC, Lewis DD *et al.*
(1996) Elbow arthrodesis in twelve
dogs. *Vet Comp Orthop Traumatol*
9:115–118.

217
Vezzoni A, Bohorquez Vanelli A,
Modenato M *et al.* (2008) Proximal
tibial epiphysiodesis to redcue tibial
plateau slope in young dogs with
cranial cruciate ligament deficient
stifle. *Vet Comp Orthop Traumatol*
21:343–348.

218
Pucheu B, Duhautois B (2008)
Surgical treatment of shoulder
instability. A retrospective study on
76 cases (1993–2007) *Vet Comp
OrthopTraumatol* **4**:368–374.

Vasseur PB (1990) Arthrodesis for
congenital luxation of the shoulder
in a dog. *J Am Vet Med Assoc*
197:501–513.

219
García-Hernández L, Déciga-Campos
M, Guevara-López U *et al.* (2007)
Co-administration of rofecoxib and
tramadol results in additive or sub-
additive interaction during arthritic
nociception in rat. *Pharmacol
Biochem Behav* **87**:331–340.

Marsolais GS, Dvorak G, Conzemius
MG (2002) Effects of postoperative
rehabilitation on limb function
after cranial cruciate ligament
repair in dogs. *J Am Vet Med Assoc*
220:1325–1330.

220
Zink C (2008) *The Agility Advantage.*
Clean Run Productions, LLC, pp.
18–21.

221
Hoffmann DE, Miller JM, Ober CP
et al. (2006) Tibial tuberosity
advancement in 65 canine stifles. *Vet
Comp Orthop Traumatol* **19**:219–
227.

222
da Silva JP, da Silva MA, Almeida APF
et al. (2010) Laser therapy in the
tissue repair process: a literature
review. *Photomed Laser Surg*
28:17–21.

Bjordal JM, Johnson MI, Iversen V *et
al.* (2006) Low-level laser therapy
in acute pain: a systematic review
of possible mechanisms of action
and clinical effects in randomized
placebo-controlled trials. *Photomed
Laser Surg* **24**:158–168.

223
Rondeau M, Walton R, Bissett S *et
al.* (2005) Suppurative, nonseptic
polyarthropathy in dogs. *J Vet Intern
Med* **19**:654–662.

References

224
Neat BC, Kowaleski MP, Litsky AS *et al.* (2006) Mechanical evaluation of pin and tension-band wire factors in an olecranon osteotomy model. *Vet Surg* 35:398–405.

225
Berg J, Lamb CR, O'Callghan MW (1990) Bone scintigraphy in the initial evaluation of 70 dogs with primary bone tumors. *J Am Vet Med Assoc* 196:917–920.

226
Eugster S, Schawalder P, Gaschen F *et al.* (2004) A prospective study of postoperative surgical site infections in dogs and cats. *Vet Surg* 33:542–550.
Marcellin-Little DJ, Papich MG, Richardson DC *et al.* (1996) Pharmacokinetic model for cefazolin distribution during total hip arthroplasty in dogs. *Am J Vet Res* 5:720–723.
Whittem TL, Johnson AL, Smith CW *et al.* (1999) Effect of perioperative prophylactic antimicrobial treatment in dogs undergoing elective orthopedic surgery. *J Am Vet Med Assoc* 15:212–216.

227
Moses PA, Lewis DD, Lanz OI *et al.* (2002) Intramedullary interlocking nail stabilization of 21 humeral fracture in 19 dogs and one cat. *Aust Vet J* 80:336–343.
Lansdowne JL, Sinnott MT, Dejardin LM *et al.* (2007) *In vitro* mechanical comparison of screwed, bolted, and novel interlocking nail systems to buttress plate fixation in torsion and mediolateral bending. *Vet Surg* 36:368–377.

Basinger RR, Suber JT (2004) Two techniques for supplementing interlocking nail repair of fractures of the humerus, femur, and tibia: results in 12 dogs and cats. *Vet Surg* 33:673–676.

228
Pozzi A, Tonks CA, Ling C (2010) Medial meniscus contact mechanics and strain following serial meniscectomies in a cadaveric dog study. *Vet Surg* 39:482–488.
Masouros SD, McDermott ID, Amis AA *et al.* (2008) Biomechanics of the meniscus-meniscal ligament construct of the knee. *Knee Surg Sports Traumatol Arthrosc* 16:1121–1132.

229
Aron DN, Crowe DT (1987) The 90-90 flexion splint for prevention of stifle joint stiffness with femoral fracture repairs. *J Am Anim Hosp Assoc* 23:447–454.

230
Tomlin J, Pead MJ, Langley-Hobbs SJ *et al.* (2001) Radial carpal bone fracture in dogs. *J Am Anim Hosp Assoc* 37:173–178.
Li A, Bennett D, Gibbs C *et al.* (2000) Radial carpal bone fractures in 15 dogs. *J Small Anim Pract* 41:74–79.

231
Muir P, Johnson KA (1994) Supraspinatus and biceps brachii tendinopathy in dogs. *J Small Anim Pract* 35:239–243.
Kriegleder H (1995) Mineralization of the supraspinatus tendon: clinical observations in seven dogs. *Vet Comp OrthopTraumatol* 8:91–97.

Lafuente MP, Fransson BA, Lincoln JD *et al.* (2009) Surgical treatment of mineralized and nonmineralized supraspinatus tendinopathy in twenty-four dogs. *Vet Surg* **38**:380–387.

232

Grundmann S, Montavon PM (2001) Stenosing tenosynovitis of the abductor pollicis longus muscle in dogs. *Vet Comp Orthop Traumatol* **14**:95–100.

Hittmair KM, Groessl V, Mayrhofer E (2011) Radiographic and ultrasonographic diagnosis of stenosing tenosynovitis of the abductor pollicis longus muscle in dogs. *Vet Radiol Ultrasound* **153**:111–116.

Moores AP, Comerford EJ (2005) What is your diagnosis? Stenosing tenosynovitis of the tendon of the abductor pollicis longus muscle. *J Small Anim Pract* **46**:41–43.

233

Cook JL, Luther JK, Beetem J *et al.* (2010) Clinical comparison of a novel extracapsular stabilization procedure and tibial plateau leveling osteotomy for treatment of cranial cruciate ligament deficiency in dogs. *Vet Surg* **39**:315–323.

Choate CJ, Pozzi A, Lewis DD *et al.* (2012) Mechanical properties of isolated loops of nylon leader material, polyethylene cord, and polyethylene tape and mechanical properties of these materials secured to cadaveric femurs via lateral femoral fabellae, toggles placed through bone tunnels, or bone anchors. *Am J Vet Res* **73**:1519–1529.

234

McLaughlin R (2002) Feline stifle disease. *Vet Clin North Am Small Anim Pract* **32**:963–982.

235

Liptak JM, Dernell WS, Rizzo SA *et al.* (2005) Partial foot amputation in 11 dogs. *J Am Anim Hosp Assoc* **41**:47–55.

Bergman PJ, McKnight J, Novosad A *et al.* (2003) Long-term survival of dogs with advanced malignant melanoma after DNA vaccination with xenogeneic human tyrosinase: a phase I trial. *Clin Cancer Res* **9**:1284–1290.

236

Schrader SC (1982) Septic arthritis and osteomyelitis of the hip in six mature dogs. *J Am Vet Med Assoc* **181**:894–898.

Hewes CA, Macintire DK (2011) Intra-articular therapy to treat septic arthritis in a dog. *J Am Anim Hosp Assoc* **47**:280–284.

Benzioni H, Shahar R, Yudelevitch S *et al.* (2008) Bacterial infective arthritis of the coxofemoral joint in dogs with hip dysplasia. *Vet Comp OrthopTraumatol* **21**:262–266.

237

Kienzle E, Bergler R, Mandernach A (1998) Comparison of the feeding behavior and the man–animal relationship in owners of normal and obese dogs. *J Nutr* **128**:2779S–2782S.

References

238

Bound N, Zakai D, Butterworth SJ *et al.* (2009) The prevalence of canine patellar luxation in three centres. Clinical features and radiographic evidence of limb deviation. *Vet Comp Orthop Traumatol* **22**:32–37.

Palmer RH, Ikuta CL, Cadmus JM (2011) Comparison of femoral angulation measurement between radiographs and anatomic specimens across a broad range of varus conformations. *Vet Surg* **40**:1023–1028.

Dudley RM, Kowaleski MP, Drost WT *et al.* (2006) Radiographic and computed tomographic determination of femoral varus and torsion in the dog. *Vet Radiol Ultrasound* **47**:546–552.

239

Roch SP, Gemmill TJ (2007) Treatment of medial patellar luxation by femoral closing wedge ostectomy using a distal femoral plate in four dogs. *J Small Anim Pract* **49**:152–158.

240

Jaeger GH, Marcellin-Little DJ, Ferretti A (2007) Morphology and correction of distal tibial valgus deformities. *J Small Anim Pract* **48**:678–682.

Altunatmaz K, Ozsoy S, Guzel O. (2007) Bilateral pes valgus in an Anatolian Sheepdog. *Vet Comp OrthopTraumatol* **20**:241–244.

Burton NJ, Owen MR (2007) Limb alignment of pes valgus in a giant breed dog by plate-rod fixation. *Vet Comp OrthopTraumatol* **20**:236–240.

241

Pettitt RA, Innes JF (2008) Arthroscopic management of a lateral glenohumeral ligament rupture in two dogs. *Vet Comp Orthop Traumatol* **21**:302–306.

242

Bergman RL, Inzana KD, Monroe WE *et al.* (2002) Dystrophin-deficient muscular dystrophy in a Labrador retriever. *J Am Anim Hosp Assoc* **38**:255–261.

243

Demko JL, Sidaway BK, Thieman KM *et al.* (2006) Toggle rod stabilization for treatment of hip joint luxation in dogs: 62 cases (2000–2005). *J Am Vet Med Assoc* **229**:984–989.

Baltzer WI, Schulz KS, Stover SM *et al.* (2001) Biomechanical analysis of suture anchors and suture materials used for toggle pin stabilization of hip joint luxation in dogs. *Am J Vet Res* **62**:721–728.

Beckham HP, Smith MM, Kern DA (1996) Use of a modified toggle pin for repair of coxofemoral luxation in dogs with multiple orthopedic injuries: 14 cases (1986–1994). *J Am Vet Med Assoc* **208**:81–84.

244

Muir P, Dubielzig RR, Johnson KA *et al.* (1996) Hypertrophic osteodystrophy and calvarial hyperostosis. *Compend Contin Educ Pract Vet* **18**:143–151.

Arnott JL, Philbey AW, Bennett D (2008) Pathological fractures secondary to metaphyseal osteopathy in a dog. *Vet Comp Orthop Traumatol* **21**:177–180.

245

Ter Haar G (1978) Basic physics of therapeutic ultrasound. *Physiotherapy* **64**:100–103.

Mason TJ (2011) Therapeutic ultrasound an overview. *Ultrason Sonochem* **18**:847–852.

246

Wiemer P, van Ryssen B, Gielen I *et al.* (2007) Diagnostic findings in a lame-free dog with complete rupture of the biceps brachii tendon. *Vet Comp Orthop Traumatol* **20**:73–77.

247

Halling KB, Lewis DD, Cross AR *et al.* (2002) Complication rate and factors affecting outcome of olecranon osteotomies repaired with pin and tension-band fixation in dogs. *Can Vet J* **43**:528–534.

McKee WM, Macias C, Innes JF (2005) Bilateral fixation of Y-T humeral condyle fractures via medial and lateral approaches in 29 dogs. *J Small Anim Pract* **46**:217–226.

248

Webb AA, Cantwell SL, Duke T *et al.* (1999) Intravenous regional anaesthesia (Bier block) in a dog. *Can Vet J* **40**:419–421.

249

Zontine WJ, Weitkamp RA, Lippincott CL (1989) Redefined type of elbow dysplasia involving calcified flexor tendons attached to the medial humeral epicondyle in three dogs. *J Am Vet Med Assoc* **194**:1082–1085.

Meyer-Lindenberg A, Heinen V, Hewicker-Trautwein M *et al.* (2004) Incidence and treatment of metaplasia in the flexor tendons attached to the medial humeral epicondyle in the dog. *Tieraerztliche Praxis* **32**:276–285.

de Bakker E, Saunders J, Gielen I *et al.* (2012) Radiographic findings of the medial humeral epicondyle in 200 canine elbow joints. *Vet Comp Orthop Traumatol* **25**:359–365.

250

Stork CK, Petite AF, Norrie RA *et al.* (2009) Variation in position of the medial fabella in West Highland white terriers and other dogs. *J Small Anim Pract* **50**:236–240.

Casale SA, McCarthy RJ (2009) Complications associated with lateral fabellotibial suture surgery for cranial cruciate ligament injury in dogs: 363 cases (1997–2005). *J Am Vet Med Assoc* **234**:229–235.

251

Devor M, Sørby R (2006) Fibrotic contracture of the canine infraspinatus muscle: pathophysiology and prevention by early surgical intervention. *Vet Comp Orthop Traumatol* **19**:117–121.

252

Gielen I, van Ryssen B, van Bree H (2007) Comparison of subchondral lesion size between clinical and non-clinical medial trochlear ridge talar osteochondritis dissecans in dogs. *Vet Comp Orthop Traumatol* **20**:8–11.

References

Gielen I, van Ryssen B, van Bree H (2005) Computerized tomography compared with radiography in the diagnosis of lateral trochlear ridge talar osteochondritis dissecans in dogs. *Vet Comp Orthop Traumatol* **18**:77–82.

253
Ganz SM, Jackson J, VanEnkevort B (2010) Risk factors for femoral fracture after canine press-fit cementless total hip arthroplasty. *Vet Surg* **39**:688–695.

Hayes G, Ramirez J, Langley Hobbs SJ (2011) Does the degree of preoperative subluxation or soft tissue tension affect the incidence of postoperative luxation in dogs after total hip replacement? *Vet Surg* **40**:6–13.

254
Macias C, McKee WM, May C (2002) Caudal proximal tibial deformity and cranial cruciate ligament rupture in small-breed dogs. *J Small Anim Pract* **43**:433–438.

Bailey CJ, Smith BA, Black AP (2007) Geometric implications of the tibial wedge osteotomy for the treatment of cranial cruciate ligament disease in dogs. *Vet Comp Orthop Traumatol* **20**:169–174.

Apelt D, Pozzi A, Marcellin-Little DJ et al. (2010) Effect of cranial tibial closing wedge angle on tibial subluxation: an ex vivo study. *Vet Surg* **39**:44–49.

255
Roch SP, Clements DN, Mitchell RAS et al. (2008) Complications following tarsal arthrodesis using bone plate fixation in dogs. *J Small Anim Pract* **49**:117–126.

Gautier E, Sommer C (2003) Guidelines for the clinical application of the LCP. *Injury* **34**(Suppl 2): B63–76.

Index

Index

Index

Index

Index

Printed and bound by CPI Group (UK) Ltd, Croydon, CR0 4YY
23/10/2024
01777696-0004